Lecture Notes in Computational Vision and Biomechanics

Volume 19

Research related to the analysis of living structures (Biomechanics) has been carried out extensively in several distinct areas of science, such as, for example, mathematics, mechanical, physics, informatics, medicine and sports. However, for its successful achievement, numerous research topics should be considered, such as image processing and analysis, geometric and numerical modelling, biomechanics, experimental analysis, mechanobiology and Enhanced visualization, and their application on real cases must be developed and more investigation is needed. Additionally, enhanced hardware solutions and less invasive devices are demanded. On the other hand, Image Analysis (Computational Vision) aims to extract a high level of information from static images or dynamical image sequences. An example of applications involving Image Analysis can be found in the study of the motion of structures from image sequences, shape reconstruction from images and medical diagnosis. As a multidisciplinary area, Computational Vision considers techniques and methods from other disciplines, like from Artificial Intelligence, Signal Processing, mathematics, physics and informatics. Despite the work that has been done in this area, more robust and efficient methods of Computational Imaging are still demanded in many application domains, such as in medicine, and their validation in real scenarios needs to be examined urgently. Recently, these two branches of science have been increasingly seen as being strongly connected and related, but no book series or journal has contemplated this increasingly strong association. Hence, the main goal of this book series in Computational Vision and Biomechanics (LNCV&B) consists in the provision of a comprehensive forum for discussion on the current state-of-the-art in these fields by emphasizing their connection. The book series covers (but is not limited to):

- Applications of Computational Vision and Biomechanics
- Biometrics and Biomedical Pattern Analysis
- Cellular Imaging and Cellular Mechanics
- Clinical Biomechanics
- Computational Bioimaging and Visualization
- Computational Biology in Biomedical Imaging
- Development of Biomechanical Devices
- Device and Technique Development for Biomedical Imaging
- Experimental Biomechanics
- Gait & Posture Mechanics
- Grid and High Performance Computing on Computational Vision and Biomechanics
- Image Processing and Analysis
- Image processing and visualization in Biofluids
- Image Understanding
- Material Models
- Mechanobiology
- Medical Image Analysis
- Molecular Mechanics
- Multi-modal Image Systems
- Multiscale Biosensors in Biomedical Imaging
- Multiscale Devices and BioMEMS for Biomedical Imaging
- Musculoskeletal Biomechanics
- Multiscale Analysis in Biomechanics
- Neuromuscular Biomechanics
- Numerical Methods for Living Tissues
- Numerical Simulation
- Software Development on Computational Vision and Biomechanics
- Sport Biomechanics
- Virtual Reality in Biomechanics
- Vision Systems
- Image-based Geometric Modeling and Mesh Generation
- Digital Geometry Algorithms for Computational Vision and Visualization

In order to match the scope of the Book Series, each book has to include contents relating, or combining both Image Analysis and mechanics. Indexed by SCOPUS and Springerlink

More information about this series at http://www.springer.com/series/8910

João Manuel R.S. Tavares • Renato Natal Jorge
Editors

Developments in Medical Image Processing and Computational Vision

Springer

Editors
João Manuel R.S. Tavares
Departamento de Engenharia Mecânica
Universidade do Porto
Faculdade de Engenharia
Porto
Portugal

Renato Natal Jorge
Departamento de Engenharia Mecânica
Universidade do Porto
Faculdade de Engenharia
Porto
Portugal

ISSN 2212-9391 ISSN 2212-9413 (electronic)
Lecture Notes in Computational Vision and Biomechanics
ISBN 978-3-319-13406-2 ISBN 978-3-319-13407-9 (eBook)
DOI 10.1007/978-3-319-13407-9

Library of Congress Control Number: 2015930828

Springer Cham Heidelberg New York Dordrecht London

Printed on acid-free paper

Springer is part of Springer Science+Business Media (www.springer.com)

Preface

This book presents novel and advanced topics in Medical Image Processing and Computational Vision in order to solidify knowledge in the related fields and define their key stakeholders.

The twenty-two chapters included in this book were written by invited experts of international recognition and address important issues in Medical Image Processing and Computational Vision, including: 3D Vision, 3D Visualization, Colour Quantisation, Continuum Mechanics, Data Fusion, Data Mining, Face Recognition, GPU Parallelisation, Image Acquisition and Reconstruction, Image and Video Analysis, Image Clustering, Image Registration, Image Restoring, Image Segmentation, Machine Learning, Modelling and Simulation, Object Detection, Object Recognition, Object Tracking, Optical Flow, Pattern Recognition, Pose Estimation, and Texture Analysis.

Different applications are addressed and described throughout the book, comprising: Biomechanical Studies, Bio-structure Modelling and Simulation, Bone Characterization, Cell Tracking, Computer-Aided Diagnosis, Dental Imaging, Face Recognition, Hand Gestures Detection and Recognition, Human Motion Analysis, Human-Computer Interaction, Image and Video Understanding, Image Processing, Image Segmentation, Object and Scene Reconstruction, Object Recognition and Tracking, Remote Robot Control, and Surgery Planning.

Therefore, this book is of crucial effectiveness for Researchers, Students, End-Users and Manufacturers from several multidisciplinary fields, as the ones related with Artificial Intelligence, Bioengineering, Biology, Biomechanics, Computational Mechanics, Computational Vision, Computer Graphics, Computer Sciences, Computer Vision, Human Motion, Imagiology, Machine Learning, Machine Vision, Mathematics, Medical Image, Medicine, Pattern Recognition, and Physics.

The Editors would like to take this opportunity to thank to all invited authors for sharing their works, experiences and knowledge, making possible its dissemination through this book.

João Manuel R.S. Tavares
Renato Natal Jorge

Contents

On the Evaluation of Automated MRI Brain Segmentations: Technical and Conceptual Tools 1
Elisabetta Binaghi, Valentina Pedoia, Desiree Lattanzi, Emanuele Monti, Sergio Balbi and Renzo Minotto

Analysis of the Retinal Nerve Fiber Layer Texture Related to the Thickness Measured by Optical Coherence Tomography 19
J. Odstrcilik, R. Kolar, R. P. Tornow, A. Budai, J. Jan, P. Mackova and M. Vodakova

Continuum Mechanics Meets Echocardiographic Imaging: Investigation on the Principal Strain Lines in Human Left Ventricle 41
A. Evangelista, S. Gabriele, P. Nardinocchi, P. Piras, P.E. Puddu, L. Teresi, C. Torromeo and V. Varano

A GPU Accelerated Algorithm for Blood Detection in Wireless Capsule Endoscopy Images 55
Sunil Kumar, Isabel N. Figueiredo, Carlos Graca and Gabriel Falcao

Automated Image Mining in fMRI Reports: a Meta-research Study 73
N. Gonçalves, G. Vranou and R. Vigário

Visual Pattern Recognition Framework Based on the Best Rank Tensor Decomposition 89
B. Cyganek

Tracking Red Blood Cells Flowing through a Microchannel with a Hyperbolic Contraction: An Automatic Method 105
B. Taboada, F. C. Monteiro and R. Lima

A 3D Computed Tomography Based Tool for Orthopedic Surgery Planning 121
João Ribeiro, Victor Alves, Sara Silva and Jaime Campos

Preoperative Planning of Surgical Treatment with the Use of 3D Visualization and Finite Element Method 139
Wojciech Wolański, Bożena Gzik-Zroska, Edyta Kawlewska, Marek Gzik, Dawid Larysz, Józef Dzielicki and Adam Rudnik

Pretreatment and Reconstruction of Three-dimensional Images Applied in a Locking Reconstruction Plate for a Structural Analysis with FEA ... 165
João Paulo O. Freitas, Edson A. Capello de Sousa, Cesar R. Foschini, Rogerio R. Santos and Sheila C. Rahal

Tortuosity Influence on the Trabecular Bone Elasticity and Mechanical Competence 173
Waldir Leite Roque and Angel Alberich-Bayarri

Influence of Beam Hardening Artifact in Bone Interface Contact Evaluation by 3D X-ray Microtomography 193
I. Lima, M. Marquezan, M. M. G. Souza, E. F. Sant'Anna and R. T. Lopes

Anisotropy Estimation of Trabecular Bone in Gray-Scale: Comparison Between Cone Beam and Micro Computed Tomography Data 207
Rodrigo Moreno, Magnus Borga, Eva Klintström, Torkel Brismar and Örjan Smedby

Fractured Bone Identification from CT Images, Fragment Separation and Fracture Zone Detection 221
Félix Paulano, Juan J. Jiménez and Rubén Pulido

On Evolutionary Integral Models for Image Restoration 241
E. Cuesta, A. Durán and M. Kirane

Colour Image Quantisation using KM and KHM Clustering Techniques with Outlier-Based Initialisation 261
Henryk Palus and Mariusz Frackiewicz

A Study of a Firefly Meta-Heuristics for Multithreshold Image Segmentation 279
H. Erdmann, G. Wachs-Lopes, C. Gallão, M. P. Ribeiro and P. S. Rodrigues

Visual-Inertial 2D Feature Tracking based on an Affine Photometric Model 297
Dominik Aufderheide, Gerard Edwards and Werner Krybus

Inferring Heading Direction from Silhouettes 319
Amina Bensebaa, Slimane Larabi and Neil M. Robertson

A Fast and Accurate Algorithm for Detecting and Tracking Moving Hand Gestures 335
Walter C. S. S. Simões, Ricardo da S. Barboza, Vicente F. de Jr Lucena and Rafael D. Lins

Hand Gesture Recognition System Based in Computer Vision and Machine Learning 355
Paulo Trigueiros, Fernando Ribeiro and Luís Paulo Reis

3D Scanning Using RGBD Imaging Devices: A Survey 379
Eduardo E. Hitomi, Jorge V. L. Silva and Guilherme C. S. Ruppert

Contributors

Angel Alberich-Bayarri Biomedical Imaging Research Group, La Fe Health Research Institute, Valencia, Spain

Victor Alves CCTC-Computer Science and Technology Center, University of Minho, Braga, Portugal

Dominik Aufderheide Division Soest, Institute for Computer Science, Vision and Computational Intelligence, South Westphalia University of Applied Sciences, Soest, Germany

Sergio Balbi Dipartimento di Biotecnologie e Scienze della Vita, Università degli Studi dell'Insubria Varese, Varese, Italy

Ricardo da S. Barboza Universidade Federal de Pernambuco, Pernambuco, Brazil

Amina Bensebaa Computer Science Department, USTHB University, Algiers, Algeria

Elisabetta Binaghi Dipartimento di Scienze Teoriche e Applicate-Sezione Informatica, Università degli Studi dell'Insubria, Varese, Italy

Magnus Borga Department of Biomedical Engineering, Linköping University, Linköping, Sweden

Center for Medical Image Science and Visualization (CMIV), Linköping University, Linköping, Sweden

Torkel Brismar Department of Radiology, Karolinska University Hospital at Huddinge, Huddinge, Sweden

A. Budai Department of Ophthalmology, University of Erlangen, Erlangen-Nuremberg, Germany

Pattern Recognition Lab and Erlangen Graduate School of Advanced Optical Technologies, University of Erlangen, Erlangen-Nuremberg, Erlangen, Germany

Jaime Campos CCTC-Computer Science and Technology Center, University of Minho, Braga, Portugal

E. Cuesta Department of Applied Mathematics, E.T.S.I. of Telecomunication, University of Valladolid, Valladolid, Spain

B. Cyganek AGH University of Science and Technology, Krakow, Poland

A. Durán Department of Applied Mathematics, E.T.S.I. of Telecomunication, University of Valladolid, Valladolid, Spain

Józef Dzielicki Medical University of Silesia, School of Medicine in Katowice, Katowice, Poland

Gerard Edwards Department of Electronic & Electrical Engineering, Faculty of Science and Engineering, The University of Chester, Chester, UK

H. Erdmann Inaciana Educational Foundation, Sao Paulo, Brazil

A. Evangelista Ospedale San Giovanni Calibita Fatebenefratelli-Isola Tiberina, Rome, Italy

Gabriel Falcao Instituto de Telecomunicações, Department of Electrical and Computer Engineering, Faculty of Science and Technology, University of Coimbra, Coimbra, Portugal

Isabel N. Figueiredo CMUC, Department of Mathematics, Faculty of Science and Technology, University of Coimbra, Coimbra, Portugal

Cesar R. Foschini Faculdade de Engenharia de Bauru, Universidade Estadual Paulista-Unesp, Bauru, São Paulo, Brazil

Mariusz Frackiewicz Silesian University of Technology, Gliwice, Poland

João Paulo O. Freitas Faculdade de Engenharia de Bauru, Universidade Estadual Paulista-Unesp, Bauru, São Paulo, Brazil

S. Gabriele Dipartimento di Architettura, LaMS-Modeling & Simulation Lab, Università Roma Tre, Rome, Italy

C. Gallão Inaciana Educational Foundation, Sao Paulo, Brazil

Gonçalves Department of Information and Computer Science, Aalto University School of Science, Aalto, Finland

Carlos Graca Instituto de Telecomunicações, Department of Electrical and Computer Engineering, Faculty of Science and Technology, University of Coimbra, Coimbra, Portugal

Marek Gzik Biomechatronics Department, Faculty of Biomedical Engineering, Silesian University of Technology, Zabrze, Poland

Bożena Gzik-Zroska Department of Biomaterials and Medical Devices Engineering, Faculty of Biomedical Engineering, Silesian University of Technology, Zabrze, Poland

Eduardo E. Hitomi Center for Information Technology Renato Archer, Campinas, SP, Brazil

J. Jan Department of Biomedical Engineering, Faculty of Electrical Engineering and Communication, Brno University of Technology, Brno, Czech Republic

Juan J. Jiménez University of Jaén, Jaén, Spain

Edyta Kawlewska Biomechatronics Department, Faculty of Biomedical Engineering, Silesian University of Technology, Zabrze, Poland

M. Kirane Laboratoire de Mathématiques, Image et Applications, Université de La Rochelle, La Rochelle Cedex, France

Eva Klintström Department of Radiology and Department of Medical and Health Sciences, Linköping University, Linköping, Sweden

Center for Medical Image Science and Visualization (CMIV), Linköping University, Linköping, Sweden

Linköping University, Linköping, Sweden

R. Kolar St. Anne's University Hospital—International Clinical Research Center (ICRC), Brno, Czech Republic

Department of Biomedical Engineering, Faculty of Electrical Engineering and Communication, Brno University of Technology, Brno, Czech Republic

Werner Krybus Division Soest, Institute for Computer Science, Vision and Computational Intelligence, South Westphalia University of Applied Sciences, Soest, Germany

Sunil Kumar CMUC, Department of Mathematics, Faculty of Science and Technology, University of Coimbra, Coimbra, Portugal

Slimane Larabi Computer Science Department, USTHB University, Algiers, Algeria

Dawid Larysz Department of Radiotherapy, Maria Sklodowska-Curie Memorial Cancer Center and Institute of Oncology, Gliwice, Poland

Desiree Lattanzi Dipartimento di Biotecnologie e Scienze della Vita, Università degli Studi dell'Insubria Varese, Varese, Italy

I. Lima Federal University of Rio de Janeiro, Ilha do Fundão, Rio de Janeiro, Brazil

R. Lima ESTiG, IPB, C. Sta. Apolonia, Bragança, Portugal

CEFT, FEUP, R. Dr. Roberto Frias, Porto, Portugal

University of Minho, Mechanical Engineering Department, Guimarães, Portugal

Rafael D. Lins Universidade Federal de Pernambuco, Pernambuco, Brazil

R. T. Lopes Federal University of Rio de Janeiro, Ilha do Fundão, Rio de Janeiro, Brazil

Vicente F. de Jr Lucena Universidade Federal do Amazonas, Amazonas, Brazil

P. Mackova Department of Biomedical Engineering, Faculty of Electrical Engineering and Communication, Brno University of Technology, Brno, Czech Republic

M. Marquezan Federal University of Rio de Janeiro, Ilha do Fundão, Rio de Janeiro, Brazil

Renzo Minotto Unità Operativa di Neuroradiologia Ospedale di Circolo e Fondazione Macchi, Varese, Italy

F. C. Monteiro ESTiG, IPB, C. Sta. Apolonia, Bragança, Portugal

Emanuele Monti Dipartimento di Biotecnologie e Scienze della Vita, Università degli Studi dell'Insubria Varese, Varese, Italy

Rodrigo Moreno Department of Radiology and Department of Medical and Health Sciences, Linköping University, Linköping, Sweden

Center for Medical Image Science and Visualization (CMIV), Linköping University, Linköping, Sweden

Linköping University, Linköping, Sweden

P. Nardinocchi Dipartimento di Ingegneria Strutturale e Geotecnica, Sapienza-Università di Roma, Rome, Italy

J. Odstrcilik St. Anne's University Hospital—International Clinical Research Center (ICRC), Brno, Czech Republic

Department of Biomedical Engineering, Faculty of Electrical Engineering and Communication, Brno University of Technology, Brno, Czech Republic

Henryk Palus Silesian University of Technology, Gliwice, Poland

Félix Paulano University of Jaén, Jaén, Spain

Valentina Pedoia Musculoskeletal Quantitative Imaging Research Group Department of Radiology and Biomedical Imaging University of California, San Francisco, USA

P. Piras Dipartimento di Ingegneria Strutturale e Geotecnica, Sapienza-Università di Roma, Rome, Italy

Dipartimento di Scienze, Università Roma Tre, Rome, Italy

Center for Evolutionary Ecology, Università Roma Tre, Rome, Italy

P. E. Puddu Dipartimento di Scienze Cardiovascolari, Respiratorie, Nefrologiche, Anestesiologiche, Sapienza Università di Roma, Rome, Italy

Rubén Pulido University of Jaén, Jaén, Spain

Sheila C. Rahal School of Veterinary Medicine and Animal Science, Universidade Estadual Paulista-Unesp, Botucatu, Sōo Paulo, Brazil

Luís Paulo Reis DSI/EEUM-Departamento de Sistemas de Informação, Escola de Engenharia, Universidade do Minho, Guimarães, Portugal

Centro Algoritmi, Universidade do Minho, Guimarães, Portugal

LIACC-Laboratório de Inteligência Artificial e Ciência de Computadores, Porto, Portugal

Fernando Ribeiro DEI/EEUM-Departamento de Electrónica Industrial, Escola de Engenharia, Universidade do Minho, Guimarães, Portugal

Centro Algoritmi, Universidade do Minho, Guimarães, Portugal

João Ribeiro CCTC-Computer Science and Technology Center, University of Minho, Braga, Portugal

M. P. Ribeiro Federal University of Viçosa, Minas Gerais, Viçosa, Brazil

Neil M. Robertson Edinburgh Research Partnership in Engineering and Mathematics, Heriot-Watt University, Edinburgh, UK

P. S. Rodrigues Inaciana Educational Foundation, Sao Paulo, Brazil

Waldir Leite Roque Department of Scientific Computation, Federal University of Paraíba, João Pessoa, Brazil

Adam Rudnik Department of Neurosurgery, Medical University of Silesia, Katowice, Poland

Guilherme C. S. Ruppert Center for Information Technology Renato Archer, Campinas, SP, Brazil

E. F. Sant'Anna Federal University of Rio de Janeiro, Ilha do Fundão, Rio de Janeiro, Brazil

Rogerio R. Santos School of Veterinary Medicine and Animal Science, Universidade Estadual Paulista-Unesp, Botucatu, São Paulo, Brazil

Jorge V. L. Silva Center for Information Technology Renato Archer, Campinas, SP, Brazil

Sara Silva CCTC-Computer Science and Technology Center, University of Minho, Braga, Portugal

Walter C. S. S. Simões Universidade Federal do Amazonas, Amazonas, Brazil

Örjan Smedby Department of Radiology and Department of Medical and Health Sciences, Linköping University, Linköping, Sweden

Center for Medical Image Science and Visualization (CMIV), Linköping University, Linköping, Sweden

Linköping University, Linköping, Sweden

Edson A. Capello de Sousa Faculdade de Engenharia de Bauru, Universidade Estadual Paulista-Unesp, Bauru, São Paulo, Brazil

M. M. G. Souza Federal University of Rio de Janeiro, Ilha do Fundão, Rio de Janeiro, Brazil

B. Taboada ESTiG, IPB, C. Sta. Apolonia, Bragança, Portugal

CEFT, FEUP, R. Dr. Roberto Frias, Porto, Portugal

L. Teresi Dipartimento di Matematica e Fisica, LaMS-Modeling & Simulation Lab, Università Roma Tre, Rome, Italy

R. P. Tornow Department of Ophthalmology, University of Erlangen, Erlangen-Nuremberg, Erlangen, Germany

Pattern Recognition Lab and Erlangen Graduate School of Advanced Optical Technologies, University of Erlangen, Erlangen-Nuremberg, Erlangen, Germany

C. Torromeo Dipartimento di Scienze Cardiovascolari, Respiratorie, Nefrologiche, Anestesiologiche, Sapienza Università di Roma, Rome, Italy

Paulo Trigueiros Insituto Politécnico do Porto, IPP, Porto, Portugal

DEI/EEUM-Departamento de Electrónica Industrial, Escola de Engenharia, Universidade do Minho, Guimarães, Portugal

Centro Algoritmi, Universidade do Minho, Guimarões, Portugal

V. Varano Dipartimento di Architettura, LaMS-Modeling & Simulation Lab, Università Roma Tre, Rome, Italy

R. Vigário Department of Information and Computer Science, Aalto University School of Science, Aalto, Finland

M. Vodakova Department of Biomedical Engineering, Faculty of Electrical Engineering and Communication, Brno University of Technology, Brno, Czech Republic

G. Vranou Department of Informatics, Technological Education Institute, Sindos, Thessaloniki, Greece

G. Wachs-Lopes Inaciana Educational Foundation, Sao Paulo, Brazil

About the Editors

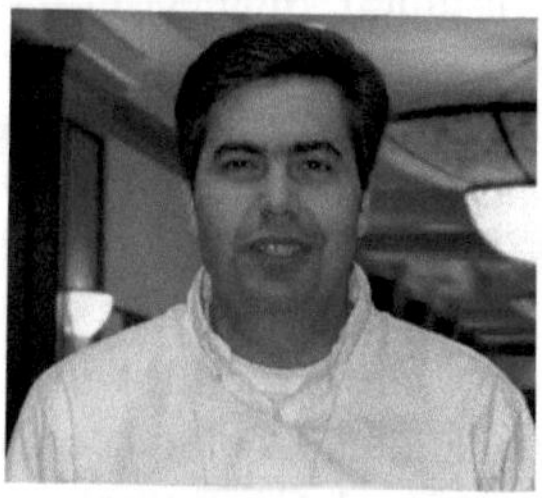

João Manuel R. S. Tavares is graduated in Mechanical Engineering from the University of Porto, Portugal (1992). He also earned his M.Sc. degree and Ph.D. degree in Electrical and Computer Engineering from the University of Porto in 1995 and 2001, respectively. He is a senior researcher and project coordinator at the Institute of Mechanical Engineering and Industrial Management (INEGI) and an Associate Professor at the Department of Mechanical Engineering of the Faculty of Engineering of the University of Porto (FEUP).

João Tavares is co-editor of more than 30 books, co-author of more than 30 book chapters, 550 articles in international and national journals and conferences, and 3 international and 2 national patents. He has been a committee member of several international and national journals and conferences, is co-founder and co-editor of the book series "Lecture Notes in Computational Vision and Biomechanics" published by Springer, founder and Editor-in-Chief of the journal "Computer Methods in Biomechanics and Biomedical Engineering: Imaging & Visualization" published by Taylor & Francis, and co-founder and co-chair of the international conference series: CompIMAGE, ECCOMAS VipIMAGE, ICCEBS and BioDental. Also, he has been (co-)supervisor of several MSc and PhD thesis and supervisor of several post-doc projects, and has participated in many scientific projects both as researcher and as scientific coordinator.

His main research areas include computational vision, medical imaging, computational mechanics, scientific visualization, human-computer interaction and new product development. (More information can be found at: www.fe.up.pt/~tavares).

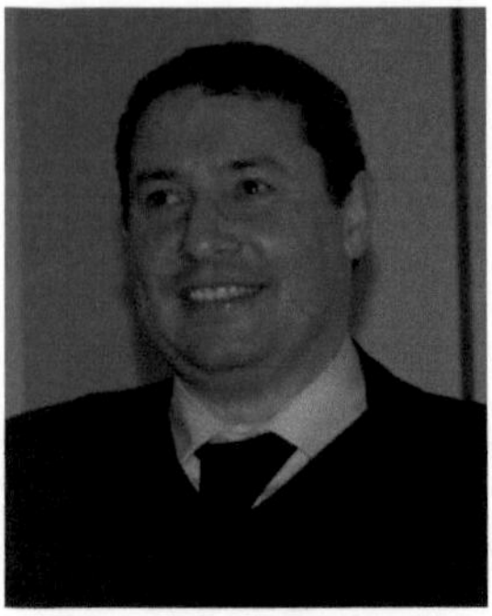

Renato Natal Jorge Associate Professor at the Faculty of Engineering, University of Porto (FEUP); Mechanical Engineer from the University of Porto, 1987; MSc from the University of Porto, 1991; PhD from the University of Porto, 1999.

Present teaching and research interests: Computational methods in applied mechanics and engineering; New product development; Biomechanics and mechanobiology; Computational vision and medical image processing.

Between 2007 and 2011 was the Director of the "Structural Integrity Unit" research group of the Institute of Mechanical Engineering at FEUP (IDMEC-a R & D non-profit, private Research Institute). Member of the executive board of IDMEC-FEUP.

Responsible for the Supervision or Co-supervision of 22 PhD students.

Co-chair of the following conferences: all issues of CompIMAGE; 14th International Product Development Management; VIPIMAGE; Fourteenth Annual Scientific Conference on WEB Technology, New Media, Communications and Telematics Theory, Methods, Tools and Applications; all issues of VIPIMAGE; all issues of BioDENTAL; all issues of IDEMi; 6th International Conference on Technology and Medical Sciences, CIBEM 2011; International Conference on Computational and Experimental Biomedical Sciences; among other mini-symposia within conferences.

Founder and Editor of the International Journal for Computational Vision and Biomechanics. Guest editor of several scientific journals.

Founder and Editor of the Book Series: Lecture Notes in Computational Vision and Biomechanics, Springer. Principal Investigator for several national and European scientific projects.

Co-author of more than 110 papers in international journals and more than 380 publications in international conferences.

On the Evaluation of Automated MRI Brain Segmentations: Technical and Conceptual Tools

Elisabetta Binaghi, Valentina Pedoia, Desiree Lattanzi, Emanuele Monti, Sergio Balbi and Renzo Minotto

Abstract The present work deals with segmentation of Glial Tumors in MRI images focusing on critical aspects in manual labeling and reference estimation for segmentation validation purposes. A reproducibility analysis was conducted confirming the presence of different sources of uncertainty involved in the process of manual segmentation and responsible of high intra-operator and inter-operator variability. Technical and conceptual solutions aimed to reduce operator variability and support in the reference estimation process are integrated in *GliMAn* (Glial Tumor Manual Annotator), an application allowing to view and manipulate MRI volumes and implementing a label fusion strategy based on fuzzy connectedness. A set of experiments was conceived and conducted to evaluate the contribution of the solutions proposed in the process of manual segmentation and reference data estimation.

1 Introduction

Magnetic Resonance (MR) imaging plays a fundamental role in scientific and clinical studies of brain pathologies. By visual inspection of MRI imagery, physicians can accurately examine and identify tissues thanks to the high spatial resolution and contrast and their enhanced differentiation. Segmentation intended as a precise

E. Binaghi (✉)
Dipartimento di Scienze Teoriche e Applicate—Sezione Informatica,
Università degli Studi dell'Insubria, Varese, Italy
e-mail: elisabetta.binaghi@uninsubria.it

V. Pedoia
Musculoskeletal Quantitative Imaging Research Group
Department of Radiology and Biomedical Imaging University of California,
San Francisco, USA

D. Lattanzi · E. Monti · S. Balbi
Dipartimento di Biotecnologie e Scienze della Vita,
Università degli Studi dell'Insubria Varese, Varese, Italy

R. Minotto
Unità Operativa di Neuroradiologia Ospedale di
Circolo e Fondazione Macchi, Varese, Italy

J. M. R. S. Tavares, R. Natal Jorge (eds.), *Developments in Medical Image Processing and Computational Vision,* Lecture Notes in Computational Vision and Biomechanics 19,
DOI 10.1007/978-3-319-13407-9_1

delineation of the pathological and healthy tissues composing the MR image is important to develop quantitative analysis, understand pathologies, evaluate the evolutionary trend, plan the best surgical approach or evaluate alternative strategies [1–3].

In some areas, such as Glial Tumor studies, it is particularly difficult to objectively establish the limits between the tumor and the normal brain tissue. However glial tumor segmentation is of great importance to plan resection, quantify the postoperative residual, identify radiotherapy margins and evaluate the therapy response based on the tumor volume evaluation. Segmentation accomplished through a complete manual tracing is a difficult, time consuming task usually affected by intra- and inter-variation that limits the stability and reproducibility of the results. Difficulties encountered in manual labeling make in some cases computer support highly desirable offering segmentation procedures with varying degrees of automation. However, the use of automated segmentation procedures poses in turn the problem of a reference standard representative of the true segmentation which is required for the assessment of accuracy of the automated results. Recent works focus the attention on methods which do not require ground truth, but rely on behavioral comparison [2, 4–6]. With this approach, the evaluation involves the design of a reliable common agreement strategy able to define a suitable reference standard through combining manually traced segmentations. Proceeding from these considerations, the contribution of the present work is twofold. Firstly a reproducibility study is proposed, aimed to experimentally assess quantitatively the extent of the operator variability in the critical context of Glial Tumor segmentation studies. The motivation of this experimental investigation lies in the fact that few studies have been recently developed to investigate the extent of the operator variability in specific MRI clinical applications. The second contribution is the design of *GliMAn* (Glial Tumor Manual Annotator), an integrated system that offers visualization tools and facilities in support to manual labeling and reference data estimation for validating automated segmentation results. The facilities offered by *GliMAn* in truth label collection for fully manual segmentation was the subject of a previous work [7]. An extended version of GliMAn is here presented implementing fuzzy connectedness algorithms [8] used to merge individual labels and generate segmentation representative of a common agreement.

2 Inter-intra-expert Variability in Fully Manual Segmentation: A Case Study

A precise volumetric computation of the pathological MRI signal has several fundamental implications in clinical practice. In fact, the accurate definition of both the topographical features and the growing pattern of the tumor is crucial in order to select the most appropriate treatment, to plan the best surgical approach and to post-operatively correctly evaluate the extent of resection and monitoring the evolution over time of any eventual residue [9]. However, it is worth noting that gliomas are characterized by constant local growth (4 mm/year) within the brain parenchyma, migration along white matter pathways both in ipsilateral and even contralateral hemisphere and unavoidable anaplastic transformation [10]. Because of their infiltrative nature, the exact boundaries of gliomas wouldn't be reflected reliably in the pathological signal revealed in MRI. On the contrary, especially in the case of slow-growing lesions, it was by taking multiple biopsy samples demonstrated that tumor cells are present in a consistent number, but not in a sufficient number to give an hyperintense signal, at a distance of at least 20 mm from the tumor landmarks shown by MR imaging [11, 12]. From these considerations it follows that radiological detection and segmentation for gliomas are critical tasks due to their histopathological features, especially at the periphery of the hyperintensity detected by MRI.

An experimental analysis is developed to quantitatively assess the reproducibility of manual segmentation of glial tumors in MRI images, measured under different variations.

2.1 *Quantitative Evaluation*

The aim of the present analysis is twofold: to assess the agreement of segmentations as performed by different experts (inter-variability) and to assess the reproducibility of the manual segmentations as performed by the same expert (intra-variability). The dataset used is composed of four FLAIR MRI gray scale volumes with the following acquisition parameters:

- gray scale
- 12 bit depth
- Volume Size $[432 \times 432 \times 300]$
- Slice Thickness 0.6 mm
- Spacing Between Slices 0.6 mm
- Pixel Spacing $(0.57, 0.57)$ mm
- Repetition Time 8000
- Echo Time 282.89

All dataset volumes are altered by the presence of glial tumors, which are heterogeneous in terms of position, dimension, intensity and shape. A team of five medical experts was asked to segment axial, sagittal and coronal slices of these volume data by employing an image annotator normally in use in clinical practice and by offering standard image viewing facilities. Figure 1 shows an example of slice-by-slice manual segmentation of glial tumor areas provided by 5 experts along the axial plane and superimposed on the original MRI slice.

MRI segmentation was performed with the purpose of determining the size of pathological tissues and their spatial distribution in two or three dimensions according to the nature of the data. Metrics adopted in the present analysis for size estimation error and spatial distribution error are described below.

Size Estimation Error Let be S_1^i S_2^i S_3^i the size estimation of the region (surface or volume) extracted from the axial, sagittal and coronal plane segmentation respectively, performed by the $i-th$ expert. The intra- and inter- size estimation errors

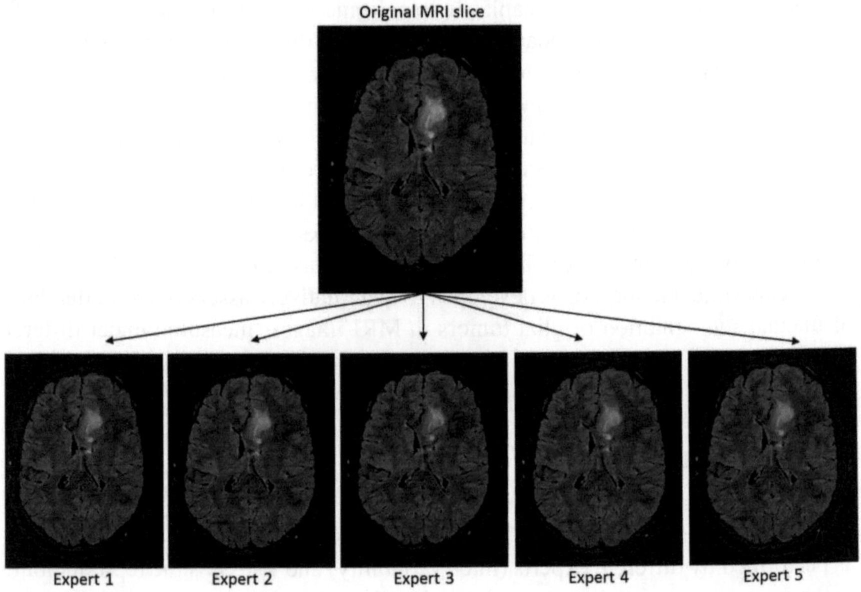

Fig. 1 Slice-by-slice manual segmentations of low grade glioma brain tumor performed by 5 medical experts

along the plane p with $p \in \{1, 2, 3\}$ and the $i - th$ expert are computed as follows:

$$intraSizeErr^i_p = \frac{S^i_p - \frac{1}{N_{seg}} \sum_{j=1}^{N_{seg}} S^i_j}{\frac{1}{N_{seg}} \sum_{j=1}^{N_{seg}} S^i_j};$$

$$interSizeErr^i_p = \frac{S^i_p - \frac{1}{N_{exp}} \sum_{j=1}^{N_{exp}} S^j_p}{\frac{1}{N_{exp}} \sum_{j=1}^{N_{exp}} S^j_p} \quad (1)$$

where N_{seg} is the number of segmentations performed by the same expert on the same volume and N_{exp} is the total number of experts.

Spatial Distribution Error Let be M^i_1 M^i_2 M^i_3 the 2D or 3D masks obtained from the segmentations along axial, sagittal and coronal plane respectively, performed by the $i - th$ expert. The intra- and inter- spatial distribution errors, evaluated in terms of Jaccard Distance [13] are computed as follows:

$$J^i_{p,t} = 1 - \frac{M^i p \cap M^i t}{M^i p \cup M^t i}; \quad J^{i,j}_p = 1 - \frac{M^i p \cap M^j p}{M^i p \cup M^j p}; \quad (2)$$

where i and j are indexes related to the experts and p and t related to the segmentation planes.

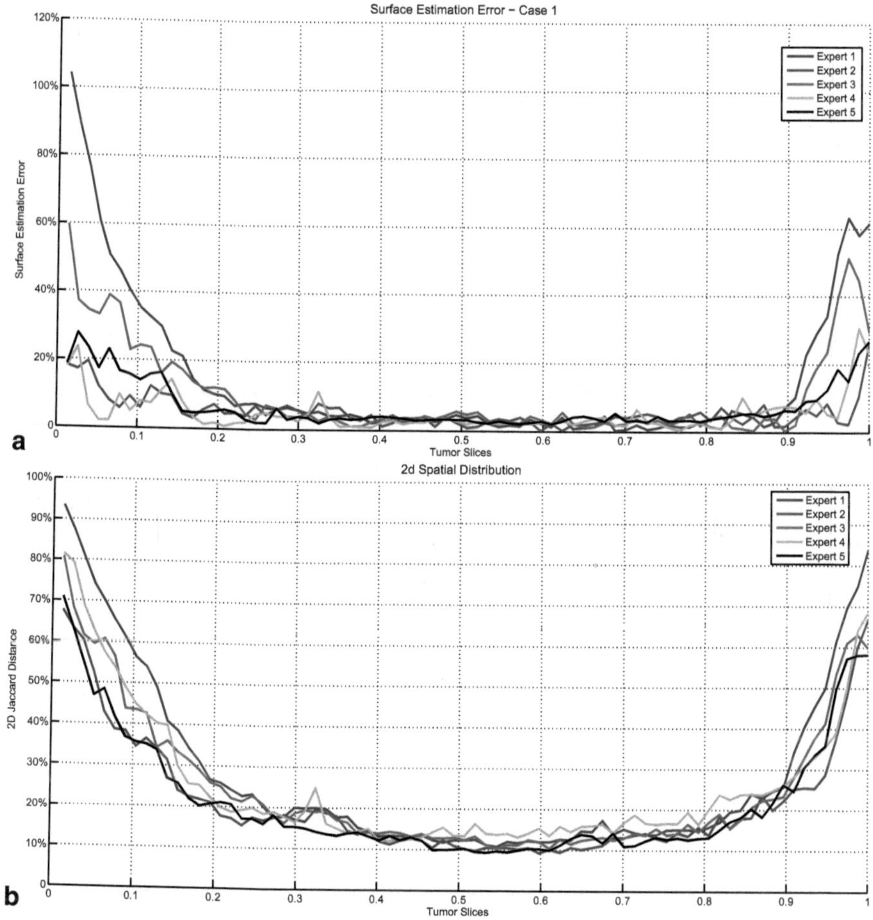

Fig. 2 2D intra-variability analysis conducted on each expert on one MRI volume: (**a**) Surface estimation error (**b**) 2D Spatial distribution error

2.1.1 2D Variability Analysis

Figure 2a shows the mean of the intra-size estimation error $intraSizeErr_p^i$ as computed varying the segmentation plane p and referring to each slice presenting a tumor of one MRI volume in the data set as operated by each varying expert.

Figure 2b shows the mean of the spatial distribution error $J_{p,t}^i$, as computed varying all the possible pairs of planes p, t and referring to each slice presenting a tumor of one MRI volume as operated by each varying expert.

The intra-variability measures confirm consistently an acceptable level of reproducibility for slices including the central part of the tumor area, with values lower than 15 and 20 % for the surface estimation error and for the Jaccard distance respectively. The intra-variability increases considerably in the slices which include

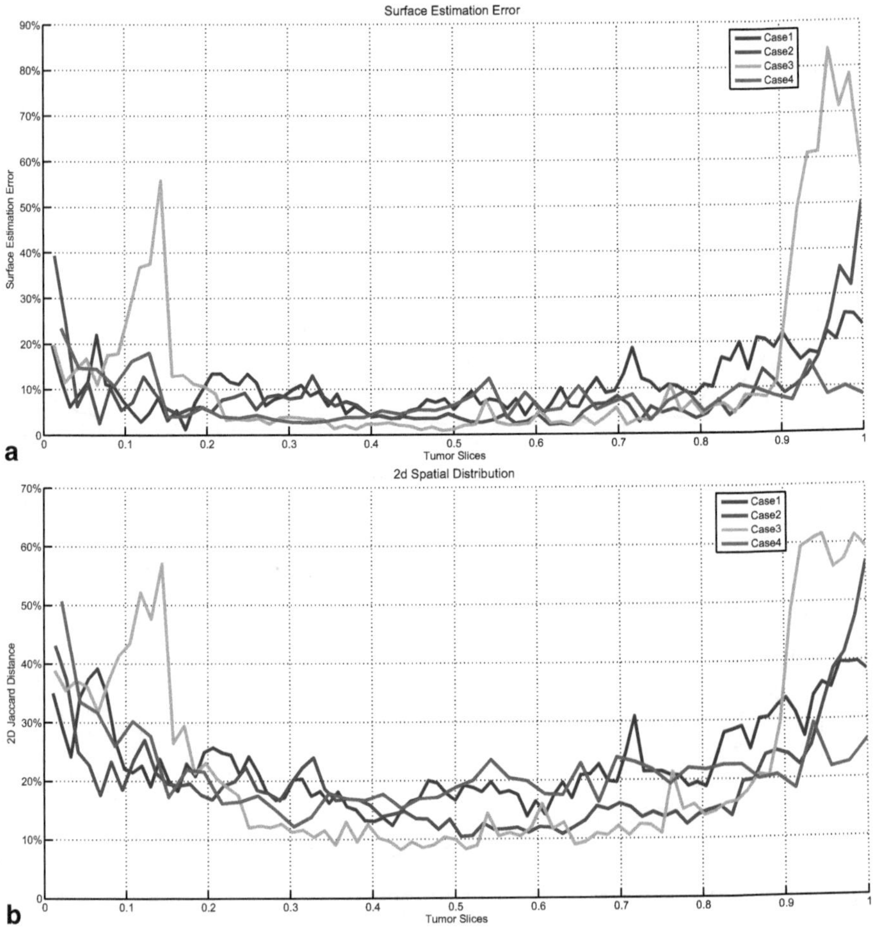

Fig. 3 2D inter-variability analysis conducted on 4 MRI volumes: (**a**)Mean of surface estimation errors (**b**) Mean of 2D spatial distribution errors

the marginal part of the tumor with peaks of 103 % in surface estimation error and 92 % in spatial distribution error. This result can be interpreted mainly in light of two facts that the boundary masks are smaller and an error computed on few pixels results in a large percentage error; secondly that the slices are difficult to segment considering the high level of infiltration in the healthy tissue.

Figure 3a shows the mean of the inter-size estimation error $interSizeErr_p^i$ as computed varying the expert i and referring to both each volume in the data set and each segmentation along the axial plane.

Figure 3b shows the mean of the spatial distribution error $J_p^{i,j}$ as computed by each varying pair of experts i, j and referring to each volume in the data set and to each segmentation along the axial plane.

Table 1 3D intra-variability analysis conducted on 4 MRI volumes

	Case 1		Cace 2	
	Volume estimation error (%)	3D jaccard Distance (%)	Volume Estimation error (%)	3D Jaccard Distance (%)
Expert 1	0.32	23.33	1.20	15.03
Expert 2	4.58	24.67	2.46	24.33
Expert 3	6.46	24.33	6.09	24.33
Expert 4	1.68	22.00	4.83	16.33
Expert 5	7.79	25.00	9.10	20.00

Table 2 3D inter-variability analysis conducted on 4 MRI volumes

	Volume Estimation error (%)	3D Jaccard Distance (%)
Case 1	7.20	21.52
Case 2	5.72	15.56
Case 3	3.00	16.08
Case 4	1.80	20.78

Both the inter- variability measures adopted confirm a high level of variability when segmenting both central and boundary slices with peaks exceeding 50 % and with definitely unacceptable results in the boundary slices.

2.1.2 3D Variability Analysis

Table 1 reports the results of intra-variability analysis both in terms of volume estimation error and of 3D spatial distribution for 2 cases of the dataset. The analysis of the volume estimation shows an acceptable level of variability. The Jaccard Distances indicate instead a high level of variability in spatial distribution. The inconsistency of the two metrics comes from the compensation of errors in volume estimation.

Table 2 reports the results of the inter-variability analysis for all the 4 cases of the dataset. The results obtained lead to the same conclusion drawn in the previous case. The low variance values equal to 0.14 and 0.10 % as computed on the volume estimation and the 3D spatial distribution errors respectively, indicates that dissimilarities are equally distributed among experts. Anomalous behaviors of individuals or sub-groups of experts (i.e. neuroradiologists and neurosurgeons) is not detected.

2.2 *Discussion of Results*

Results obtained were discussed and interpreted through a close dialogue between physicians and computer scientists during joint meetings. Our analysis confirms the well known result that a validation procedure based on interactive drawing of the desired segmentation by domain experts which is often considered the only acceptable approach, suffers from intra-expert and inter-expert variability. In addition the analysis allows to conclude that the extent of the problem in the specific context of MRI brain tumor segmentation strongly affects the reliability of manual labeling as a source of reference standard in segmentation studies.

Dissimilarities among experts can be traced back to two main sources. A first source of uncertainty is identified in the lack of information during the visual inspection phase. Considering the trend of the areas of tumor sections manually annotated by each expert and reported in Fig. 4 we notice large transitions between consecutive slices indicating non-compliance with the constraint of continuity. We concluded that physicians should explore a resonance volume through subsequent axial coronal and sagittal slices and the inspection on a given slice must be contextually related to the inspection of previous and subsequent slices.

The second source of uncertainty originates within the process of assigning a region under a given category, based on complex and vague clinical signs. The assignment of crisp labels is accomplished arbitrarily reducing uncertainty and forcing a boolean decision.

We assume that such an intrinsic uncertainty can be properly managed within the fuzzy set framework. Images are fuzzy by nature, and object intensities come from different factors such as the material heterogeneity of the object and the degradation introduced by the imaging device. Under these critical conditions, the labeling process has to be properly modeled as a matter of degrees in order to completely represent the expert decisional attitudes in connecting heterogeneous image elements forming objects.

3 *GliMAn* Design and Architecture

GliMAn is an application designed to support glial tumor segmentation studies improving reproducibility of manual labeling and contributing to generate reference standards for segmentation validation purposes. It was conceived and developed basing on conclusions reached in the operator variability analysis described in section 2. As detailed in Fig. 5, The *GliMAn* architecture includes modules for viewing, managing and processing MRI volumes supporting the following main tasks:

1. fully manual labeling of glial tumors by experts
2. semi-automatic generation of segmented reference data through the use of Fuzzy Connectedness-based truth estimation.

The conceptual design phase of *GliMAn* proceeds from the conclusion that experts should explore a resonance volume for subsequent axial, coronal and sagittal slices and that decisions on the given slice must be contextually related on the inspection of previous and subsequent slices.

The main feature of *GliMAn* is then the preservation of the volumetric nature of the data through the simultaneous display of the three orthogonal planes (axial,

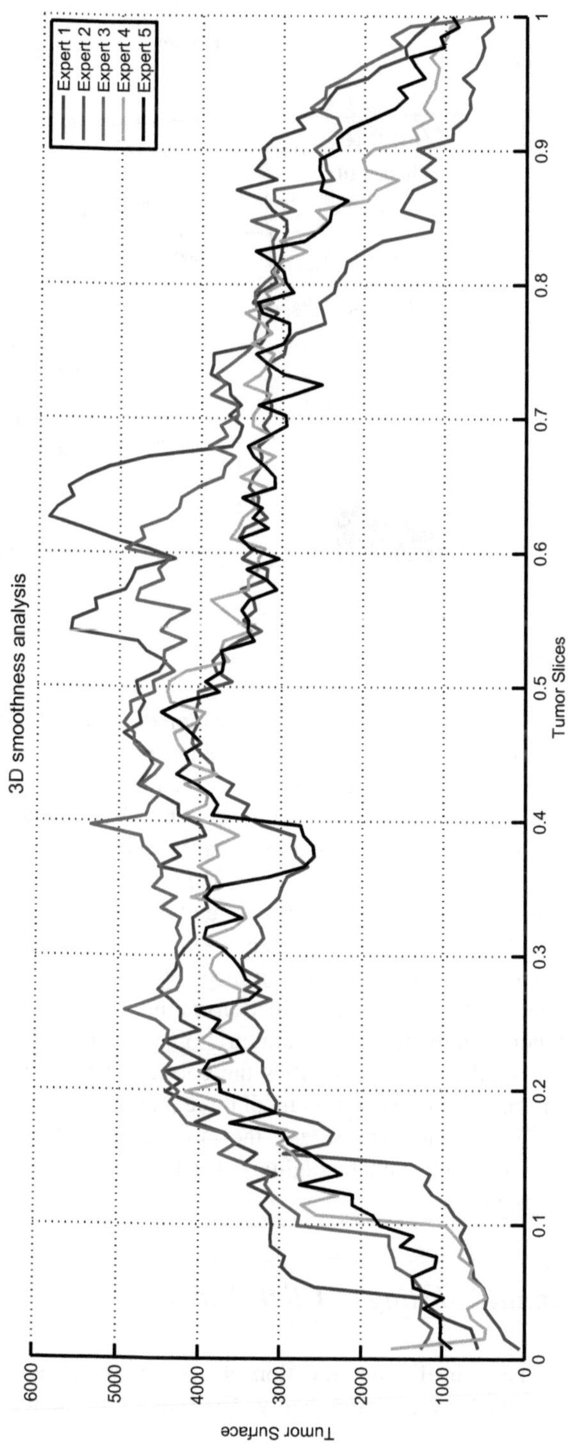

Fig. 4 Trends of the areas of tumor sections manually segmented along the axial direction by the experts

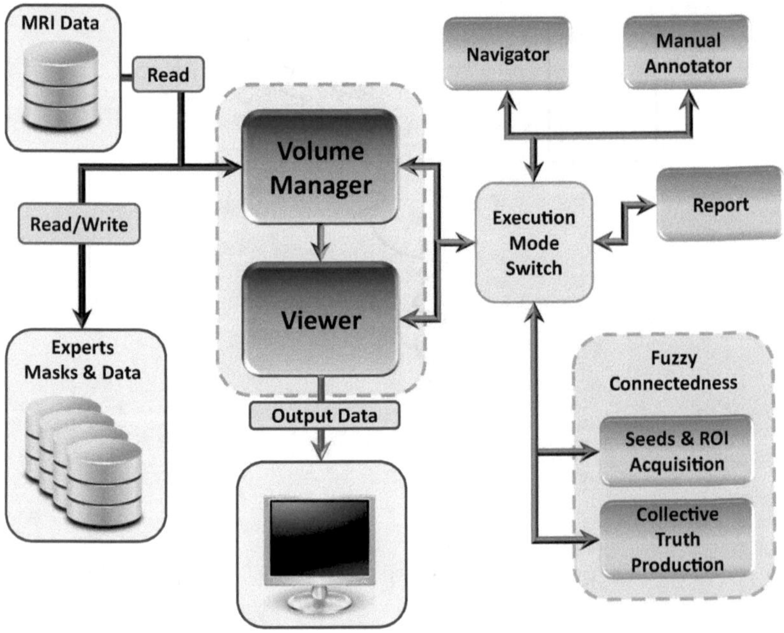

Fig. 5 *GliMAn* architecture diagram

sagittal and coronal) and the synchronized visualization of the input labels. Human-computer interaction principles and usability guidelines have been strictly observed in the *GliMAn* physical design, in order to limit eyestrain and ambiguities that can undermine the effectiveness of conceptual solutions in the GUI interaction. The GUI is composed of 3 principal areas (Fig. 4): upper, central and lateral. The upper zone includes standard I/O features of an image viewer and management tools, the central zone shows orthogonal planes and the lateral zone allows to change the execution mode. Plan layout has been designed in accordance with solutions adopted in standard image processing and viewer environments for medical applications.

Moreover the method of orthogonal projections is universally used to represent objectively and dimensionally accurate volumetric object. The essential feature of this visualization method is that it preserves the correct proportions between the elements of the volume. The visualization in all three planes is synchronized: when choosing a point of coordinates $(x_0; y_0; z_0)$, the three images represented are the intersection of the MRI volume with the sagittal coronal and axial planes respectively passing through the point.

3.1 *Fully Manual Labeling of Glial Tumors*

Manual labeling consists in the identification of a series of points on one of the three planes done by each expert individually. The remaining planes are inspected

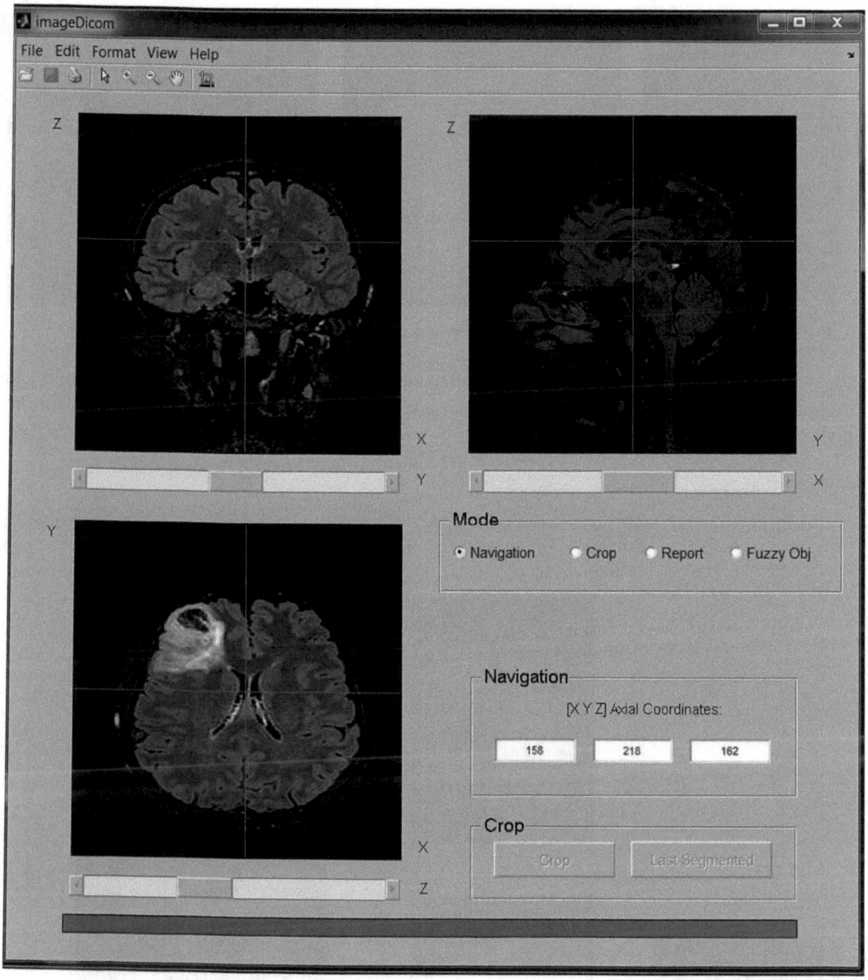

Fig. 6 *GliMAn* Graphical User Interface(GUI): Central zone in navigation mode

by experts to get contextual feedback. The boundary detection task is accomplished element by element and it is organized as follows:

- the user points and selects a candidate point in a given plane;
- the same point is reported in the other two planes and analyzed;
- the expert confirms the decision by re-selecting the same point or decides to examine another point.

Figure 7 shows a crop of axial, sagittal and coronal sections of brain MRI with the presence of glial tumor. In the given case the high degree of infiltration makes tumor boundary identification a very difficult and uncertain task. The analysis of the axial section alone is not enough to make a reliable decision on the point identified with

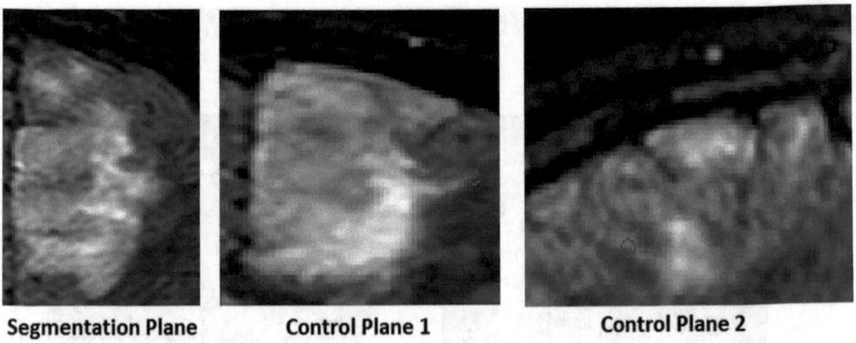

Fig. 7 Crop of brain MRI axial, sagittal and coronal sections with presence of Low Grade Glial Tumor; label assignement considering axial section alone is made under a high level of uncertainty that can be reduced considering the label position in the other two planes

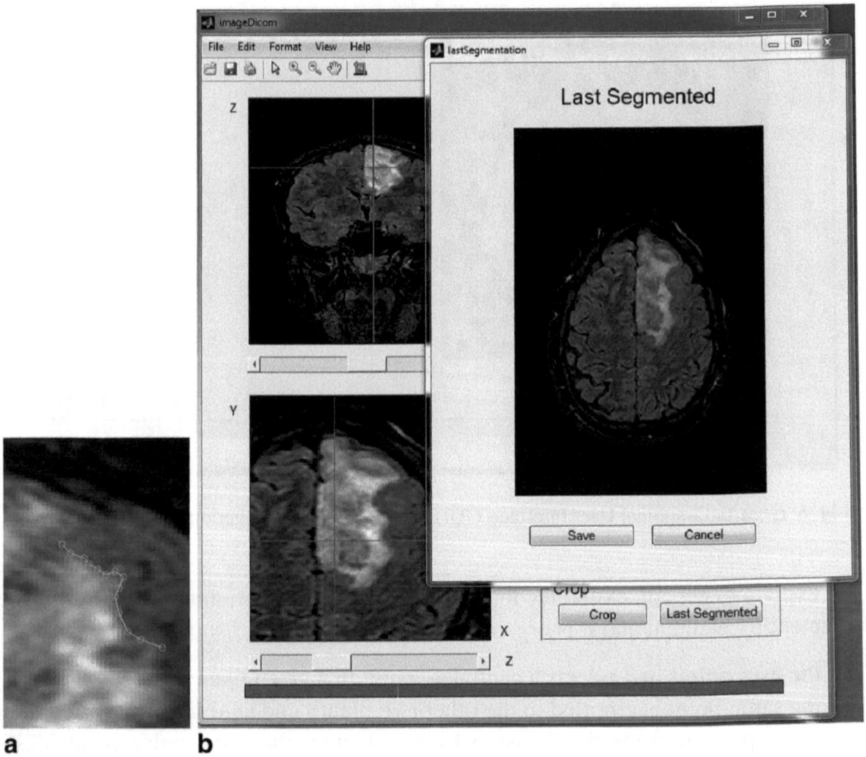

Fig. 8 *GliMAn* Manual Segmentation interactive procedure: (**a**) broken line joining selected points (**b**)segmentation mask superimposed on the original image MRI

the red circle to the edge of the tumor. The visualization of the orthogonal control planes in *GliMAn* interface reduces the uncertainty in the assignment of the point to the boundary. The selected points are then joined by a broken line (Figure 8a). Clicking on the first point the broken line becomes a polygon that encloses the area of interest. Figure 8b shows a segmentation superimposed to the original MRI image. During the segmentation of the $N - th$ slice the segmentation performed on the slice $(N - 1) - th$ is visualized.

3.2 Simultaneous Truth Estimation Using Fuzzy Connectedness

GliMAn implements a reference data estimation method which uses Fuzzy Connectedness principles to merge individual labels and generate segmentation representative of a common agreement [14]. Labels are provided by the experts who are asked to manually identify few highly reliable points belonging to the objects of interest. Points collected by each experts are conceived as multiple seeds and starting from them, the Fuzzy Connectedness algorithm computes the segmentation. The proposed strategy, rooted in the fuzzy set theory, is able to deal with uncertain information and then to manage dissimilarity among manually identified labels. The operator intervention is drastically limited with respect to a complete manual tracing and the formal fuzzy framework supports in the overall process of estimation.

The overall session is organized in two phases:

- collection of information by each expert,
- fusion of the information.

In the first phase, *GliMAm* provides a specific execution mode *Fuzzy Obj*, which imposes a change of visualization based on Maximum Intensity Projection Images [15]. The Maximum Projection Intensity Images (MIP) computed in axial, sagittal and coronal direction are shown on the 3 plans (Fig. 9).

The experts surround the region of interest on each plane containing the tumor. With the intersection of the three projections a *Volume of Interest* (VoI) is identified and the display of orthogonal planes moves in the VoI extracted from the original MRI.

In a second step users identify a set of objects and background seeds together with two regions characterizing the same object and background.

As in a manual labeling session the selection of seed points and regions made by experts is supported with the synchronized visualization in all of the three planes. The set of parameters provided by each expert is then stored using a own identifer. In a subsequent phase the total set of parameters is loaded and the Fuzzy Connectedness is with it initialized and executed.

Segmentation results can be represented in two different ways corresponding to two different display modes. In the *absolute* mode, fuzzy grades of membership associated to an absolute fuzzy object are hardened according to a threshold value provided by experts and the resulting crisp object is display. In the *relative* mode, object elements for which the grades of membership are higher than the grades of the background are computed and displayed.

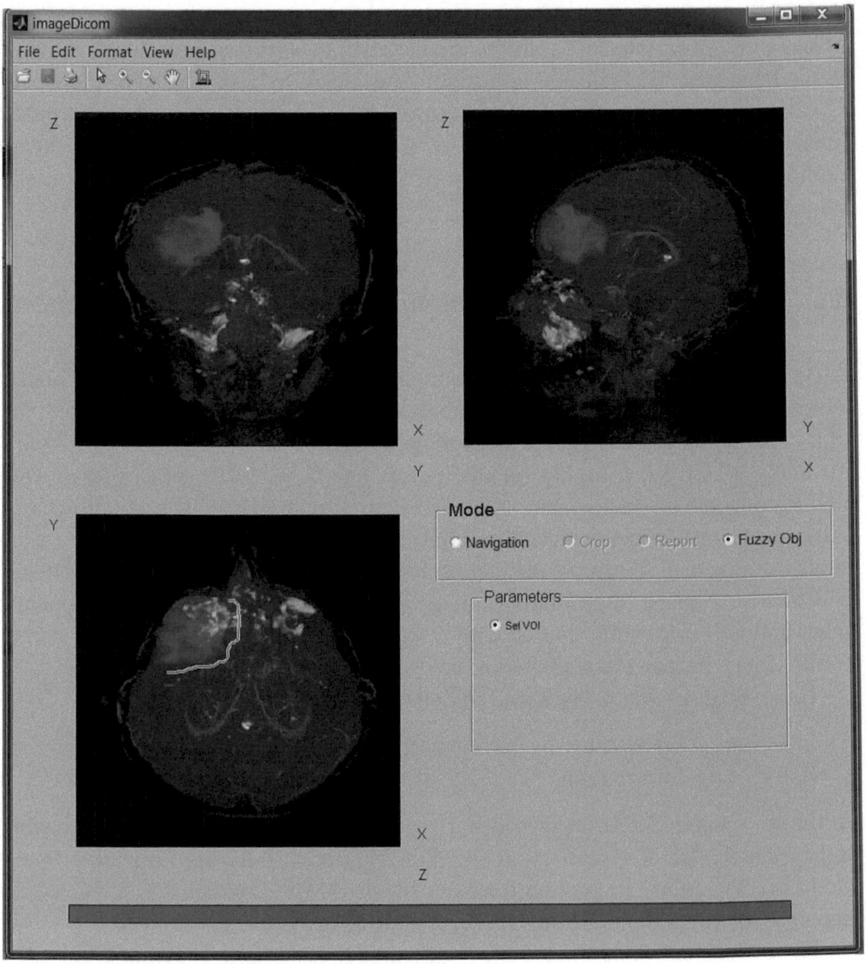

Fig. 9 Axial Sagittal and Coronal Maximun Intensity Projection (MIP) Images shown by *GliMAn* for the Volume Of Interest(VoI) identification

4 Experiments

A set of experiments is conducted to assess how *GliMAn* contributes to the reduction of operation variability in the context of Glial brain tumor segmentation and support the validation of automated segmentation results.

4.1 Experiments in Fully Manual Labeling Using GliMAn

The same group of experts who worked in the operation variability analysis, has been involved again to segment, 4 slices for each of the 4 MRI volumes (case 1-4) of our

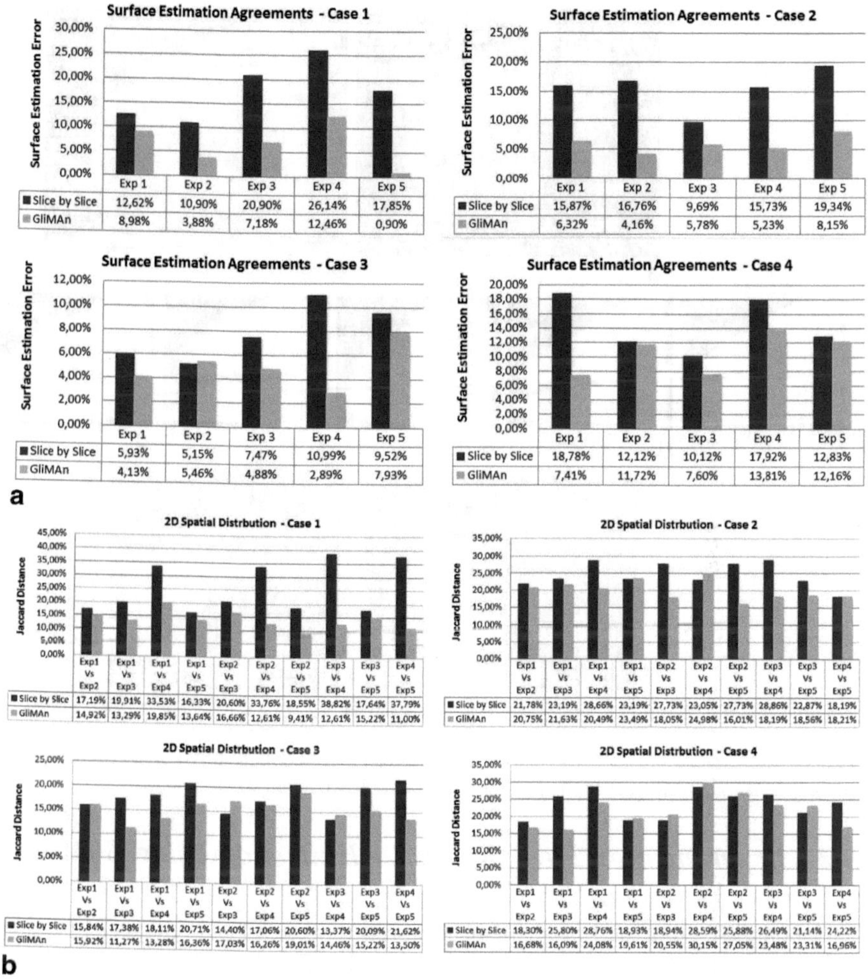

Fig. 10 Mean of the Surface Errors (**a**) and 2D Jaccard distances computed for each expert, varying the 4 slices segmented using conventional and *GliMAn* tools

dataset with the support of *GliMAn*. We measured the 2D inter- variability using the metrics described in section 2 and we compared results with those obtained using the conventional annotator (see Fig. 10a and b). Results are expressed in terms of mean of the surface estimation error and mean of the Jaccard distance respectively, each varying 4 slices and expert. The use of *GliMAn* has determined a significant reduction of the surface estimation error, with a maximum value equal to 16.95 % for case 1 expert 5 and minimum value equal to −0.30 % for case 3 expert 2. The average reduction of the Jaccard distance is equal to 5.14 %, with a maximum value equal to 26.79 % for case 1 between experts 4 and 5; and minimum value equal to −2.63 % for case 3 between experts 2 and 3.

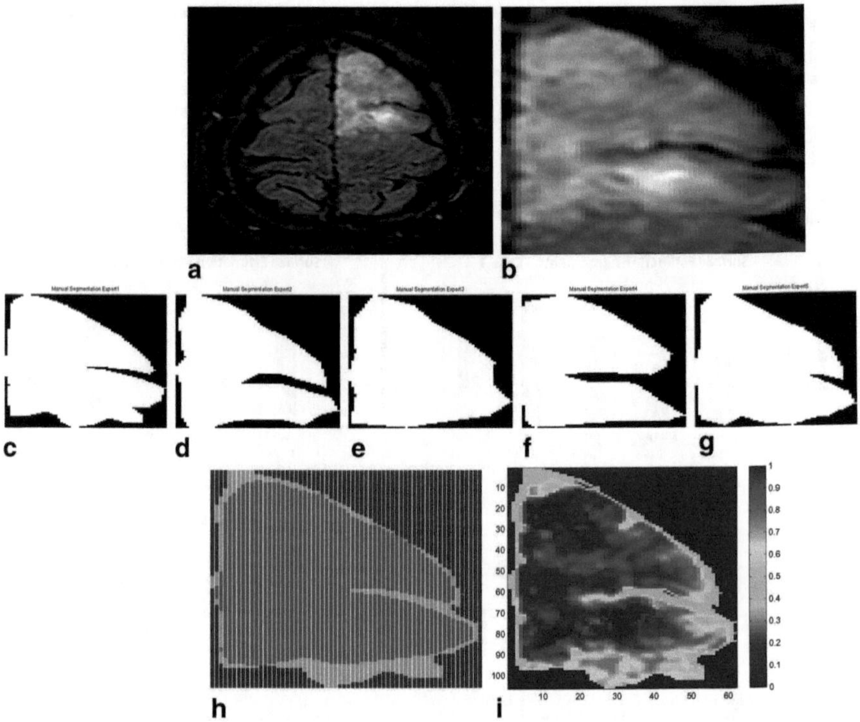

Fig. 11 Reference segmentations of source slice 1-case2 (*a,b*) obtained by Fuzzy Connectedness (i) and by majory voting (*h*) applied on the individual fully manual labels (*c–g*)

4.2 Experiments in Fuzzy Reference Estimation Using GliMAn

To accomplish this experiments medical experts to were asked to manually segment axial slices of volume data and to provide the initialization information necessary to the proposed label fusion strategy. Fuzzy Connectedness-based segmentations are compared with those obtained by applying label fusion by majority voting rule, which is one generally used fusion rules [16]. Figure 11 shows an axial slice of one MRI volume of our dataset (a–b), the resulting segmentations obtained with Fuzzy Connectedness (i), and by majory voting rule (h) applied on the individual fully manual labels (c–g). Some dissimilarities can be observed among the segmentations manually produced by the experts. These differences are conservatively reduced by majority voting that inevitably implies a loss of information. In the fuzzy segmentation output dissimilarities are preserved and accommodated in terms of grades. Looking into the detail of Fig. 11, dissimilarities are particularly evident at the top left, middle right and bottom of the individual segmentation outputs. These regions are included in the fuzzy output but simply discarded by the majority voting fusion process. In the middle right region characterized by a high level of heterogeneity, grades are assessed reflecting the decision attitude of the experts.

5 Conclusion

This paper analyzes and meaures the inter-intra-operator variability in glial tumor segmentation. Based on the results obtained, a strategy for label collection and reference data estimation was designed and implemented in the system *GliMAn*. As seen in our experimental context, fully manual labeling benefits from the use of *GliMAn* facilities that preserves the volumetric nature of image data. The reference data estimation based on fuzzy connectedness allows to estimate consensus segmentation with improved reproducibility and low requirements on operator time.

References

1. Clarke L, Velthuizen R, Camacho M, Heine J, Vaidyanathan M, Hall L, Thatcher R, Silbiger M (1995) MRI segmentation: methods and applications. Magn Reson Imaging 13(3):343
2. Bouix S, Martin-Fernandez M, Ungar L, Koo MNMS, McCarley RW, Shenton ME (2007) On evaluating brain tissue classifiers without a ground truth. Neuroimage, 36:1207–1224
3. Balafar MA Ramli AR, Saripan MI, Mashohor S Review of brain MRI image segmentation methods. Artif Intell Rev 33(3):261–274 (2010)
4. Warfield SK, Zou KH, Wells WM (2004) Simultaneous truth and performance level estimation (STAPLE): an algorithm for the validation of image segmentation. IEEE Transactions Medical Imaging 23(7):903–921. http://view.ncbi.nlm.nih.gov/pubmed/15250643.
5. Rohlfing T, Maurer CR Jr (2007) Shape-based averaging. IEEE Trans Image Process 61:153–161
6. Robitaille N, Duchesne S (2012) Label fusion strategy selection. Int J Biomed Imaging 2012:431095. doi:10.1155/2012/431095
7. Pedoia V, De Benedictis A, Renis G, Monti E, Balbi S, Binaghi E (2012) Proceedings of the 1st International Workshop on Visual Interfaces for Ground Truth Collection in Computer Vision Applications. (ACM, New York, NY, USA, 2012), VIGTA '12, pp 8:1–8:4. doi:10.1145/2304496.2304504. http://doi.acm.org/10.1145/2304496.2304504
8. Udupa J, Samarasekera S (1996) Fuzzy connectedness and object definition: theory, algorithms, and applications in image segmentation. Gr Models Image Process 58(3):246–261
9. Duffau H (2009) Surgery of low-grade gliomas: towards a 'functional neurooncology'. Curr Opin Oncol 21:543–549
10. Duffau H (2005) Lessons from brain mapping in surgery for low-grade glioma: insights into associations between tumour and brain plasticity. Lancet Neurol 4(8):476–486
11. Pallud J, Varlet P, Devaux B, Geha S, Badoual M, Deroulers C (2010) Diffuse low-grade oligodendrogliomas extend beyond MRI-defined abnormalities. Neurology 74(21):1724
12. Kelly PJ, Daumas-Duport C, Kispert DB, Kall BA, Scheithauer BW, Illig JJ (1987) Imaging-based stereotaxic serial biopsies in untreated intracranial glial neoplasms. Journal of Neurosurgery 66(6):865–875
13. Jaccard P (1912) New Phytologist 11(2):37
14. Binaghi E, Pedoia V, Lattanzi D, Balbi S, Monti E, Minotto R (2013) Proceedings Vision And Medical Image Processing, VipIMAGE.
15. Wallis J, Miller T, Lerner C, Kleerup E (1989) Three-dimensional display in nuclear medicine. IEEE Trans Med Imagin 8(4):297–230. doi:10.1109/42.41482
16. Heckemann RA, Hajnal JV, Aljabar P, Rueckert D, Hammers A (2006) Automatic anatomical brain MRI segmentation combining label propagation and decision fusion. Neuroimage 33(1):115–126. doi:10.1016/j.neuroimage.2006.05.061. http://www.sciencedirect.com/science/article/pii/S1053811906006458

Analysis of the Retinal Nerve Fiber Layer Texture Related to the Thickness Measured by Optical Coherence Tomography

J. Odstrcilik, R. Kolar, R. P. Tornow, A. Budai, J. Jan, P. Mackova and M. Vodakova

Abstract The retinal nerve fiber layer (RNFL) is one of the most affected retinal structures due to the glaucoma disease. Progression of this disease results in the RNFL atrophy that can be detected as the decrease of the layer's thickness. Usually, the RNFL thickness can be assessed by optical coherence tomography (OCT). However, an examination using OCT is rather expensive and still not widely available. On the other hand, fundus camera is considered as a common and fundamental diagnostic device utilized at many ophthalmic facilities worldwide. This contribution presents a novel approach to texture analysis enabling assessment of the RNFL thickness in widely used colour fundus photographs. The aim is to propose a regression model based on different texture features effective for description of changes in the RNFL textural appearance related to the variations of RNFL thickness. The performance evaluation uses OCT as a gold standard modality for validation of the proposed approach. The results show high correlation between the models predicted output and RNFL thickness directly measured by OCT.

1 Introduction

Glaucoma is one of the most common causes of permanent blindness worldwide with mean prevalence of 2.4 % for all ages and of 4.7 % for ages above 75 years [1]. One of the glaucoma symptoms is progressive atrophy of the retinal nerve fiber

J. Odstrcilik (✉) · R. Kolar
St. Anne's University Hospital—International Clinical Research Center (ICRC), Brno, Czech Republic
e-mail: odstrcilik@feec.vutbr.cz

J. Odstrcilik · R. Kolar · J. Jan · P. Mackova · M. Vodakova
Department of Biomedical Engineering, Faculty of Electrical Engineering and Communication, Brno University of Technology, Brno, Czech Republic

R. P. Tornow · A. Budai
Department of Ophthalmology, University of Erlangen, Erlangen-Nuremberg, Germany

Pattern Recognition Lab and Erlangen Graduate School of Advanced Optical Technologies, University of Erlangen, Erlangen-Nuremberg, Germany

J. M. R. S. Tavares, R. Natal Jorge (eds.), *Developments in Medical Image Processing and Computational Vision,* Lecture Notes in Computational Vision and Biomechanics 19,
DOI 10.1007/978-3-319-13407-9_2

layer (RNFL) resulting in decrease of the layer's thickness. Degeneration of the nerve fibers starts many years before any changes in the patient's vision can be registered. Unfortunately, pathological changes in the RNFL cannot be revitalized by current medicine. Only, an immediate treatment can help to stop progression of the disease. Hence, it is extremely desirable to detect the disease as soon as possible. The RNFL thickness can be measured by optical coherence tomography (OCT), which is relatively new approach and it is still not widely available due to the high costs. In comparison, fundus camera is considered as a common diagnostic device currently available at many ophthalmic clinics around the world. Moreover, in contrast with OCT, examination by fundus camera is much faster, reducing workload of specialists, and cheaper. Hence, it brings an idea to use this widely available device for the RNFL assessment, especially for screening purposes.

Since the RNFL atrophy is one of the first signs of glaucoma disease that can be visible in fundus images, many researchers try to assess the visual appearance of RNFL. Historically, an attempt to utilize fundus cameras for glaucoma detection by evaluation of the RNFL appearance has been first introduced by Hoyt et al. [2]. The authors qualitatively revealed that the funduscopic signs of the RNFL pattern provide the earliest objective evidence of the RNFL atrophy in the retina. Other authors followed this subjective evaluation of fundus photographs afterwards. Airaksinen et al. [3] investigated the RNFL pattern visually and scored glaucomatous damage in a numerical scale. Peli et al. [4] performed one of the first semi-automatic analysis of the RNFL texture using digitized black-and-white fundus photographs. Yogesan et al. [5] made preliminary analysis of digitized fundus photographs via texture analysis based on gray level run length matrices. In addition, an intensity information about the RNFL texture was utilized again by Dardjat et al. [6] and Lee et al. [7]. Beside these older articles, recent authors have been investigating fundus photographs in more or less similar way. In the case of glaucomatous damage, the RNFL appears darker in fundus images. Therefore, many authors tried to involve intensity criteria for the glaucoma assessment [8–11]. A pilot study to search the RNFL thinning in digital colour fundus images was recently presented by Oliva et al. [10]. The article presents semi-automatic method to texture analysis based on evaluation of the RNFL pattern intensity. Hayashi et al. [8] used an approach with Gabor's filters to enhance certain regions with the RNFL pattern and to cluster these regions towards glaucoma detection. The paper presented preliminary results that were further followed up by the same group in [9]. The authors extended the earlier concept to analysis and performed evaluation using larger dataset. Furthermore, Prageeth et al. [11] published a method for glaucoma detection using intensity criterion as well. Although, the results seemed to be promising, utilization of intensity criteria used alone is probably not a good solution. Intensity changes in the RNFL pattern can be detected only if the RNFL atrophy is so distinctive than the patient has rather large vision loss already. Moreover, image intensity can be influenced by many factors as non-homogenous illumination, reflection of the retina, (in) homogeneity of light power used for image acquisition, etc.

Although, there is a considerable range of articles focused on analysis of fundus images aimed at glaucoma diagnosis, a complex methodology for the RNFL assessment in colour fundus images is still missing. Many published articles present methods based on evaluation of the RNFL intensity. As discussed above, utilization of intensity as a feature for detection of changes in the RNFL is less robust and unsuitable due to many physical as well as physiological reasons. Moreover, testing of the published methods is based mainly on low-resolution images. Thus, subtle variations in the RNFL thickness cannot be easily handled, since the RNFL texture is not detailed enough due to the low-resolution. The RNFL pattern is much more detailed and easily observed in current high-resolution fundus images. This offers a potential application of advanced texture analysis techniques taking into account not only the intensity criteria, but also various spatial characteristics of adjacent pixels in the texture [12–17].

As presented in this contribution, we have utilized our previous methods [13, 15, 16] to RNFL texture analysis using commonly available high-resolution colour fundus images. We extended the potential of these methods in order to show usability of the proposed texture features and their combination. Our approach utilizes Gaussian Markov random field (GMRF) texture modeling and local binary patterns (LBP) to generate features useful for description of changes in the RNFL texture. Different regression models are tested as the predictors of the RNFL thickness using the proposed features. The models are satisfactorily validated utilizing direct measurement of the RNFL thickness via OCT. The results proved that the model predicted output is closely correlated with the RNFL thickness, thus enabling detection of possible RNFL thinning.

2 Image Database

The database contains a number of 19 fundus image sets of healthy subjects and a number of 8 image sets of glaucomatous subjects with distinctive focal wedge-shaped RNFL loss. Only one eye of each subject was images. Each image set contains images acquired by a common non-mydriatic digital fundus camera CANON CR–1 (EOS 40D) with 60-degree field of view (FOV). The images have size of 3504 × 2336 pixels. Standard CANON raw data format (CR2) was used for storage of the images (Fig. 1).

The database also contains three-dimensional volume data and circular scans, acquired by spectral domain OCT system (Spectralis HRA—OCT, Heidelberg Engineering) for each of the 27 subjects. Infrared reflection images (scanning laser ophthalmoscope—SLO) and OCT B–scan (cross-sectional) images were acquired simultaneously. Acquisition of the OCT image volume (Fig. 2a) was performed within the peripapillary area. Circular scan pattern (Fig. 2b) is usually used for glaucoma diagnosis via OCT. A circle with diameter 3.4 mm is placed in the center of the optic disc (OD) and one B-scan is measured along this circle [18].

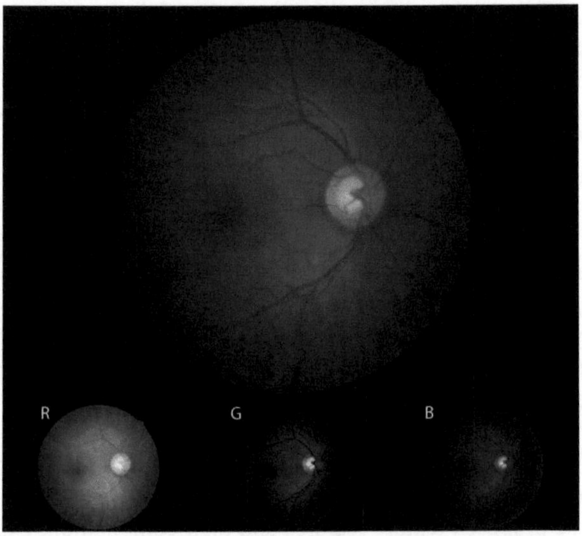

Fig. 1 An example of an original RGB fundus image of the healthy eye and individual colour channels of the image. In standard fundus image, the red (*R*) channel appears oversaturated, while the green (*G*), and the blue (*B*) channels show the blood vessels and retinal nerve fiber layer highly contrasted

3 Methods

An illustrative schematic diagram of the proposed RNFL assessment methodology is depicted in Fig. 3. The texture analysis is carried out within the peripapillary area at the locations without the blood vessels only. Our previously published matched filtering approach [19] is used for the blood vessel segmentation. Various regression models are tested towards prediction of the RNFL thickness using the proposed texture features. The regression models are trained on small square image regions (ROIs) selected from fundus images in the database and known measurement of the RNFL thickness. Circular profiles are extracted from the predicted images provided by the regression models. The resulted profiles are further validated with respect to the real RNFL thickness measured via OCT. The following subsections deal with the description of particular processing steps as well as evaluation of the approach.

3.1 Data Preprocessing

3.1.1 Preprocessing of Fundus Images

The fundus images are preprocessed in several steps. First, standard uncompressed TIFF format is reconstructed from the raw data, whereas a linear gamma transfer function is applied in the reconstruction process. Secondly, non-uniform illumination

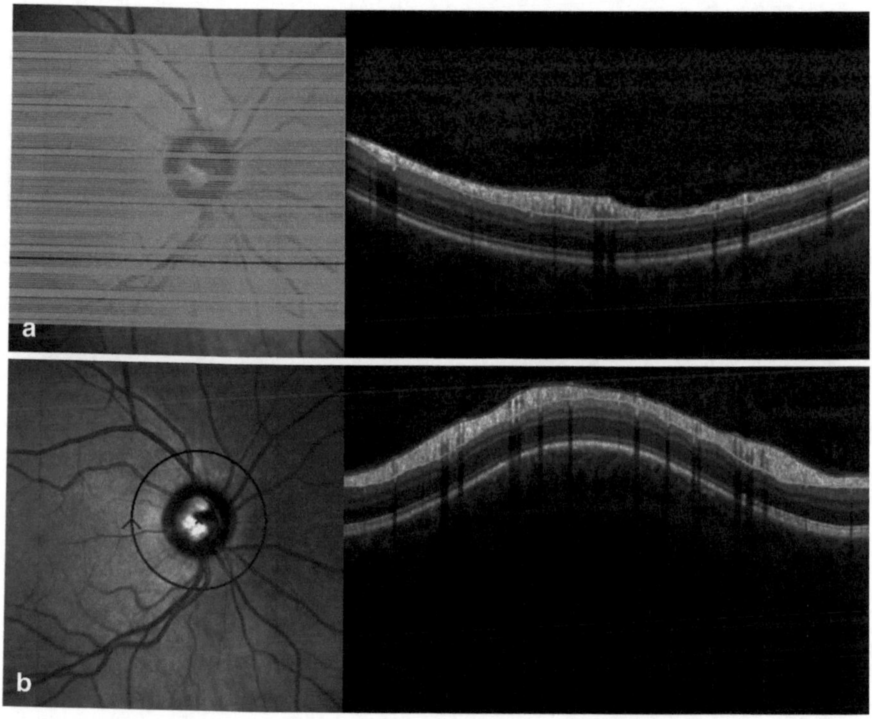

Fig. 2 An example of OCT volume and circular scans. **a** SLO image (*left*) with the volume scan pattern allocated by the *green lines* and one B-scan (*right*) measured at the position depicted by the *blue line* in SLO image; **b** SLO image (*left*) with the circular scan pattern defined by the *blue circle* and the B-scan (*right*) measured along this circle in direction given by the *arrow*. The curves in individual B-scans define segmentation of the RNFL

of fundus images is corrected together with the increase of image contrast using CLAHE (Contrast Limited Adaptive Histogram Equalization) technique [20]. The RNFL texture is the most contrasted in the green (G) and the blue (B) channels of the input RGB image (Fig. 1). Therefore, an average of G and B channel (called GB image) is computed for each fundus image after CLAHE. Further, only the GB images are used for processing.

In the first step, we manually selected small square-shaped image regions of interest (ROIs) with size of 61 × 61 pixels from all fundus images included in the group of normal subjects. Extraction of ROIs was performed uniformly in the peripapillary area to the maximum distance not exceeding 1.5 × diameter of the OD; whereas only locations without the blood vessels were considered (Fig. 4). In this way, a total number of 354 ROIs was collected. Particular ROIs then represent the typical RNFL pattern depending on the position in the peripapillary area for normal subjects without any signs of glaucoma disease.

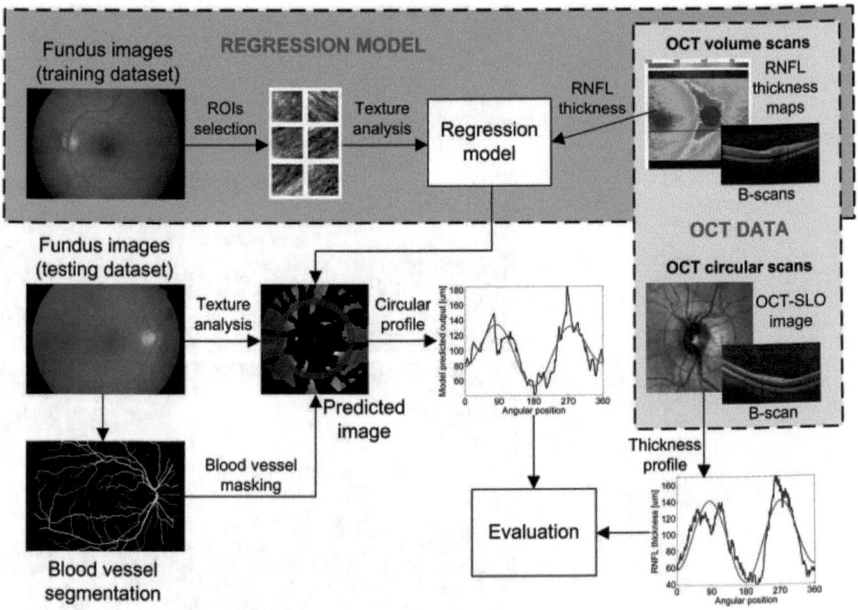

Fig. 3 Schematic diagram of the proposed methodology

3.1.2 Preprocessing of OCT Data

The OCT volume data were preprocessed in order to obtain the RNFL thickness in the peripapillary area of each subject in the database. Hence, the RNFL was segmented and the corresponding RNFL thickness map was created using freely available research software [21]. Segmentation of the RNFL layer was done automatically with very good precision so that only subtle manual corrections had to be performed in some B-scans using this software package (see segmentation of the RNFL in Fig. 2), especially in the area of large blood vessels (shadow artifacts in the B-scans). The final RNFL thickness map can be seen in Fig. 5.

3.1.3 Fundus-OCT Image Registration

Our previously published [22] landmark-based retinal image registration approach with manually selected landmarks and second-order polynomial transformation model was applied for registration of fundus to OCT–SLO image data. This registration step was necessary to be able to compare the proposed texture features with the RNFL thickness at various positions on the retina. However, different registration approaches could be used for this purpose as well, e.g. as in [23].

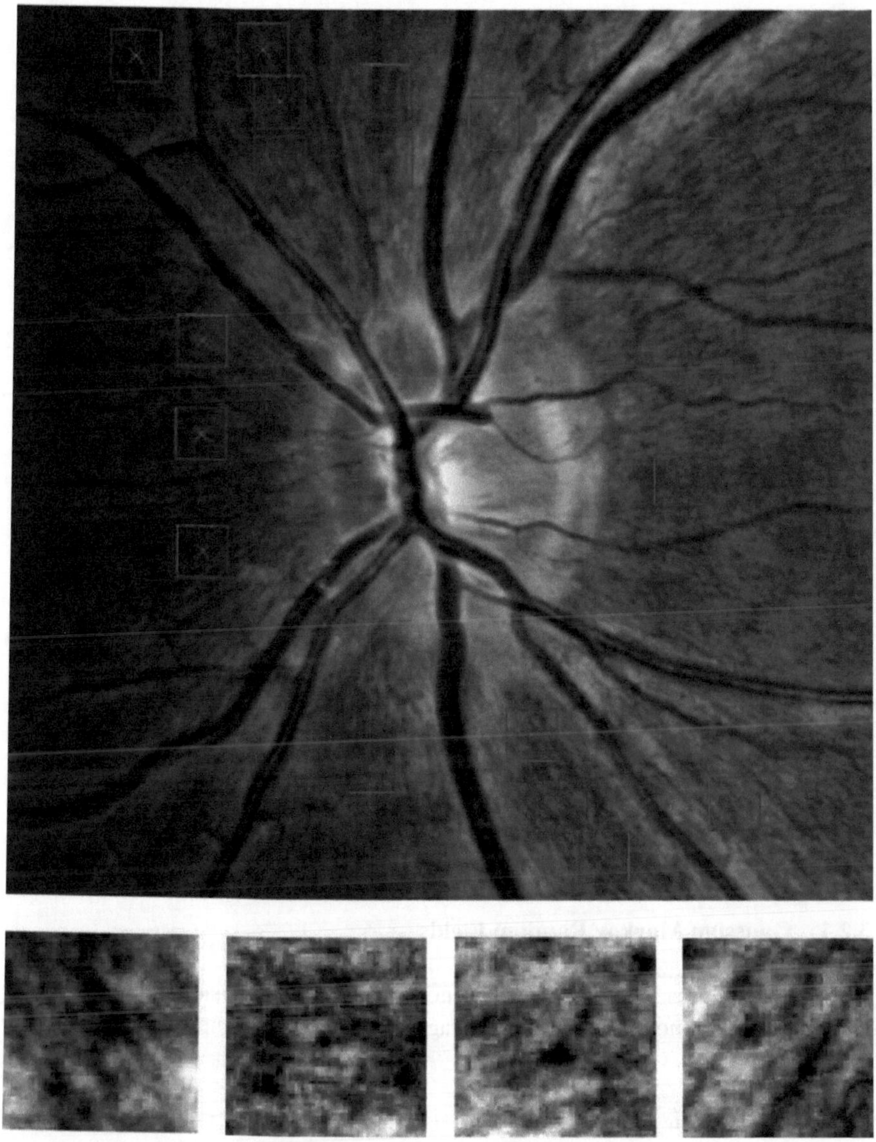

Fig. 4 At the top: section of the GB image after CLAHE processing with depiction of ROI positions; at the bottom: few examples of magnified ROIs with the RNFL texture taken in different positions in the peripapillary area (around the OD)

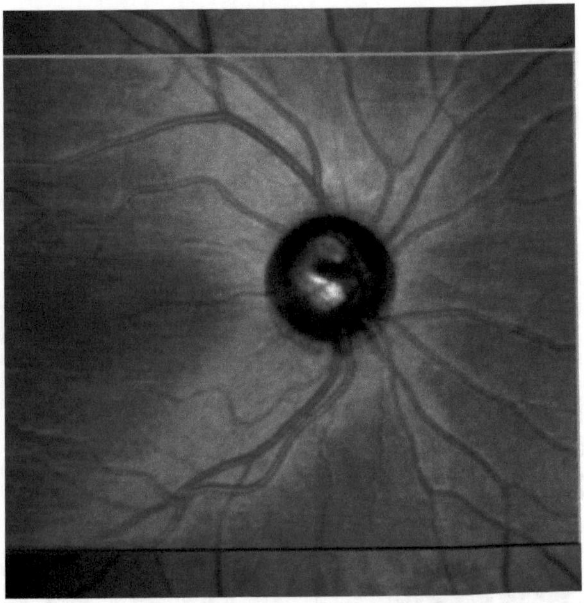

Fig. 5 The RNFL thickness map mapped on the SLO image of a normal subject. The colour spectral scale represents the changes of RNFL thickness approx. from 20 μm (*red*) to 180 μm (*green*)

3.2 Feature Extraction

The advance texture analysis methods, namely Gaussian Markov random field (GMRF) [24] and local binary patterns (LBP) [25] were used for the description of RNFL texture. These approaches were selected due to their rotation- and illumination-invariant properties as well as noise robustness.

3.2.1 Gaussian Markov Random Fields

First set of features is given by GMRF non/causal two/dimensional autoregressive model [24]. The model assumes the image texture is represented by a set of zero mean observations $y(s)$ [24]:

$$y(s), s \in \Omega, \Omega = \{s = (i, j) : 0 \leq i, j \leq M - 1\} \tag{1}$$

for a rectangular $M \times M$ image lattice Ω. An individual observation is then represented by the following difference Eq. [24]:

$$y(s) = \sum_{r \in N_s} \phi_r y(s + r) + e(s) \tag{2}$$

where N_s is a neighborhood set centered at pixel s,ϕ_r is the model parameter of a particular neighbor r, and $e(s)$ is a stationary Gaussian noise process with zero mean and unknown variance σ. A neighborhood structure depends directly on the

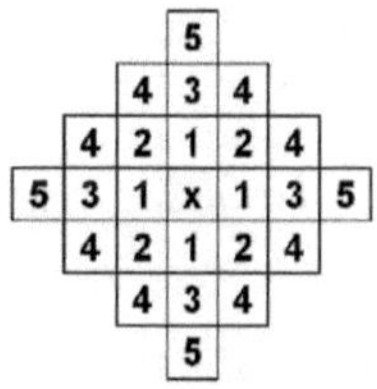

Fig. 6 A fifth-order symmetric rotation-invariant neighborhood structure

order and type of the model. We assume a fifth-order symmetric rotation-invariant neighborhood structure as shown in Fig. 6. The structure considers five parameters expressed by particular numbers. These five parameters describe the relationship between central pixel and its neighbors. Gaussian variance σ is the sixth parameter of the model. Then, these 6 parameters represent features, which are used for the RNFL texture description.

The least square error (LSE) estimation method is used for estimation of the GMRF model's parameters according to the following equations [24]:

$$\phi = \left[\sum_{\Omega} q(s) q^T(s) \right]^{-1} \left(\sum_{\Omega} q(s) y(s) \right), \tag{3}$$

$$\sigma = \frac{1}{M^2} \sum_{\Omega} (y(s) - \phi^T q(s))^2, \tag{4}$$

where

$$q(s) = col \left[\sum_{r \in N_i} y(s+r);\ i = 1, ..., I \right], \tag{5}$$

for an i-th–order neighborhood structure.

3.2.2 Local Binary Patterns

The second applied method—LBP is based on conversion of the local image texture into the binary code using rotation-invariant and uniform LBP operator [25]. The local image texture around the central pixel (x_c, y_c) can be characterized by the LBP code, which is derived via the Eq. [25]:

$$LBP_{P,R}^{riu2}(x_c, y_c) = \begin{cases} \sum_{p=0}^{P-1} s(g_p - g_c) & U(G_P) \leq 2, \\ P+1 & otherwise \end{cases} \tag{6}$$

where $U(G_p)$ means:

$$U(G_P) = |s(g_{P-1} - g_c) - s(g_0 - g_c)| + \sum_{p=1}^{P-1} |s(g_P - g_c) - s(g_{p-1} - g_c)| \quad (7)$$

In Eqs. 6 and 7, g_c corresponds to the grey value of the central pixel (x_c, y_c) of a local neighborhood and $g_p(p=0, \ldots, P\text{–}1)$ corresponds to the grey values of P equally spaced pixels on a circle of radius R ($R > 0$) that form a circularly symmetric neighborhood structure. The LPB operator expressed by Eg. 6 assumes uniform patterns. The "uniformity" of a pattern is ensured by the term $U(G_P)$. Patterns with U value of less than or equal to two are considered as "uniform" [25]. It means these patterns have at most two 0–1 or 1–0 transitions in the circular binary code.

Two variants of LBP were utilized in the proposed approach. Both variants are based on the rotation-invariant and uniform $\mathrm{LBP}_{16,2}$ operator (i.e. $P=16$, $R=2$). One variant uses only LBP distribution computed from an input GB image. Then, the grey-level histogram of such parametric image is computed and extraction of 6 statistical features follows [25]: mean value, standard deviation, skewness, kurtosis, total energy and entropy. In the second variant, standard LBP distribution is supplemented with computation of local contrast $C_{P,R}$:

$$C_{P,R} = \frac{1}{P}\sum_{p=0}^{P-1}(g_p - \mu)^2, \text{ where } \mu = \frac{1}{P}\sum_{p=0}^{P-1} g_p \quad (8)$$

Then, in turn, a joint histogram of $LBP_{P,R}^{riu2}$ and $C_{P,R}$ (LBP/C) is computed. A feature vector is then obtained from LBP/C joint histogram by extraction of 14 texture features proposed by Haralick et al. [26] and Othmen et al. [27] (energy, contrast, homogeneity, entropy, correlation, sum average, sum variance, sum entropy, difference variance, difference entropy, two information measures of correlation, cluster shade, and cluster prominence).

3.2.3 Pyramidal Decomposition

Finally, a 26-dimensional feature vector assembled via connection of particular texture analysis approaches (GMRF, LPB, and LBP/C) is obtained. In addition, the features are computed for an original image resolution and even for each of the two levels of Gaussian pyramid decomposed images. Let the original image be denoted as $G_0(i,j)$, which is zero level of the Gaussian pyramid. Then, the l-th level of the pyramid is defined as follows:

$$G_l(i, j) = \sum_m \sum_n w(m, n) G_{l-1}(2i + m, 2j + n), \quad (9)$$

where $w(m,n)$ is a two-dimensional weighting function, usually called as "generating kernel". According to, [28] recommended symmetric 5 × 5 kernel, written in

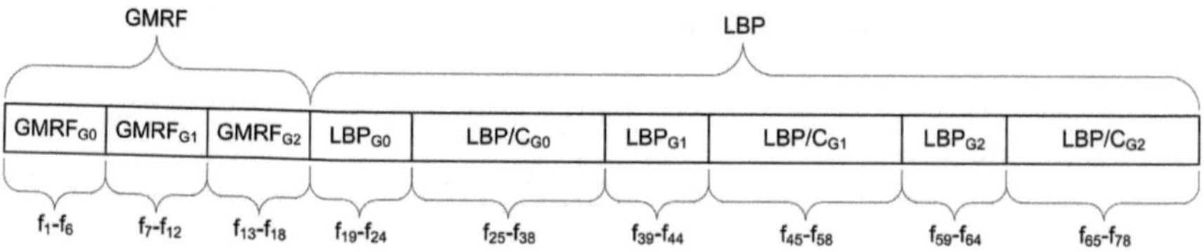

Fig. 7 Schematic diagram of the final feature vector

separated form as $w = \left[\frac{1}{4} - \frac{a}{2}, \frac{1}{4}, a, \frac{1}{4}, \frac{1}{4} - \frac{a}{2}\right]$, where $a = 0.4$, is utilized. Finally, a 78-dimensional feature vector is obtained via extraction of the features from $G_0(i,j)$, $G_1(i,j)$, and $G_2(i,j)$. Composition of the final feature vector is depicted schematically in Fig. 7.

3.2.4 Feature Selection and Regression

The aim of this work is to propose the utilization of texture analysis in fundus images for description of changes in the RNFL pattern related to variations in the RNFL thickness. The ability of the proposed texture analysis methods, in connection with several regression models, to predict the RNFL thickness has been investigated. Different regression models—linear regression (LinReg) [29], two types of support vector regression (ν-SVR, ε-SVR) [30], and multilayer neural network (NN) [31] have been tested to predict values of the RNFL thickness using the proposed texture features. In addition, different feature selection approaches [32] have been tested towards identification of the most relevant feature subset of the original feature set. Finally, we have chosen a popular wrapper-based feature selection strategy with a sequential forward search method (SFS) that provided the most accurate prediction of the RNFL thickness using various regression models. In SFS strategy, standard forward hill-climbing procedure is utilized. The procedure starts with an empty feature set and sequentially adds a feature that yields in the best improvement of a subset. This proceeds until there is no improvement in performance of a particular feature subset. In each iteration of the wrapper approach (for each feature subset), a cross-validation procedure is used to evaluate model output via a chosen evaluation criterion (e.g. mean squared error).

4 Results and Discussion

4.1 Evaluation Methodology

Spearman's rank correlation coefficient (ρ) and root mean squared error of prediction (*RMSEP*) were used as evaluation criteria of the models output. ρ is computed between the model predicted output y and the target variable c as follows [33]:

$$\rho = 1 - \frac{6\sum_{i=1}^{n}(c_i - y_i)^2}{n(n^2 - 1)}, \tag{10}$$

where n is number of samples. The values of y and c are separately ranked from 1 to n in increasing order. y_i and c_i in Eq. 10 represent the ranks of particular observations $i = 1, \ldots, n$ of the respective variables. Spearman's rank correlation coefficient was chosen because of two main properties: (i) it can measure a general monotonic relationship between two variables, even when the relationship is not necessarily linear, and (ii) it is robust to outliers due to ranking of values.

Even when the correlation between y and c can be strong, the predicted values can still differ from the target values with some error. In order to evaluate model accuracy in the error sense, a frequently used heuristic criterion is utilized:

$$RMSEP = \sqrt{\frac{\sum_{i=1}^{n}(c_i - y_i)^2}{n}}. \tag{11}$$

Evaluation of the proposed approach was carried out in two stages. In the first stage, ability of the proposed features to predict the RNFL thickness with particular regression models was evaluated. A feature vector was computed for each of the 354 ROIs. The target variable, i.e. the vector of the RNFL thicknesses at particular locations on the retina, was derived from the interpolated RNFL thickness map provided by the OCT volume data. The repeated random sub-sampling cross-validation technique was used for performance evaluation. This random sub-sampling procedure was repeated 100 times. In each cross-validation run, 70 and 30 % of randomly selected ROIs was utilized for training and testing the model, respectively. Parameters ρ and *RMSEP*, computed between the predicted output and the vector of RNFL thicknesses, were used to evaluate the models performance.

In the second stage, the proposed method was evaluated utilizing entire fundus images. Usually, the OCT device acquires a circular scan (with diameter 3.4 mm) around the ONH and the RNFL thickness is then evaluated in this single scan [18]. Hence, evaluation of the RNFL in fundus images was performed similarly as in OCT in a predefined peripapillary area. First, the blood vessels in fundus images were extracted via our match filtering approach [19] to be able to conduct an analysis in the *non-vessel* areas only. A circular scan pattern was placed manually into the ONH center for each fundus image. This scan pattern consists of five particular circles (to make the scan reasonably thick). Scanning was performed for individual circles and the final profile was interpolated. The same interpolation technique was used to interpolate final profile in the *non-vessel* areas as well.

Table 1 Averaged cross-validation results of particular regression models using the wrapper-based SFS search strategy

Model	ρ[–]	*RMSEP* [μm]
LinReg (5,6,9,11,37,39,48,49,54,64,69,71,78)	0.7430 ± 0.0370	20.0054 ± 1.4542
ν-SVR (5,6,10,32,37,39,44,58,78)	0.7450 ± 0.0379	19.9746 ± 1.3609
ε-SVR (5,6,12,32,37,39,44,49,78)	0.7437 ± 0.0375	20.0587 ± 1.3689
NN (1,6,19,40,44,46,78)	0.6497 ± 0.0469	24.5163 ± 1.7310

All values of ρ are statistically significant with p–values $\ll 0.05$

4.2 Evaluation of the Approach via Cross-Validation

In the first step, the regression models were evaluated using above-mentioned set of 354 ROIs. An optimal feature subset was identified for individual models by an iterative wrapper algorithm (as mentioned in a previous section) minimizing the error between the model output and the RNFL thickness. This way, different subsets were selected for particular models (Table 1). As the best subsets were identified, both ρ and *RMSEP* were evaluated for particular models. Cross-validation results are presented graphically in Figs. 8 and 9, along with their averaged values in Table 1. The selected features are numerically listed below the name of particular models in this table.

4.3 Evaluation of the Method Using Circular Scan Patterns

Previous cross-validation stage revealed that the performance of ν-SVR is slightly over other approaches so it was considered for further testing. Figure 10 shows a significant statistical relation between the RNFL thickness and the model trained on the whole dataset of ROIs ($\rho = 0.7850$, $RMSEP = 18.9402$ μm).

As described earlier, evaluation was carried out in a diagnostically interesting area around the optic disc as can be seen from Figs. 11 and 12. Results of the proposed method (Figs. 11a and 12a) are compared with the RNFL thickness measured by the OCT circular scans (Figs. 11b and 12b). Approximated regression curves are depicted for each scan showing typical double-peak circular scan profiles of the RNFL. Evaluation parameters ρ and *RMSEP* were computed for each circular scan extracted from the images of normal and glaucomatous subjects at the *non-vessel* areas only (Tables 2 and 3).

The results show that there is a significant statistical relation between the values obtained via the proposed texture analysis and the RNFL thickness measured

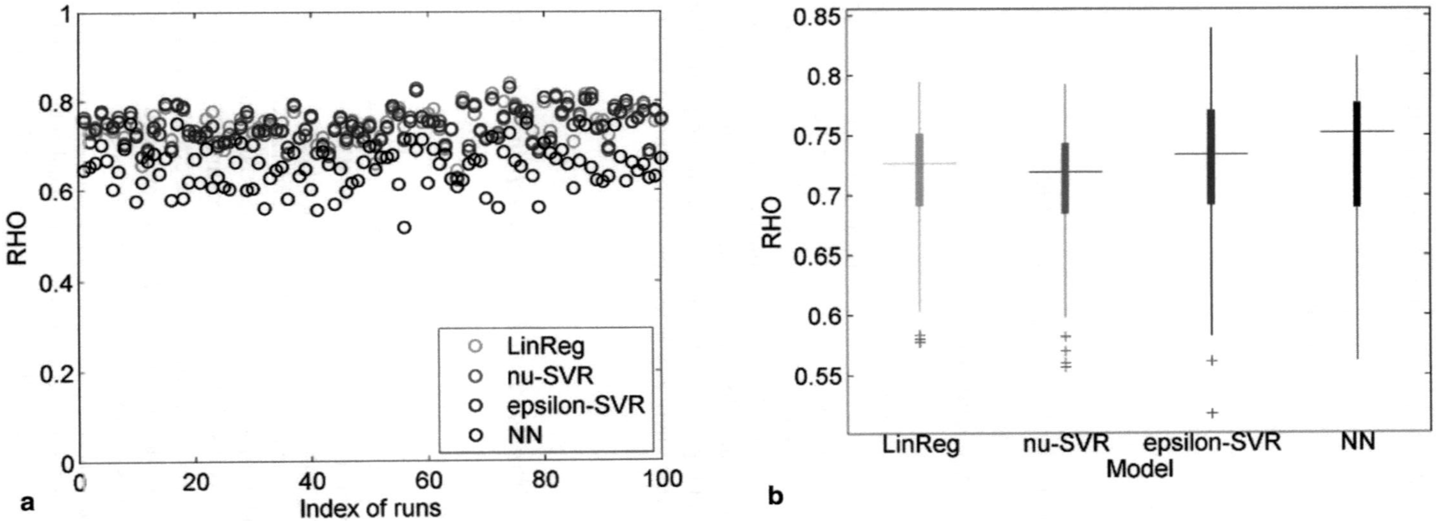

Fig. 8 Cross-validation results of particular models with the wrapper-based SFS search strategy—ρ computed between the models predicted output and the RNFL thickness. The results are depicted graphically in terms of **a** particular cross-validation runs and **b** statistical boxplot diagrams

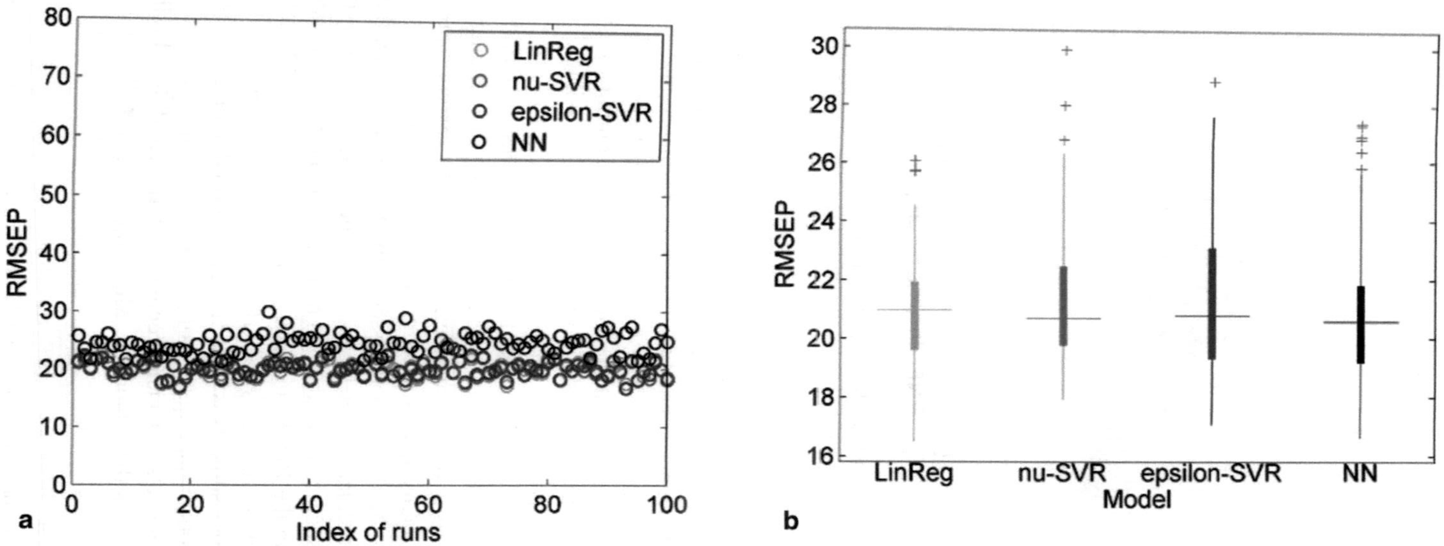

Fig. 9 Cross-validation results for particular models using the wrapper-based SFS search strategy—*RMSEP* computed between the models predicted output and the RNFL thickness. The results are depicted graphically in terms of **a** particular cross-validation runs and **b** statistical boxplot diagrams

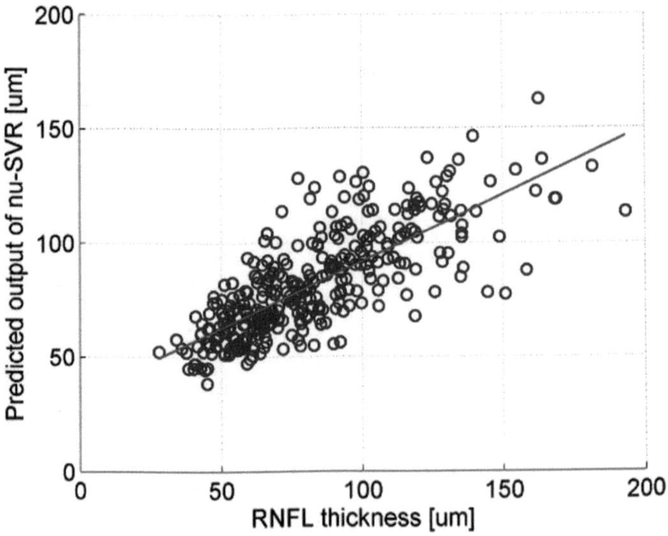

Fig. 10 Relation between the ν-SVR predicted output and the RNFL thickness for a feature subset identified via the wrapper-based SFS approach. The model output was computed for each of the 354 ROIs

by OCT[1]. Examples of the results are shown in Fig. 11–12 to demonstrate major outcomes and drawbacks of the proposed approach. Particularly, Fig. 11 shows results of the image that achieved one of the highest performance in terms of ρ along with one of the lowest error of prediction (image no. 1 in Table 2). Inspecting the result in detail, one can reveal that the model predicted output follows correctly the RNFL thickness profile with subtle differences only. Possible deviations can be caused probably by variations in image quality (blurring and presence of noise in a couple of images). In addition, one drawback concerns the blood vessels that cover rather large area of the retina, especially in the OD surroundings. At the locations of blood vessels and their near neighborhood, the texture representing the RNFL is missing in fundus images. Hence, the texture analysis needs to be carried out at the locations without the blood vessels only. Due to this issue, the predicted values are reduced particularly at the locations of major blood vessel branches. However, even in the worst case, the evaluation revealed that the results are still relevant capturing variations in the RNFL thickness significantly. Figure 12 then shows an example of glaucomatous subject. The performance of the method evaluated using images of glaucomatous subjects is lower than for normal subjects. Generally, this is probably due to worse image quality of glaucomatous subjects that were tested (possibly caused by cataracts and unclear ocular media). In addition, limited number of patients also influences the evaluation. Mean values of *RMSEP* (Table 2 and 3)

[1] Significance of the results was statistically validated by t-test at the 5 % significance level.

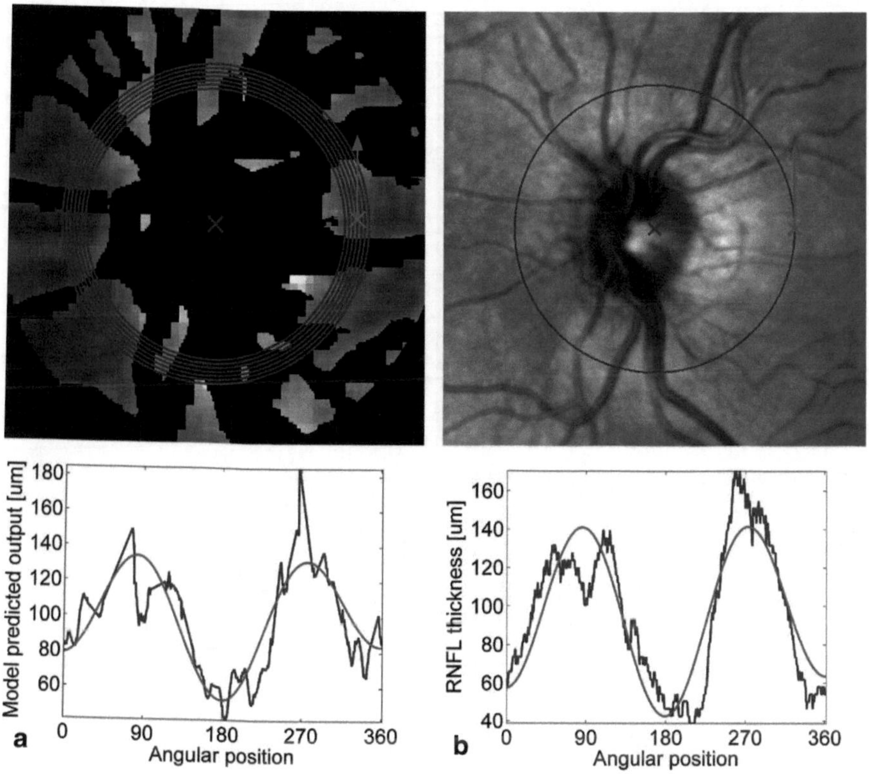

Fig. 11 Images of circular scans of the normal subject and corresponding profiles: **a** ν-SVR model output with the corresponding profile, **b** SLO image with circular scan pattern and the RNFL thickness profile. *Red curves* represent polynomial approximation of each profile. The *red arrow* indicates direction of scanning

could signalize limited precision of the proposed methodology. However, these error values are probably acceptable (especially for screening purposes), since they are comparable with the general difference between normal and glaucomatous RNFL thickness (~20–25 μm) [34]. Despite the drawbacks mentioned, the evaluation part revealed that the proposed methodology could satisfactorily contribute to the RNFL assessment based only on fundus camera. The proposed texture analysis approach is able to capture continues variations in the RNFL thickness and thus can be used for possible detection of the RNFL thinning caused by pathological changes in the retina. Additional advantage of this texture approach is that the proposed features are invariant to changes of illumination and light reflection.

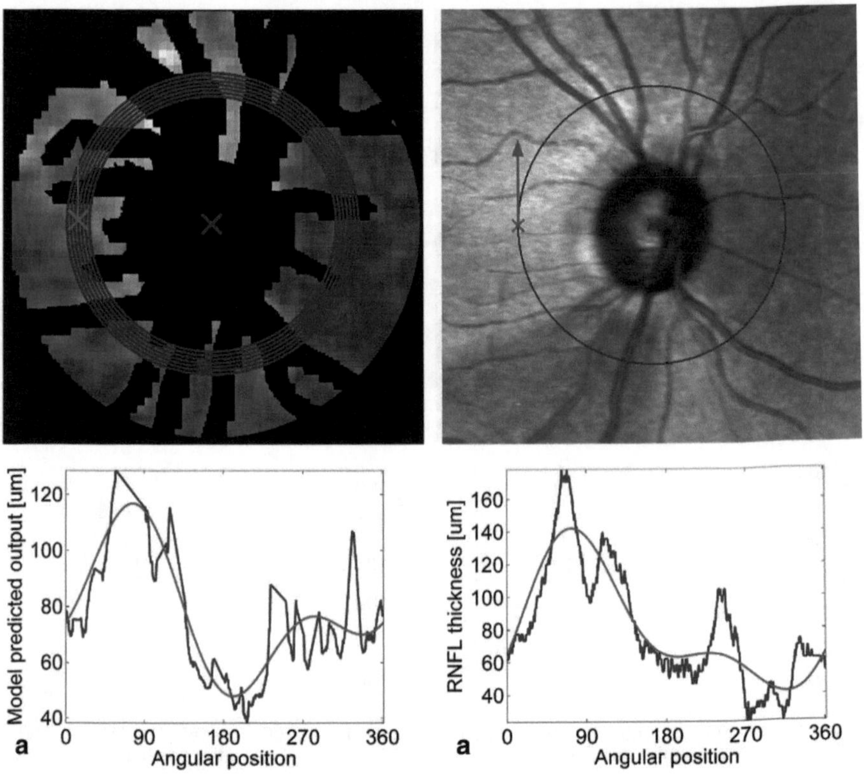

Fig. 12 Images of circular scans of the glaucomatous subject and corresponding profiles: **a** ν-SVR model output with corresponding profile, **b** SLO image with circular scan pattern and the RNFL thickness profile. *Red curves* represent polynomial approximation of each profile. The *red arrow* indicates direction of scanning. The RNFL loss can be seen approx. at the angular position of 270-degrees

5 Conclusions

The complex approach to texture analysis of the RNFL in colour fundus images is presented. The results revealed that the proposed texture features can be satisfactorily applied for quantitative description of continues variations in the RNFL thickness. Obtained values of ρ and *RMSEP* confirmed usability of the proposed approach for prediction of the RNFL thickness using only colour fundus images. Thus, it promises applicability of this approach for detection of the RNFL thinning caused by pathological changes in the retina.

One limitation of the proposed texture approach may be requirement of high quality fundus images with sufficient resolution and sharpness. However, many recent fundus cameras are able to take images with sufficient resolution and it will be no longer a problem due to progressive development of fundus imaging in the future. In addition, some preprocessing approaches could be considered for enhancement

Table 2 Evaluation of the method on the images of normal subjects. The values in brackets deal with approximated profiles (the red curves in Fig. 11). The values are computed for the non-vessel locations only. Minimum and maximum values are boldfaced in each column

Image no.	ρ [−]		*RMSEP* [μm]	
1	**0.90**	(0.98)	15.85	(10.50)
2	0.81	(0.82)	16.51	(24.89)
3	0.69	(0.88)	18.23	(14.59)
4	0.83	(0.98)	16.34	(16.25)
5	0.85	(0.96)	22.37	(22.48)
6	**0.60**	(0.92)	22.11	(12.75)
7	0.67	(0.91)	17.50	(11.34)
8	0.82	(0.97)	23.08	(23.50)
9	0.79	(0.90)	18.65	(12.02)
10	0.72	(0.92)	**25.65**	(17.81)
11	**0.90**	**(0.99)**	24.36	(24.29)
12	0.80	(0.98)	24.73	**(25.49)**
13	0.80	(0.92)	22.10	(22.13)
14	0.79	**(0.80)**	21.66	(20.43)
15	0.64	(0.90)	23.69	(15.18)
16	0.70	(0.90)	22.67	(20.71)
17	0.71	(0.95)	21.12	(17.86)
18	0.83	(0.94)	**14.56**	(10.58)
19	0.65	**(0.99)**	16.15	**(13.57)**
mean	**0.76**	**(0.93)**	**20.39**	**(17.70)**
std	**0.09**	**(0.05)**	**3.48**	**(5.18)**

All values of ρ are statistically significant with p–values $\ll 0.05$

of the RNFL in fundus images (e.g. as in [35]) or for improving an image quality using some image restoration techniques (e.g. as in [36]). Moreover, using a contrast enhancing optical filter may also help to enhance appropriate colour channels and improve visibility of the RNFL pattern [37].

The proposed methodology is not limited for utilization of presented texture analysis methods, namely GMRF and LBP. Other approaches, with respect to noise robustness and rotation- and illumination- invariant properties, can be probably used as well. Then, different feature sets could be used as an input for regression models. Hence, in the further development, possible addition of other texture features could be considered.

The performance evaluation has been so far performed with limited sample size (especially of glaucomatous subjects). Nevertheless, evaluation on normal subjects is

Table 3 Evaluation of the method on the images of glaucomatous subjects. The values in brackets deal with approximated profiles (the red curves in Fig.12). The values are computed for the non-vessel locations only. Minimum and maximum values are boldfaced in each column

Image no	ρ [–]		RMSEP [μm]	
1	0.66	(0.71)	20.08	(19.49)
2	0.59	(0.68)	20.44	(18.05)
3	0.57	**(0.82)**	**12.63**	**(10.48)**
4	**0.36**	**(0.36)**	24.23	(21.30)
5	0.37	(0.41)	**32.05**	**(28.91)**
6	**0.69**	(0.75)	27.45	(25.24)
7	0.53	**(0.82)**	18.97	(12.91)
8	0.45	(0.43)	23.71	(18.12)
mean	**0.53**	**(0.62)**	**22.44**	**(19.31)**
std	**0.13**	**(0.19)**	**5.86**	**(6.02)**

All values of ρ are statistically significant with p–values $\ll 0.05$

equally important in comparison to evaluation on pathological retinas of glaucomatous subjects. Also in the healthy eyes, the range of the RNFL thicknesses is sufficient enough (approx. 20–200 μm) to evaluate an ability of the proposed approach aimed to capture continues variations in the RNFL thickness. However, a study using larger dataset of colour fundus images with corresponding OCT thickness measurement still need to be carried out in a future. Further development can lead to clinical validation of the proposed approach and creating an extensive normative database. A normative database can then allow performing classification of the RNFL (similarly as is used in OCT).

Acknowledgments This work has been supported by European Regional Development Fund—Project FNUSA-ICRC (No.CZ.1.05/1.1.00/02.0123). In addition, the authors gratefully acknowledge funding of the Erlangen Graduate School in Advanced Optical Technologies (SAOT) by the German Research.

References

1. Bock R, Meier J, Nyul L et al (2010) Glaucoma risk index: automated glaucoma detection from color fundus images. Med Image Anal 14:471–481
2. Hoyt WF, Frisen L, Newman NM (1973) Fundoscopy of nerve fiber layer defects in glaucoma. Invest Ophthalmol Vis Sci 12:814–829
3. Airaksinen JP, Drance MS, Douglas RG et al (1984) Diffuse and localized nerve fiber loss in glaucoma. Am J Opthalmol 98(5):566–571
4. Peli E, Hedges TR, Schwartz B (1989) Computer measurement of the retina nerve fiber layer striations. Appl Optics 28:1128–1134

5. Yogesan K, Eikelboom RH, Barry CJ (1998) Texture analysis of retinal images to determine nerve fibre loss. Proceedings of the 14th International Conference on Pattern Recognition, vol 2, Aug. 16–20, Brisbane, Australia, pp 1665–1667
6. Dardjat MT, Ernastuti E (2004) Application of image processing technique for early diagnosis and monitoring of glaucoma. Proceedings of KOMMIT, Aug. 24–25, Jakarta, pp 238–245
7. Lee SY, Kim KK, Seo JM et al (2004) Automated quantification of retinal nerve fiber layer atrophy in fundus photograph, Proceedings of 26th IEEE IEMBS, pp 1241–1243
8. Hayashi Y, Nakagawa T, Hatanaka Y et al (2007) Detection of retinal nerve fiber layer defects in retinal fundus images using Gabor filtering. Proceedings of SPIE, vol 6514, pp 65142Z
9. Muramatsu Ch, Hayashi Y, Sawada A et al (2010) Detection of retinal nerve fiber layer defects on retinal fundus images for early diagnosis of glaucoma. J Biomed Opt 15(1):1–7
10. Oliva AM, Richards D, Saxon W (2007) Search for color–dependent nerve–fiber–layer thinning in glaucoma: a pilot study using digital imaging techniques. Proc Invest Ophthalmol Vis Sci 2007 (ARVO), May 6–10, 2007, Fort Lauderdale, USA, E-Abstract 3309
11. Prageeth P, Sukesh K (2011) Early detection of retinal nerve fiber layer defects using fundus image processing. Proc. of IEEE Recent Advances in Intelligent Computational Systems (RAICS), Sept. 22–24, Trivandrum, India, pp 930–936
12. Kolar R, Jan J (2008) Detection of glaucomatous eye via color fundus images using fractal dimensions. Radioengineering 17(3):109–114
13. Novotny A, Odstrcilik J, Kolar R et al (2010) Texture analysis of nerve fibre layer in retinal images via local binary patterns and Gaussian Markov random fields, Proceedings of 20th International EURASIP Conference (BIOSIGNAL 2010), Brno, Czech Republic, pp 308–315
14. Acharya UR, Dua S, Du X, Sree SV et al (2011) Automated diagnosis of glaucoma using texture and higher order spectra features. IEEE Trans Inf Technol Biomed 15:449–455
15. Odstrcilik J, Kolar R, Jan J et al (2012) Analysis of retinal nerve fiber layer via Markov random fields in color fundus images, Proceedings of 19th International Conference on Systems, Signals and Image Processing (IWSSIP 2012), Vienna, Austria, pp 518–521
16. Odstrcilik J, Kolar R, Tornow RP et al (2013) Analysis of the retinal nerve fiber layer texture related to the thickness measured by optical coherence tomography, Proceedings of VIPimage 2014 conference, Funchal-Madeira, Portugal, pp 105–110
17. Jan J, Odstrcilik J, Gazarek J et al (2012) Retinal image analysis aimed at blood vessel tree segmentation and early detection of neural–layer deterioration. Comput Med Imag Graph 36:431–441
18. Bendschneider D, Tornow RP, Horn F et al (2010) Retinal nerve fiber layer thickness in normal measured by spectral domain OCT. J Glaucoma 19(7):475–482
19. Odstrcilik J, Kolar R, Budai A et al (2013) Retinal vessel segmentation by improved matched filtering: evaluation on a new high-resolution fundus image database. IET Image Process 7(4):373–383
20. Pizer SM, Amburn EP, Austin JD (1987) Adaptive histogram equalization and its variations. Comput Vis Graph Image Proc 39:355–368
21. Mayer M, Hornegger J, Mardin CY, Tornow RP (2010) Retinal nerve fiber layer segmentation on FD–OCT scans of normal subjects and glaucoma patients. Biomed Opt Express 1:1358–1383
22. Kolar R, Harabis V, Odstrcilik J (2013) Hybrid retinal image registration using phase correlation. Imaging Sci J 61(4):269–384
23. Ghassabi Z, Shanbehzadeh J, Sedeghat A, Fatemizadeh E (2013) An efficient approach for robust multimodal retinal image registration based on UR-SIFT features and PIIFD descriptors. EURASIP J Image Video Proc 25:1–16
24. Porter R, Canagarajah N (1997) Robust rotation–invariant texture classification: wavelet, Gabor filter and GMRF based schemes. IEEE Proc Vis–Image Signal Proc 144(3):180–188
25. Ojala T, Pietikäinen M, Mäenpää T (2002) Multiresolution gray-scale and rotation invariant texture classification with Local Binary Patterns. IEEE Trans Pattern Anal Mach Intell 24(7):971–987

26. Haralick RM, Shanmugan K, Dinstein I (1973) Textural Features for Image Classification. IEEE Trans Syst, Man, Cybern 3(6):610–621
27. Othmen MB, Sayadi M, Fnaiech F (2008) A multiresolution approach for noised texture classification based on co–occurrence matrix and first–order statistics. World Acad Sci, Eng Tech 39:415–421
28. Burt P (1983) The Laplacian pyramid as a compact image code. IEEE Trans Commun 31(4):532–540
29. Murphy KP (2012) Machine learning: a probabilistic perspective. The MIT Press, Cambridge, p 1067
30. Chang Ch, Lin Ch (2011) LIBSVM: a library for support vector machines. ACM Trans Intell Syst Technol 27(2):1–27
31. Mandic DP, Chambers JA (2001) Recurrent neural networks for prediction. Wiley, New York, p 285
32. Liu H, Motoda H (2007) Computational methods of feature selection. Chapman Hall/CRC Data Mining and Knowledge Discovery Series, Boca Raton, p 440
33. Indrayan A (2008) Medical biostatistics, 2nd ed. Chapman and Hall/CRC, Boca Raton, p 771
34. Madeiros FA, Zangwill LM, Bowd C, Vessain RM, Susanna R et al (2005) Evaluation of retinal nerve fiber layer, optic nerve head, and macular thickness measurements for glaucoma detection using optical coherence tomography. Am J Ophthalmol 139:44–55
35. Frisén L (2007) Anisotropic enhancement of the retinal nerve fiber layer. Neuro-Ophthalmology 31(4):99–103.
36. Marrugo AG, Šorel M, Šroubek F et al (2011) Retinal image restoration by means of blind deconvolution. J Biomed Optics 16(11):1–11
37. Tornow RP, Laemmer R, Mardin C et al (2007) Quantitative imaging using a fundus camera. Proceeding of Invest Ophthalmol Vis Sci (ARVO), Fort Lauderdale, USA, vol 48, E-Abstract 1206

Continuum Mechanics Meets Echocardiographic Imaging: Investigation on the Principal Strain Lines in Human Left Ventricle

A. Evangelista, S. Gabriele, P. Nardinocchi, P. Piras, P.E. Puddu, L. Teresi, C. Torromeo and V. Varano

Abstract We present recent investigations on the state of strain in human left ventricle based on the synergy between continuum mechanics and echocardiographic imaging. When data from three-dimensional Speckle Tracking Echocardiography are available, special strain directions can be detected on the epicardial and endocardial surfaces, which are well-known in continuum mechanics as principal strain lines (PSLs), further classified into primary and secondary strain lines. An appropriate investigation on PSLs can help to identify lines where strains are largest as primary and smallest as secondary. As PSLs change when cardiac diseases appear, the challenge is that the analysis may allow for the identification of new indicators of cardiac function.

P. Nardinocchi (✉) · P. Piras
Dipartimento di Ingegneria Strutturale e Geotecnica, Sapienza—Università di Roma, Rome, Italy
e-mail: paola.nardinocchi@uniroma1.it

A. Evangelista
Ospedale San Giovanni Calibita Fatebenefratelli-Isola Tiberina, Rome, Italy

S. Gabriele · V. Varano
Dipartimento di Architettura, LaMS—Modeling & Simulation Lab, Università Roma Tre, Rome, Italy

P. Piras
Dipartimento di Scienze, Università Roma Tre, Rome, Italy

Center for Evolutionary Ecology, Università Roma Tre, Rome, Italy

P. E. Puddu · C. Torromeo
Dipartimento di Scienze Cardiovascolari, Respiratorie, Nefrologiche, Anestesiologiche, Sapienza Università di Roma, Rome, Italy

L. Teresi
Dipartimento di Matematica e Fisica, LaMS—Modeling & Simulation Lab, Università Roma Tre, Rome, Italy

J. M. R. S. Tavares, R. Natal Jorge (eds.), *Developments in Medical Image Processing and Computational Vision*, Lecture Notes in Computational Vision and Biomechanics 19,
DOI 10.1007/978-3-319-13407-9_3

1 Introduction

The heart is a specialised muscle that contracts regularly and pumps blood to the body and the lungs. The center of the pumping function are the ventricles; due to the higher pressures involved, the left ventricle (LV) is especially studied. On a simplistic level, LV is a closed chamber, whose thick walls are composed of muscle fibres. It is the *contraction* originated in the muscles that translates into pressure and/or volume changes of the chamber. Moreover, the helicoidal fibres make relevant the torsion of the chamber with respect to the longitudinal axis due to both pressure changes and muscle contraction. The LV cycle may be schematized as the sequence of four steps: filling-the *diastolic* phase; isovolumetric contraction; ejection-the *systolic* phase; isovolumetric relaxation [1].

During the cycle, both pressure and volume vary in time, and a quite useful determinant of the cardiac performance is the plot representing the pressure-volume relationship in the LV during the entire cycle, that is, the PV loop; some of the many clues contained in the plot (see Fig. 1) are briefly summarized in the following. Point 1 defines the end of the diastolic phase and is characterized by the end-diastolic volume (EDV) and pressure (EDP); at this point the mitral valve closes and cardiac muscle starts to *contract* in order to increase the blood pressure. At point 2 the systolic phase begins: the aortic valve opens and blood is ejected outside the LV; muscle keeps on contracting in order to further the ejection, while volume decreases to a minimum. Point 3 defines the end of the systolic phase, and is characterized by the end-systolic volume (ESV) and pressure (ESP); starting from here, LV undergoes an isovolumic *relaxation* until point 4, where mitral valve opens and filling begins.

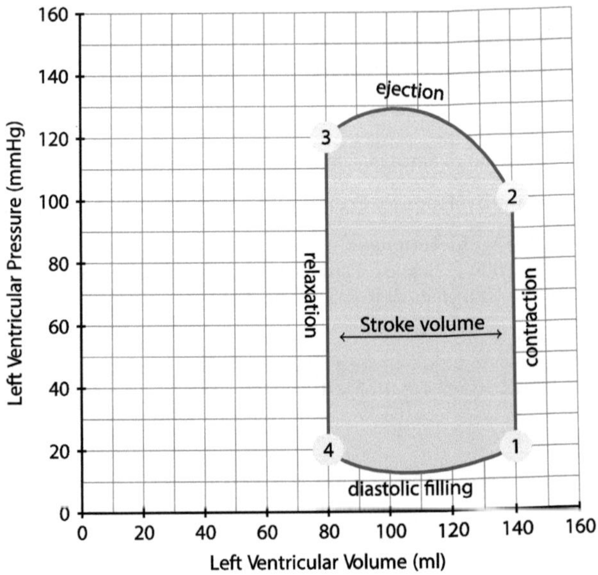

Fig. 1 Cartoon sketching the phases of the cardiac cycle of a normal human subject. *1* Mitral valve closes; isovolumetric contraction. *2* Aortic valve opens; ejection. *3* Aortic valve closes; relaxation. *4* Mitral valve opens, filling. The green area represents the stroke work

During the filling phase, muscle keeps on relaxing in order to accomodate a large increase in blood volume, while maintaining the pressure at a quite low level. Filling is completed at point 1. The difference between maximum and minimum volume is called stroke volume (SV): $SV := EDV - ESV$. From a mechanical point of view, the most intense work is performed along the pattern from point 2 to point 3, that is, along the systolic phase, when pressures are high and muscle contraction too. Typically, critical behaviors of the ventricular function are evidenced in this phase, and mechanics can suggest which are good indicators of cardiac function. A relevant condition about these indicators is the possibility to catch them through noninvasive analyses.

A well-known example is ventricular torsion [23]. The role played by the LV torsional rotation with respect to LV ejection and filling was only recently recognized by application of speckle tacking echocardiography, whose output includes, among the other things, the pattern of ventricular torsion along the cardiac cycle [4, 5, 10–12, 16]. As ventricular torsion is altered when a few pathologies are present (see [3, 13, 18, 22, 24, 28]), it can be used as an indicator of cardiac function which can be noninvasively investigated through 3-dimensional speckle tracking echocardiography (3DSTE).

Detection of principal strain lines in LV may emerge as another possible noninvasive tool to discriminate among different LVs as well as a tool that can help clinicians to identify cardiac diseases at the early stages. On the other hand, and differently from ventricular torsion, PSLs are not delivered as output by 3DSTE devices, and a post-processing analysis of 3DSTE data is needed to identify them, based on concepts borrowed from continuum mechanics. In [17, 20], it was initially proposed to look at PSLs to identify muscle fiber architecture on the endocardial surface. Therein, the echocardiographic analysis was limited to the endocardial surface, and it was noted as due to the high contractions suffered by muscle fibres along the systolic phase, PSLs may well determine just muscle fiber directions. Successively, in [8] an accurate protocol of measurement of PSLs was proposed, tested, and succesfully verified through a computational model. The conclusions of this last work were partially in contrast with the ones in [20]. It was demonstrated, firstly, that on the endocardial surface of healthy LVs, primary strain lines identify circumferential material directions; secondly, that on the epicardial surface primary strain lines are similar to muscle fiber directions. In [6, 8, 9], a comparison between a real human LV and a corresponding model was implemented by the same Authors; the conclusions of [8] were confirmed, and made precise through a statistical analysis involving real and computational data.

What is emerging, even if further investigations are needed, is that endocardial PSLs coincide with circumferential material lines, due to the relevant stiffening effect of the circumferential material lines when high pressures are involved, as it occurs along the systolic phase, and to the capacity of the same material fibers to contrast the LV dilation. It would mean that these visible functional strain lines are related to the capacity of elastic response of the cardiac tissue to the high systolic pressure, and that it might be important to follow this pattern when, due to pathological conditions, this capacity is missing.

2 Continuum Cardio-Mechanics

Typically, when mechanics is applied to biology, it is named biomechanics; we use cardio-mechanics to mean that specific branch of mechanics which has been successfully applied to the analysis and investigation of the cardiovascular system, whose center is the heart pump. Discuss the contribution of cardio-mechanics to clinics is beyond our aims (refer to [7] for extended references); we only aim to shortly discuss two different approaches of mechanics to clinics, with specific reference to the heart pump.

The first approach is based on the continuum analysis of the heart, aimed to model the cardiac activity. It starts from the construction of anatomical models of the heart and of constitutive model describing the passive and active material response of cardiac tissues. Electromechanical interaction are sometimes accounted for, if one has interest to also investigate cardiac electrophysiology. Typically, these models are implemented within a finite element code. Critical points are the constitutive models of the tissue, being cardiac tissue highly non homogeneous and contracting, due to an electrophysiological stimulus, and anatomical data about muscle architecture, which strongly influences the mechanical performances of the heart [14, 15, 27]. Once the model is complete, specific cardiac diseases can be included within the modeling, and the consequences on the heart activity studied. Typical examples are given by the investigations on the heart remodeling due to left anterior descending artery occlusion, to ventricular hypertrophy, to aortic stenosis, well discussed in literature [10, 18, 24]. Likewise, the model can be improved to account consequences of an infarct in different places of the left ventricular walls, with the aim of studying the ability of the pump to get on or not its work [13].

Here, we are more interested in the second approach, which starts from an analysis of real data extracted from the heart through appropriate tools such as Magnetic Risonance Image (MRI) and 3DSTE. Of course, such data are only concerning heart kinematics, and say nothing about stresses within heart walls. However, as it is recently shown, an accurate and careful analysis of real data allows to deeply investigate on heart. Let us note that the interest in in-vivo myocardial deformation dates back to ′80; in [26], the normal in-vivo three-dimensional finite strains were studied in dogs, through the application of appropriate markers whose coordinated were followed along the cardiac cycle through high-speed biplane cineradiography. Of course, the analysis was highly invasive. The recent techniques of visualization realized by 3DSTE make possible follow the coordinates of natural markers, automatically identified by the device, appropriately supported by an operator.

A typical example of the outcomes of a deep analysis on 3DSTE real data comes from PSLs, which are the core of this contribution. In mechanics, it is well-known that stresses and strains within a body are limited above and below by their principal counterparts; this allows for the discussion and verification of the mechanical state of that body. Moreover, the principal stress and strain lines (which are the same only when special symmetry conditions are verified) determine the directions where the largest strains and/or stresses are to be expected. Due to these characteristics, the mechanics of fiber-reinforced bodies are often based on the detection of the principal strain lines and, wherever needed, fiber architecture is conceived in order to make the fiber lines coincide with the PSLs. Fibers make a tissue highly anisotropic; hence, principal strain and stress lines may be distinct. Whereas principal strains can be measured starting with the analysis of tissue motion, being only dependent on the three-dimensional strain state of the tissue, principal stresses can only be inferred. Thus, the PSL have a predominant role where the analysis of the mechanics of a body is concerned, and can reveal which are the lines where largest strains are expected, and how they change when diseases occur.

Key point is the evaluation at any place within the body of the nonlinear strain tensor **C**, whose eigenpairs (eigenvalues-eigenvectors) deliver principal strains and PSLs, respectively. Fixed a body, identified with the region $\mathcal{B}$ of the three-dimensional Euclidean space $\mathcal{E}$ it occupies at a time t_o denoted as reference configuration of the body, we are interested in following the motion of the body at any time $t \in \mathcal{I} \subset \mathcal{R}$, with the time interval $\mathcal{I}$ identifying the duration of a human cardiac cycle (hence, different from subject to subject, as it is discussed later). The displacement field **u**, that is a map from $\mathcal{B} \times \mathcal{T} \rightarrow \mathcal{V} = T\mathcal{E}$, delivers at any time and for any point $y \in \mathcal{B}$ the position $p(y,t)$ of that point at that time: $p(y,t) = y + \mathbf{u}(y,t)$. Strains are related to displacement gradients within the body; precisely, it can be shown as, introduced the deformation gradient $\mathbf{F} = \nabla p = \mathbf{I} + \nabla \mathbf{u}$, the nonlinear Cauchy-Green strain tensor is

$$\mathbf{C} = \mathbf{F}^T\mathbf{F} = \mathbf{I} + \nabla\mathbf{u} + \nabla\mathbf{u}^T + \nabla\mathbf{u}^T\nabla\mathbf{u}\,, \tag{1}$$

being **I** the identity tensor in $\mathcal{V}$. In general, **C** is a three-dimensional tensor, describing the strain state at any point y and time t of the body. If there is within the body a distinguished surface $\mathcal{S}$, whose unit normal field is described by the unit vector field **n**, the corresponding surface strain tensor $\hat{\mathbf{C}}$ can be obtained through a preliminary projection of **C** onto that surface. The projector $\mathbf{P} = \mathbf{I} - \mathbf{n} \otimes \mathbf{n}$, leads to the following definition:

$$\hat{\mathbf{C}} = \mathbf{PCP}\,. \tag{2}$$

It is expected that $\hat{\mathbf{C}}$ will represent a plane strain state, hence, that it will have a zero eigenvalue corresponding to the eigenvector **n**. The primary strain lines on the surface will be the streamlines of the eigenvector $\mathbf{c}_2$, which lies on the surface and corresponds to the smallest non-zero eigenvalues; the secondary strain lines are the streamlines corresponding to the eigenvector $\mathbf{c}_3$. Of course, when the strain tensor **C** is ab initio evaluated from surface deformation gradients $\check{\mathbf{F}} = \mathbf{PFP}$, it naturally arises as a plane tensor.

3 Speckle Tracking Echocardiography

Speckle tracking echocardiography (STE) is an application of pattern-matching technology to ultrasound cine data and is based on the tracking of the 'speckles' in a 2D plane or in a 3D volume (2DSTE and 3DSTE, respectively). Speckles are disturbances in ultrasounds caused by reflections in the ultrasound beam: each structure

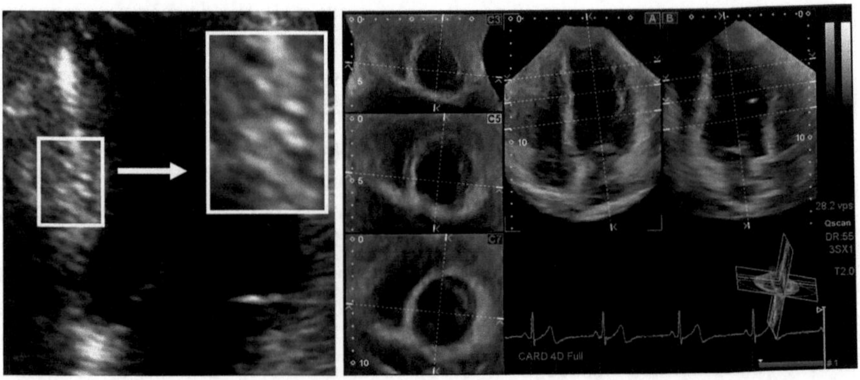

Fig. 2 Speckles moving with tissue as viewed through STE (*left*); the apical four chamber view (*A*); the second apical view orthogonal to plane A (*B*); three short-axis planes (*C*), in the apical region (*C1*), in the mid-ventricle (*C2*), and at the basal portion of the LV (C3) (*right*) (unmodified from the original ARTIDA image)

in the body has a unique speckle pattern that moves with tissue (Fig. 2, left panel). A square or cubic template image is created using a local myocardial region in the starting frame of the image data. The size of the template image is around 1 cm^2 in 2D or 1 cm^3 in 3D. In the successive frame, the algorithm identifies the local speckle pattern that most closely matches the template (see [29] for further details). A displacement vector is created using the location of the template and the matching image in the subsequent frame. Multiple templates can be used to observe displacements of the entire myocardium. By using hundreds of these samples in a single image, it is possible to provide regional information on the displacement of the LV walls, and thus, other parameters such as strain, rotation, twist and torsion can be derived.

Echocardiographic examinations were performed with an Aplio-Artida ultrasound system (Toshiba Medical Systems Co, Tochigi, Japan). Full-volume ECG-gated 3D data sets were acquired from apical positions using a 1–4 MHz 3D matrix array transducer to visualize the entire LV in a volumetric image. To obtain these 3D data sets, four or six sectors were scanned from consecutive cardiac cycles and combined to provide a larger pyramidal volume covering the entire LV. The final LV geometry was reconstructed by starting from a set of 6 homologous landmarks (see Fig. 2), manually detected by the operator for all subjects under study. The manual detection for a given set of landmarks is crucial because it allows recording spatial coordinates in perfectly comparable anatomical structures of different subjects (following a homology principle). The results of our 3DSTE system is a time-sequence of shapes, each constituted by 1297 landmarks, assumed to be homologous, for both the epicardial and endocardial surfaces, positioned along 36 horizontal circles, each comprised of 36 landmarks, plus the apex (see Fig. 3).

Typically, the results of the 3D-wall motion analysis are presented to the user as averaged values for each segment identified by the device according to the American

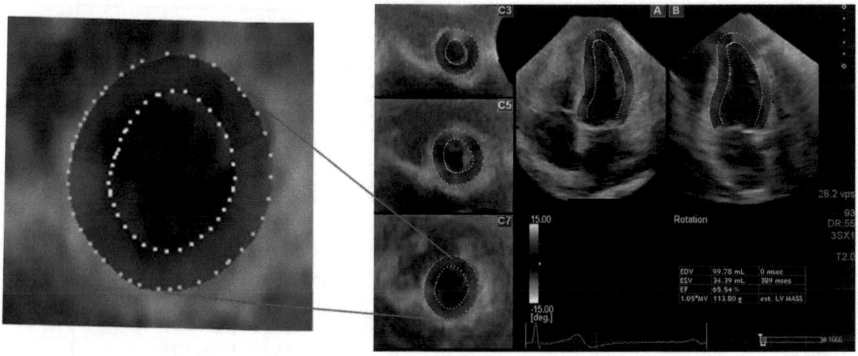

Fig. 3 The markers automatically set by the software supporting 3DSTE are shown as small yellow points on both three planes taken perpendicularly to the LV axis (*left panel*) and on two vertical sections (*right panel*). In particular, in the figure the color code corresponds to the torsional rotation of the LV at the beginning of the cardiac cycle (as evidenced by the small bar at the right bottom corner of the figure)

Heart Association standards for myocardial segmentation [2]: 6 basal segments (basal anterior (BA), basal antero-septum (BAS), basal infero-septum (BS), basal inferior (BI), basal posterior (BP), basal lateral (BL)); 6 middle segments (middle anterior (MA), middle antero-septum (MAS), middle infero-septum (MS), middle inferior (MI), middle posterior (MP), middle lateral (ML)); 4 apical segments (apical anterior (AA), apical septal (AS), apical inferior (AI), apical lateral (AL)). Hence, in each frame of the cardiac cycle time-curves graphs are generated, showing the mean values over the six middle segments, as the ones shown in Fig. 4, and representing the mean circumferential strains at any time along the cardiac cycle on each middle segment, and the overall mean value over the left ventricle's middle part, for a human subject.

3.1 Speckle Tracking Echocardiographic Data

In our case, it was possible to obtain the landmark clouds (upon which the standard rotational, torsional and strain parameters are computed and outputted by each Artida machine) by an unlocked version of the software equipping our PST25SX Artida device, thanks to a special opportunity provided in the context of an official research and development agreement between the Dipartimento di Scienze Cardiovascolari, Respiratorie, Nefrologiche Anestesiologiche e Geriatriche (Sapienza Università di Roma) and Toshiba Medical System Europe (Zoetermeer, The Netherland).

Our 3DSTE data were based on the acquisition made on a group of volunteers, who were randomly selected from the local list of employees at a single University Hospital Department. Individuals were subjectively healthy without a history of hypertension or cardiac disease and were not taking medications. They all had normal ECG and blood pressure below 140/90 mmHg [25]. Being the aim of the present

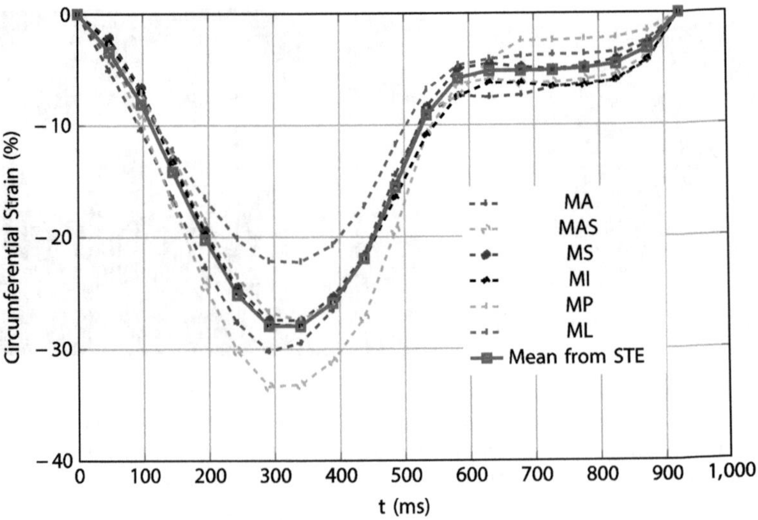

Fig. 4 Circumferential strains versus time: mean values of the circumferential strains on the six segments of the mid-myocardium identified by their acronyms (MA for middle-anterior, MAS for middle antero-septum, MS for middle infero-septum, MI for middle inferior, MP for middle posterior, ML for middle lateral); (*dashed* lines); mean value at mid-myocardium (solid, magenta)

work the analysis of the primary and secondary strain-line patterns in the LV walls, rough data from 3DSTE are played through MatLab, as prescribed by the protocol of measurement proposed and tested in [8], and shortly summed up in the next section.

3.2 *MatLab Post-Processing Code*

Starting from 3DSTE data on walls's motion and using the protocol proposed and verified in [8], the surface nonlinear strain tensor **C** on the LV epicardium and endocardium can be evaluated. Precisely, **C** is evaluated in correspondence of the landmarks (see Fig. 3), at each time along the cardiac cycle.

As already written, the real LV is identified by a cloud of $36 \times 36 \times 2 + 1$ points (called markers p_i) whose motion is followed along the cardiac cycle: the position of each of the $(36 \times 36) \times 2$ points p_i $(i = 1, 36 \times 36 \times 2)$ is registered by the device at each time frame j of the cardiac cycle, and represented through the set of its Cartesian coordinates. These coordinates refer to a system represented by the $\mathbf{i}_3$ axis defined by the longitudinal LV axis and the $(\mathbf{i}_1, \mathbf{i}_2)$ axes on the orthogonal planes. The clouds of markers are intrinsically ordered. Figure 5 shows the endocardial (left panel) and epicardial (right panel) clouds $\mathcal{S}_{endo}$ and $\mathcal{S}_{epi}$ of points corresponding to our representative individual within the sample survey. To each point $P \in \mathcal{S}_{endo}$ ($\mathcal{S}_{epi}$), identified within the intrinsic reference system by the pairs of 3DSTE coordinates z and ϕ, corresponds a set of n positions within the Cartesian coordinate system, where

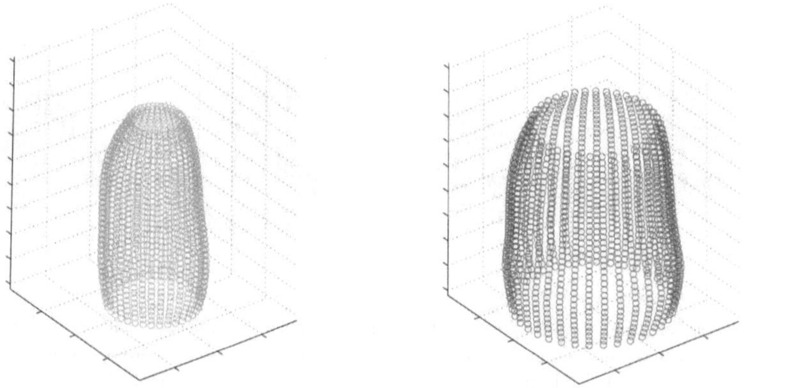

Fig. 5 Cloud of 1296 points automatically identified by the software on the endocardial (*left* panel, green empty dots) and epicardial (*right* panel, violet empty dots) surface, so as rendered by MatLab for a human subject within our group

n is the number of equally spaced frames registered by the device along the cardiac cycle. Moreover, let $P_z \in \mathcal{S}_{endo}$ and $P_\phi \in \mathcal{S}_{endo}$ be the points close to the point P in the 3DSTE topology, *i.e.* identified within the intrinsic reference system by the pair $(z + h_z, \phi)$ and $(z, \phi + h_\phi)$ of 3DSTE coordinates, where $h_z = H(LV)/36$, $h_\phi = 2\pi/10$, and $H(LV)$ the height of the LV model. The vectors $P_z - P$ and $P_\phi - P$ span a non-orthonormal covariant basis $(\mathbf{a}_1, \mathbf{a}_2)$ which corresponds to the 3DSTE coordinate system. The corresponding controvariant basis $(\mathbf{a}^1, \mathbf{a}^2)$ can be easily evaluated. Let p, p_z, and p_ϕ denote the positions occupied by the points P, P_z, and P_ϕ respectively at the frame j; they define the covariant basis $\tilde{\mathbf{a}}_1 = p_z - p$ and $\tilde{\mathbf{a}}_2 = (p_\phi - p)$.

Both $\mathbf{a}_\alpha$ and $\tilde{\mathbf{a}}_\alpha$ are known in terms of their Cartesian coordinates. Thus, the following holds:

$$\tilde{\mathbf{a}}_1 = \lambda_i^z(j)\,\mathbf{i}_i \quad \text{and} \quad \tilde{\mathbf{a}}_2 = \lambda_i^\phi(j)\,\mathbf{i}_i, \tag{3}$$

where j refers to the frame along the cardiac cycle;

$$\mathbf{a}_1 = \lambda_i^z\,\mathbf{i}_i \quad \text{and} \quad \mathbf{a}_2 = \lambda_i^\phi\,\mathbf{i}_i, \tag{4}$$

where $\lambda_i^\phi = \lambda_i^\phi(0)$ and $\lambda_i^z = \lambda_i^z(0)$.

At each point, the nonlinear strain tensor $\mathbf{C}$ can be evaluated through its components

$$\mathbf{C}_{\beta\delta} = \mathbf{F}^\alpha_\beta\,\mathbf{F}^\gamma_{\ \delta}\,(\mathbf{a}_\alpha \cdot \mathbf{a}_\gamma), \quad \alpha, \beta = 1, 2, \tag{5}$$

with

$$\mathbf{F}^\alpha_\beta = \mathbf{F}\,\mathbf{a}_\beta \cdot \mathbf{a}^\alpha = \tilde{\mathbf{a}}_\beta \cdot \mathbf{a}^\alpha. \tag{6}$$

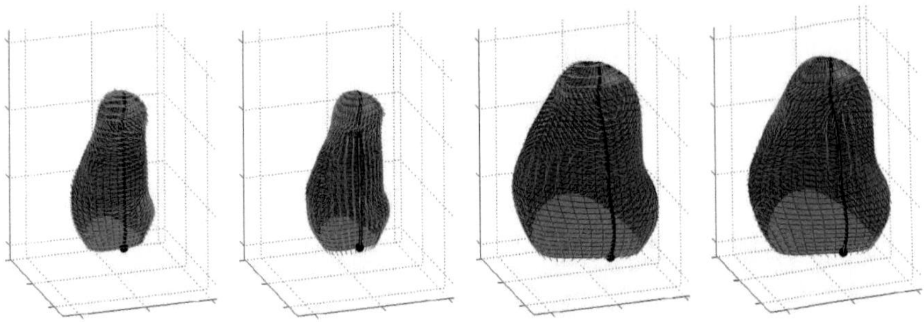

Fig. 6 Representation, in one subject, of the endocardial primary and secondary strain lines (from *left* to *right*: panel 1 and 2); and of the epicardial primary and secondary strain lines (from *left* to *right*: panel 3 and 4). It can be appreciated the behavior of primary strain lines in the middle (*green*) part of the LV

The eigenvalue analysis on **C** reveals a plane strain state, thus delivering the expected results concerning the primary and secondary strain lines. The corresponding eigenvalue-eigenvector pairs are denoted as $(\bar{\gamma}_\alpha, \bar{\mathbf{c}}_\alpha)$, where $\alpha = 2, 3$.

4 Principal Strain Lines in Real Human Left Ventricle

Through the protocol shortly summed up in the previous section, we can evaluate PSLs corresponding to different subjects. We started with the evaluation of primary and secondary strains and strain lines at the systolic peak. As cardiac cycle's duration is different from subject to subject, we needed at first to fix a few points along the cardiac cycle identifying homologous times, that is, times corresponding to the occurrences of special mechanical and electrical events which can be identified along any cardiac cycles. With this, we associate to the real-time scale based on the finite number of times caught by the 3DSTE device along the cardiac cycle, a new time scale, based on 6 homologous times which are the same along any cardiac cycle. The systolic time was identified as the one corresponding to the end systolic volume. Other homologous times before the systolic one are those corresponding to the peak of R wave and to the end of T wave; homologous times after the systolic one are those corresponding to the mitral-valve opening, to the end of rapid filling (beginning of diastasis), and to the onset of Q wave.

Figures 6 and 7 show endocardial and epicardial primary and secondary strain lines corresponding to the homologous systolic times and to two different human LVs, chosen among our data as representative of the group. The colors identify different parts of the LVs: grey for the apical part, green for the middle part, and orange for the basal part. Each line identifies the direction of the primary and secondary strain line at a point of the endocardial and epicardial cloud defined by 3DSTE. The endocardial and epicardial surfaces which in the figure represent the support for the strain lines correspond to the images of those surfaces at the systolic time.

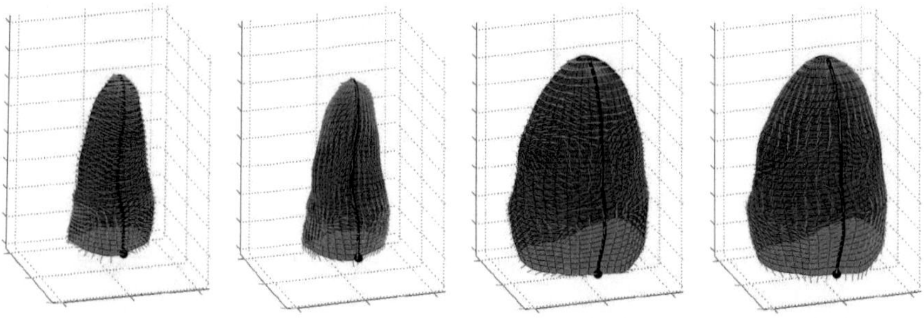

Fig. 7 Representation, in another subject, of the endocardial primary and secondary strain lines (from *left* to *right*: panel 1 and 2); and of the epicardial primary and secondary strain lines (from *left* to *right*: panel 3 and 4). It can be appreciated the behavior of primary strain lines in the middle (*green*) part of the LV

As Figs. 6 and 7 show, the LV endocardial primary strain lines (first panel from left to right in both figures) have the same circumferential pattern evidenced in the model we studied in [8], even if in the basal part of the LV, the influence of the stiffer structure of the mitral annulus alter the circumferential pattern. Even if volumes and shapes are different one from another, endocardial primary strain lines are almost the same and circumferential. The first and second panels (from left to right) in both Figs. 6 and 7 are referred to the endocardial primary and secondary strain lines, which appear prevalently longitudinal in the middle part of the ventricle, according to the prevalent circumferential orientation of the primary strain lines there. The third and fourth panels show instead epicardial primary and secondary strain lines. The pattern of primary strain lines is less regular, even over the middle part of the ventricle, which should not be much influenced by the stiffer structure of the mitral annulus. However, in both cases, different zones are evident where epicardial primary strain lines follow lines which resemble muscle fiber directions. The results we got from our investigations, even if they need be supported by further data, allowed us to make a conjecture based on the pattern of endocardial primary strain lines. We conjecture that the inflation-induced dilation due to blood pressure is more effective for subendocardial layers, which dilating reduce the circumferential shortening induced by muscle contraction. Better is the capacity of the elastic response of the endocardial surface, smaller is the dilation induced by blood pressure.

It means that the capacity to contrast blood pressure is reduced in patients with volume overload, hence the primary strain values which correspond to the circumferential principal strain lines are smaller It follows that the behavior of primary strain lines when special remodeling effects take place in the left ventricle, due to the onset of cardiac pathologies is one of our future objectives [21].

Importantly, the noninvasive analysis of this kind of data may be easily supported within a 3DSTE device, through the post-processing method we proposed in [8] and shortly summed up here. As an example, and with reference to the same human subject whose 3DSTE circumferential strain were shown in Fig. 4, we pictured in Fig. 8, the endocardial and epicardial mean values, taken over the middle part of the

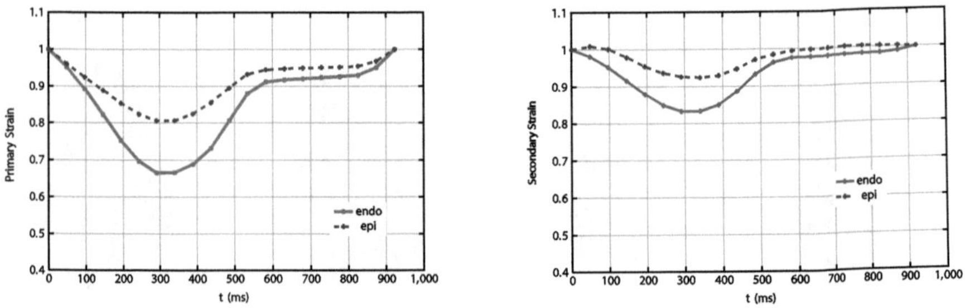

Fig. 8 Representation of the pattern of the mean values, over the middle part of the left ventricle, of the primary (*left panel*) and secondary (*right panel*) epicardial and endocardial strains along the cardiac cycle

left ventricle, of the primary and secondary strains. It might be possible to infer from a large scale investigation appropriate confidence intervals for these values, when referred to healthy situations.

Acknowledgements The work is supported by Sapienza Università di Roma through the grants N. C26A11STT5 and N. C26A13NTJY. The authors wish to express their gratitude to Willem Gorissen, Clinical Market Manager Cardiac Ultrasound at Toshiba Medical Systems Europe, Zoetermeer, The Netherland, for his continuous support and help.

References

1. Burkhoff D, Mirsky I, Suga H (2005) Assessment of systolic and diastolic ventricular properties via pressure-volume analysis: a guide for clinical, translational, and basic researchers. AJP-Heart 289:501–512
2. Cerqueira MD, Weissman NJ, Dilsizian V, Jacobs AK, Kaul S, Laskey WK, Pennel DJ, Rumberger JA, Ryan T, Verani MS (2002) Standardized myocardial segmentation and nomenclature for tomographic imaging of the heart: a statement for healthcare professionals from the Cardiac Imaging Committee of the Council on Clinical Cardiology of the American Heart Association. Circulation 105:539–542
3. DeAnda A, Komeda M, Nikolic SD, Daughters GT, Ingels NB, Miller DC (1995) Left ventricular function, twist, and recoil after mitral valve replacement. Circulation 92:458–466
4. Evangelista A, Nesser J, De Castro S, Faletra F, Kuvin J, Patel A, Alsheikh-Ali AA, Pandian N (2009) Systolic wringing of the left ventricular myocardium: characterization of myocardial rotation and twist in endocardial and midmyocardial layers in normal humans employing three-dimensional speckle tracking study. (Abstract) J Am Coll Cardiol 53(A239):1018–268
5. Evangelista A, Nardinocchi P, Puddu PE, Teresi L, Torromeo C, Varano V (2011) Torsion of the human left ventricle: experimental analysis and computational modelling. Prog Biophys Mol Biol 107(1):112–121
6. Evangelista A, Gabriele S, Nardinocchi Piras P, Puddu PE, Teresi L, Torromeo C, Varano V (2015) On the strain-line pattern in the real human left ventricle. J Biomech. doi:10.1016/j.jbiomech.2014.12.028. published on line: 15 Dec 2015

7. Evangelista A, Gabriele S, Nardinocchi P, Piras P, Puddu PE, Teresi L, Torromeo C, Varano V (2014) A comparative analysis of the strain-line pattern in the human left ventricle: experiments vs modeling. Comput Method Biomech Biomed Eng Imaging Vis. doi:10.1080/21681163.2014.927741. Published online: 23 Jun 2014
8. Fung YC (1993). Biomechanics, 2rd edn. Springer, New–York
9. Gabriele S, Nardinocchi P, Varano V (2015) Evaluation of the strain-line patterns in a human left ventricle: a simulation study. Computer Methods in Biomechanics and Biomedical Engineering 18(7), 790–798.
10. Gabriele S, Teresi L, Varano V, Evangelista A, Nardinocchi P, Puddu PE, Torromeo C (2014) On the strain line patterns in a real human left ventricle. In: Tavares JMRS, Jorge RMN (eds) Computational vision and medical image processing IV. CRC Press, Boca Raton
11. Geyer H, Caracciolo G, Abe H, Wilansky S, Carerj S, Gentile F, Nesser HJ, Khandheria B, Narula J, Sengupta PP (2010) Assessment of myocardial mechanics using speckle tracking echocardiography: fundamentals and clinical applications. J Am Soc Echo 23:351–369
12. Goffinet C, Chenot F, Robert A, Pouleur AC, le Polain de Waroux JB, Vancrayenest D, Gerard O, Pasquet A, Gerber BL, Vanoverschelde JL (2009) Assessment of subendocardial vs. subepicardial left ventricular rotation and twist using two dimensional speckle tracking echocardiography comparison with tagged cardiac magnetic resonance. Eur Heart J 30:608–617
13. Helle–Valle T, Crosby J, Edvardsen T, Lyseggen E, Amundsen BH, Smith HJ, Rosen BD, Lima JAC, Torp H, Ihlen H, Smiseth OA (2005) New noninvasive method for assessment of left ventricular rotation: speckle tracking echocardiography. Circulation 112:3149–3156
14. Helle–Valle T, Remme EW, Lyseggen E, Petersen E, Vartdal T, Opdahl A, Smith HJ, Osman NF, Ihlen H, Edvardsen T, Smiseth OA (2009) Clinical assessment of left ventricular rotation and strain: a novel approach for quantification of function in infarcted myocardium and its border zones. Am J Physiol Heart Circ Physiol 297:H257–H267
15. Nash MP, Hunter PJ (2000) Computational mechanics of the heart: from tissue structure to ventricular function. J Elast. 61:113–141
16. Humphrey JD (2002) Cardiovascular solid mechanics: cells, tissues, organs. Springer, New York
17. Maffessanti F, Nesser HJ, Weinert L, Steringer–Mascherbauer R, Niel J, Gorissend W, Sugeng L, Lang RM, Mor–Avi V (2009) Quantitative evaluation of regional left ventricular function using three-dimensional speckle tracking echocardiography in patients with and without heart disease. Am J Cardiol 104:1755–1762
18. Mangual JO, De Luca A, Toncelli L, Domenichini F, Galanti G, Pedrizzetti G (2012) Three–dimensional reconstruction of the functional strain–line patterns in the left ventricle from 3-dimensional echocardiography. Circ Cardiovasc Imaging 5:808–809
19. Nagel E, Stuber M, Burkhard B, Fischer SE, Scheidegger MB, Boesiger P, Hess OM (2000) Cardiac rotation and relaxation in patients with aortic valve stenosis. Eur Heart J 21:582–589
20. Pedrizzetti G, Kraigher-Krainer E, De Luca A, Caracciolo G, Mangual JO, Shah A, Toncelli L, Domenichini F, Tonti G, Galanti G, Sengupta PP, Narula J, Solomon S (2012) Functional strain-line pattern in the human left ventricle. PRL 109:048103
21. Piras P, Evangelista A, Gabriele S, Nardinocchi P, Teresi L, Torromeo C, Varano V, Puddu PE (2014) 4D-analysis of left ventricular cycle in healthy subjects using procrustes motion analysis. PlosOne 9: e86896
22. Rüssel IK, Götte MJW, Bronzwaer JC, Knaapen P, Paulus WJ, van Rossum AC (2009) Left ventricular torsion. An expanding role in the analysis of myocardial dysfunction. JACC 2(5):648–655
23. Shaw SM, Fox DJ, Williams SG (2008) The development of left ventricular torsion and its clinical relevance. Int J Cardiol 130:319–325
24. Tibayan FA, Lai DT, Timek TA, Dagum P, Liang D, Daughters GT, Ingels NB, Miller DC (2002) Alterations in left ventricular torsion in tachycardia–induced dilated cardiomyopathy. J Thorac Cardiovasc Surg 124(1):43–49

25. Torromeo C, Evangelista A, Pandian NG, Nardinocchi P, Varano V, Gabriele S, Schiariti M, Teresi L, Piras P, Puddu PE (2014) Torsional correlates for end systolic volume index in adult healthy subjects. Int J Appl Sci Technol 4(4):11–23.
26. Waldman LK, Fung YC, Covell JW (1985) Transmural myocardial deformation in the canine left ventricle. Normal in vivo three-dimensional finite strains. Circ Res 57:152–163
27. Wang VY, Hoogendoorn C, Frangi AF, Cowan BR, Hunter PJ, Young AA, Nash MP (2013) Automated personalised human left ventricular FE models to investigate heart failure mechanics. In: Camara et al. (eds) Statistical atlases and computational models of the heart. Imaging and modelling challenges. Lecture Notes in Computer Science, vol 7746, pp 307–316
28. Weiner RB, Hutter AM, Wang F, Kim J, Weyman AE, Wood MJ, Picard MH, Baggish AL (2010) The impact of endurance exercise training on left ventricular torsion. J Am Coll Cardiol Img 3:1001–1009
29. Yeung F, Levinson SF, Parker KJ (1998) Multilevel and motion model-based ultrasonic speckle tracking algorithms. Ultrasound Med Biol 24:427–441

A GPU Accelerated Algorithm for Blood Detection in Wireless Capsule Endoscopy Images

Sunil Kumar, Isabel N. Figueiredo, Carlos Graca and Gabriel Falcao

Abstract Wireless capsule endoscopy (WCE) has emerged as a powerful tool in the diagnosis of small intestine diseases. One of the main limiting factors is that it produces a huge number of images, whose analysis, to be done by a doctor, is an extremely time consuming process. Recently, we proposed (Figueiredo et al. An automatic blood detection algorithm for wireless capsule endoscopy images. In: Computational Vision and Medical Image Processing IV: VIPIMAGE 2013, pp. 237–241. Madeira Island, Funchal, Portugal (2013)) a computer-aided diagnosis system for blood detection in WCE images. While the algorithm in (Figueiredo et al. An automatic blood detection algorithm for wireless capsule endoscopy images. In: Computational Vision and Medical Image Processing IV: VIPIMAGE 2013, pp. 237–241. Madeira Island, Funchal, Portugal (2013)) is very promising in classifying the WCE images, it still does not serve the purpose of doing the analysis within a very less stipulated amount of time; however, the algorithm can indeed profit from a parallelized implementation. In the algorithm we identified two crucial steps, segmentation (for discarding non-informative regions in the image that can interfere with the blood detection) and the construction of an appropriate blood detector function, as being responsible for taking most of the global processing time. In this work, a suitable GPU-based (graphics processing unit) framework is proposed for speeding up the segmentation and blood detection execution times. Experiments show that the accelerated procedure is on average 50 times faster than the original one, and is able of processing 72 frames per second.

S. Kumar (✉) · I. N. Figueiredo
CMUC, Department of Mathematics, Faculty of Science and Technology, University of Coimbra, Coimbra, Portugal
e-mail: isabelf@mat.uc.pt

C. Graca · G. Falcao
Instituto de Telecomunicações, Department of Electrical and Computer Engineering, Faculty of Science and Technology, University of Coimbra, Coimbra, Portugal

J. M. R. S. Tavares, R. Natal Jorge (eds.), *Developments in Medical Image Processing and Computational Vision,* Lecture Notes in Computational Vision and Biomechanics 19,
DOI 10.1007/978-3-319-13407-9_4

1 Introduction

Wireless capsule endoscopy (WCE), also called capsule endoscopy (CE), is a non-invasive endoscopic procedure which allows visualization of the small intestine, without sedation or anesthesia, which is difficult to reach by conventional endoscopies. As the name implies, capsule endoscopy makes use of a swallowable capsule that contains a miniature video camera, a light source, batteries, and a radio transmitter (see Fig. 1). This takes continual images during its passage down the small intestine. The images are transmitted to a recorder that is worn on a belt around the patient's waist. The whole procedure lasts 8 h, after which the data recorder is removed and the images are stored on a computer so that physicians can review them and analyze the potential source of diseases. Capsule endoscopy is useful for detecting small intestine bleeding, polyps, inflammatory bowel disease (Crohn's disease), ulcers, and tumors. It was first invented by Given Imaging in 2000 [12]. Since its approval by the FDA (U.S. Food and Drug Administration) in 2001, it has been widely used in hospitals.

Although capsule endoscopy demonstrates a great advantage over conventional examination procedures, some improvements remain to be done. One major issue with this new technology is that it generates approximately 56,000 images per examination for one patient, whose analysis is very time consuming. Furthermore, some abnormalities may be missed because of their size or distribution, due to visual fatigue. So, it is of great importance to design a real-time computerized method for the inspection of capsule endoscopic images. *Given Imaging Ltd.* has also developed the so called RAPID software for detecting abnormalities in CE images. But its sensitivity and specificity, respectively, were reported to be only 21.5 and 41.8 % [10], see also [19]. Recent years have witnessed some development on automatic inspection of CE images, see [1, 4–6, 7, 9, 14, 15, 18, 20].

The main indication for capsule endoscopy is obscure digestive bleeding [5, 9, 14, 18, 20]. In fact, in most of these cases, the source of the bleeding is located in the small bowel. However, often, these bleeding regions are not imaged by the capsule endoscopy. This is why the blood detection is so important when we are dealing with capsule endoscopy. The current work is an extension of the paper [8], where an automatic blood detection algorithm for CE images was proposed. Utilizing Ohta color channel (R+G+B)/3 (where R, G and B denote the red, green and blue channel, respectively, of the input image), we employed analysis of eigenvalues of the image Hessian matrix and multiscale image analysis approach for designing a function to discriminate between blood and normal frames. The experiments show that the algorithm is very promising in distinguishing between blood and normal frames. But, the algorithm is not able to process huge number of images produced by WCE examination of a patient, within a very less stipulated amount of time. However, the computations of the algorithm can indeed be parallelized, and thus, can process the huge number of images within a very less stipulated amount of time. In the algorithm we identified two crucial steps, segmentation (for discarding non-informative regions in the image that can interfere with the blood detection) and the construction of an

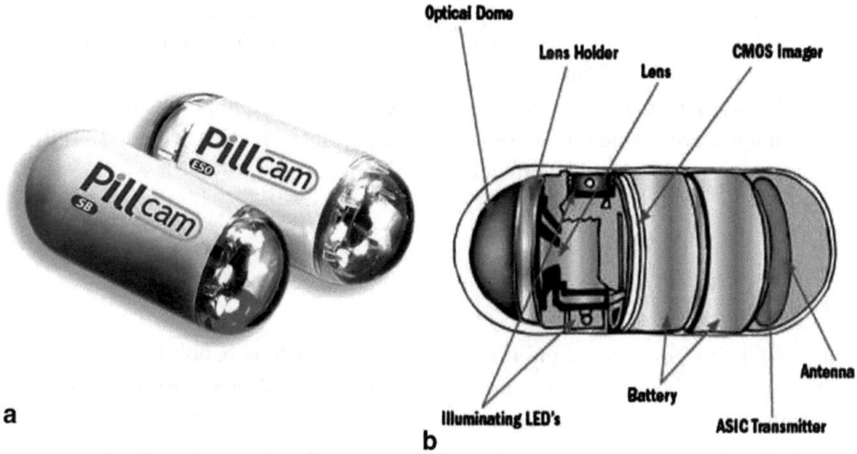

Fig. 1 **a** Image of the capsule. **b** Interior of the capsule

appropriate blood detector function, as being responsible for taking most of the global processing time. We propose a suitable GPU-based framework for speeding up the segmentation and blood detection execution times, and hence the global processing time. Experiments show that the accelerated procedure is on average 50 times faster than the original one, and is able of processing 72 frames per second.

This chapter is structured as follows. A choice of the suitable color channel is made in Sect. 2.1 and segmentation of informative regions is done in Sect. 2.2. A blood detector function is introduced in Sect. 2.3. The outline of the the algorithm is given in Sect. 2.4. Validation of the algorithm on our current data set is provided in Sect. 3. The GPU procedure for speeding up the segmentation and blood detection is described in Sect. 4. Finally, the chapter ends with some conclusions in Sect. 5.

2 Blood Detection Algorithm

Notation Let Ω be an open subset of R^2, representing the image (or pixel) domain. For any scalar, smooth enough, function u defined on Ω, $\|u\|_{L^1(\Omega)}$ and $\|u\|_{L^\infty(\Omega)}$, respectively, denote the L^1 and L^∞ norms of u.

2.1 Color Space Selection

Color of an image carries much more information than the gray levels. In many computer vision applications, the additional information provided by color can aid image analysis. The Ohta color space [17] is a linear transformation of the RGB color space. Its color channels are defined by $A_1 = (R + G + B)/3$, $A_2 = R - B$, and

$A_3 = (2G - R - B)/2$. We observe that channel A_1 has the tendency of localizing quite well the blood regions, as is demonstrated in Fig. 3. The first row corresponds to the original WCE images with blood regions and the second row exhibits their respective A_1 channel images. We also observe that, before computing the A_1 channel of the images, we applied an automatic illumination correction scheme [22] to the original images, to reduce the effect of illumination.

2.2 Segmentation

Many WCE images contain uninformative regions such as bubbles, trash, dark regions and so on, which can interfere with the detection of blood. More information on uninformative regions can be found in [1]. We observe that the second component (which we call henceforth a-channel) of the CIE Lab color space has the tendency of separating these regions from the informative ones. More precisely, for better removal of the uninformative regions, we first decompose the a-channel into geometric and texture parts using the model described in [2, Sect. 2.3], and perform the two phase segmentation. This latter relies on a reformulation of the Chan and Vese variational model [2, 3], over the geometric part of the a-channel.

The segmentation method is described as follows: We first compute the constants c_1 and c_2 (representing the averages of I in a two-region image partition). We then solve the following minimization problem

$$\min_{u,v} \left\{ TV_g(u) + \frac{1}{2\theta} \|u - v\|^2_{L^2(\Omega)} + \int_\Omega \big(\lambda\, r(I, c_1, c_2)\, v + \alpha\, \nu(v)\big)\, dx\, dy \right\} \tag{1}$$

where $TV_g(u) := \int_\Omega g(x, y)|\nabla u|\, dx\, dy$ is the total variation norm of the function u, weighted by a positive function g; $r(I, c_1, c_2)(x, y) := (c_1 - I(x, y))^2 - (c_2 - I(x, y))^2$ is the fitting term, $\theta > 0$ is a fixed small parameter, $\lambda > 0$ is a constant parameter weighting the fitting term, and $\alpha\, \nu(v)$ is a term resulting from a reformulation of the model as a convex unconstrained minimization problem (see [2, Theorem 3]). Here, u represents the two-phase segmentation and v is an auxiliary unknown. The segmentation curve, which divides the image into two disjoint parts, is a level set of u, $\{(x, y) \in \Omega : u(x, y) = \mu\}$, where in general $\mu = 0.5$ (but μ can be any number between 0 and 1, without changing the segmentation result, because u is very close to a binary function).

The above minimization problem is solved by minimizing u and v separately, and iterated until convergence. In short we consider the following two steps:
1. v being fixed, we look for u that solves

$$\min_{u} \left\{ TV_g(u) + \frac{1}{2\theta} \|u - v\|^2_{L^2(\Omega)} \right\}. \tag{2}$$

2. u being fixed, we look for v that solves

$$\min_{v} \left\{ \frac{1}{2\theta} \|u - v\|^2_{L^2(\Omega)} + \int_\Omega \big(\lambda\, r(I, c_1, c_2)\, v + \alpha\, \nu(v)\big)\, dx\, dy \right\}. \tag{3}$$

It is shown that the solution of (2) is ([2, Proposition 3])

$$u = v - \theta \operatorname{div} p,$$

where div represents the divergent operator, and $p = (p_1, p_2)$ solves

$$g\nabla(\theta \operatorname{div} p - v) - |\nabla(\theta \operatorname{div} p - v)|p = 0.$$

The problem for p can be solved using the following fixed point method

$$p^0 = 0, \; p^{n+1} = \frac{p^n + \delta t \nabla(\operatorname{div} p^n - v/\theta)}{1 + \frac{\delta t}{g}|\nabla(\operatorname{div} p^n - v/\theta)|}.$$

Again from [2, Proposition 4], we have

$$v = \min\{\max\{u - \theta\lambda r(I, c_1, c_2), 0\}, 1\}.$$

The segmentation results for some of the WCE images are shown in Fig. 2. The first row corresponds to the original images, the second row shows the segmentation masks, and the third row displays the segmentation curves superimposed on the original images.

In these experiments (and also in the tests performed in Sect. 3) the values chosen for the parameters involved in the definition of (1), are those used in [2], with g the following edge indicator function $g(\nabla u) = \frac{1}{1+\beta\|\nabla u\|^2}$ and $\beta = 10^{-3}$.

2.3 Detector Function

We now introduce the detector function that is designed to discriminate between blood and non-blood frames. We resort to the analysis of eigenvalues of the image Hessian matrix and multiscale image analysis approach. Based on the eigenvalues, both blob-like and tubular-like structures can be detected. For a scalar image $I : \Omega \subseteq \mathbb{R}^2 \rightarrow \mathbb{R}$, we define the Hessian matrix of one point (x, y), and at a scale s, by

$$H_s(x, y) = \begin{pmatrix} I_{xx}^s & I_{xy}^s \\ I_{xy}^s & I_{yy}^s \end{pmatrix},$$

where I_{xx}^s, I_{xy}^s and I_{yy}^s are the second-order partial derivatives of I and the scale s is involved in the calculation of these derivatives. The Hessian matrix describes the second order local image intensity variations around the selected point. Suppose $\lambda_{s,1}$ and $\lambda_{s,2}$ are two eigenvalues of the Hessian matrix H_s. Further, suppose that $|\lambda_{s,1}| \leq |\lambda_{s,2}|$. Setting $F_s = \lambda_{s,1}^2 + \lambda_{s,2}^2$, we define

$$F(x, y) = \max_{s_{min} \leq s \leq s_{max}} F_s(x, y), \tag{4}$$

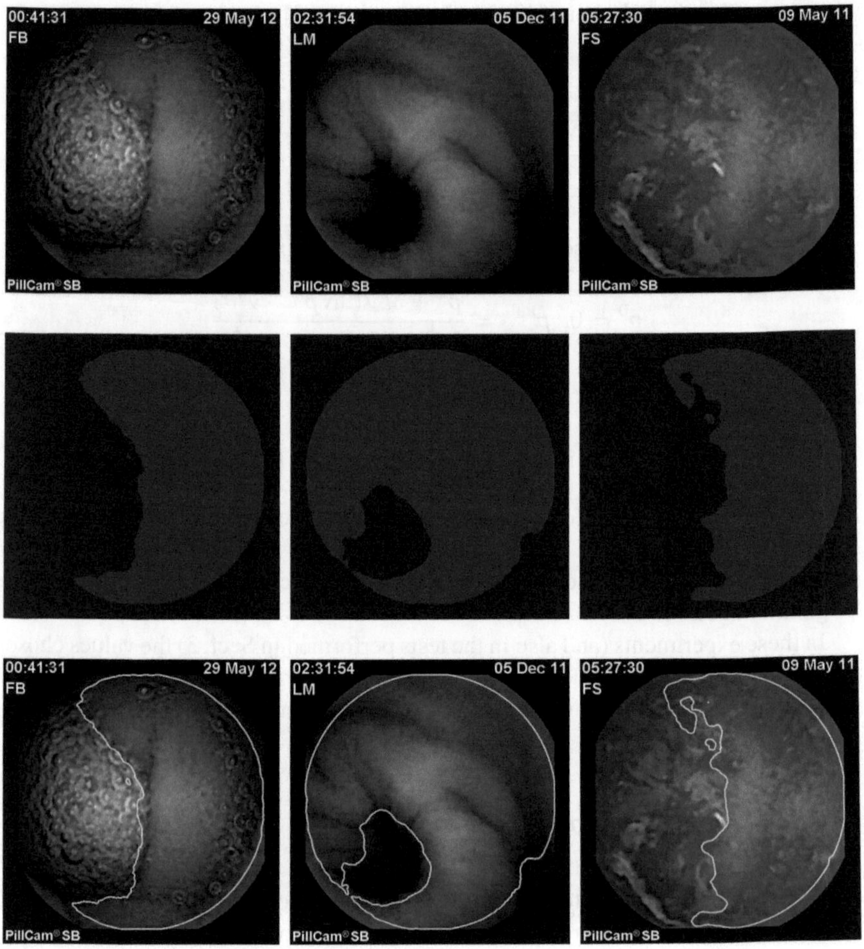

Fig. 2 *First row*: Original image. *Second row*: Segmentation mask. *Third row*: Original image with segmentation curve superimposed

where s_{min} and s_{max} are the minimum and maximum scales at which the blood regions are expected to be found. We remark that they can be chosen so that they cover the whole range of blood regions.

Setting now

$$f_1 = \exp\left(-\beta F_s^2\right) \quad \text{and} \quad f_2 = \left(1 - \exp\left(-\alpha\left(\frac{\lambda_{s,1}}{\lambda_{s,2}}\right)^2\right)\right),$$

and motivated from [11], we define the blob (B_s) and ridge (R_s) detectors (at each point of the domain)

$$B_s = \begin{cases} 0, & \text{if} \quad \lambda_{s,1}\lambda_{s,2} < 0 \quad \text{or} \quad |\lambda_{s,2} - \lambda_{s,1}| > \delta \\ (1 - f_1)f_2, & \text{otherwise,} \end{cases} \tag{5}$$

and

$$R_s = \begin{cases} 0, & \text{if} \quad \lambda_{s,2} > 0, \\ (1 - f_1)(1 - f_2), & \text{otherwise.} \end{cases} \tag{6}$$

Here α and β are the parameters which control the sensitivity of the functions and δ is an user chosen threshold. We then compute the maximum for each scale

$$B(x, y) = \max_{s_{min} \le s \le s_{max}} B_s(x, y) \quad \text{and} \quad R(x, y) = \max_{s_{min} \le s \le s_{max}} R_s(x, y),$$

In the computations, we take $s = 8, 10, 12, 14$. The results of the functions F and the sum $B + R$, for blood and non-blood images are displayed in Figs. 3 and 4, respectively.

We denote by $\widetilde{\Omega}$, in the image domain, the segmented region of I, that is, $\widetilde{\Omega} = \Omega \cap \Omega_{seg}$, where Ω_{seg} is the segmented sub-domain of I containing the blood. We use the intensity and gradient information of the above functions for designing our detector function, DF, which is defined by

$$DF = \frac{||F||_{L^\infty(\widetilde{\Omega})} ||B + R||_{L^\infty(\widetilde{\Omega})}}{||B + R||_{L^1(\widetilde{\Omega})}}.$$

2.4 *Algorithm Outline*

For each WCE image the algorithm consists of the following four steps:

1. Firstly, we remove additional details (such as patient name, date and time) from the original image. For this purpose, we clip around the circular view of the original image. Next, we apply an automatic illumination correction scheme [22], for reducing the effect of illumination.
2. We then consider the Ohta color channel $(R + G + B)/3$ for the illumination corrected image.
3. We next apply the two-phase segmentation method [2] for removing uninformative regions (such as bubbles, trash, liquid, and so on) over the geometric part of the second component of the CIE Lab color space.
4. Finally, we compute the functions F, $B + R$ and the blood detector function DF.

3 Validation of the Algorithm

We test the performance of the algorithm on a data set prepared by medical the experts. *Given Imaging*'s Pillcam SB capsule was used to collect the videos in the University Hospital of Coimbra. To make the data set representative, the images

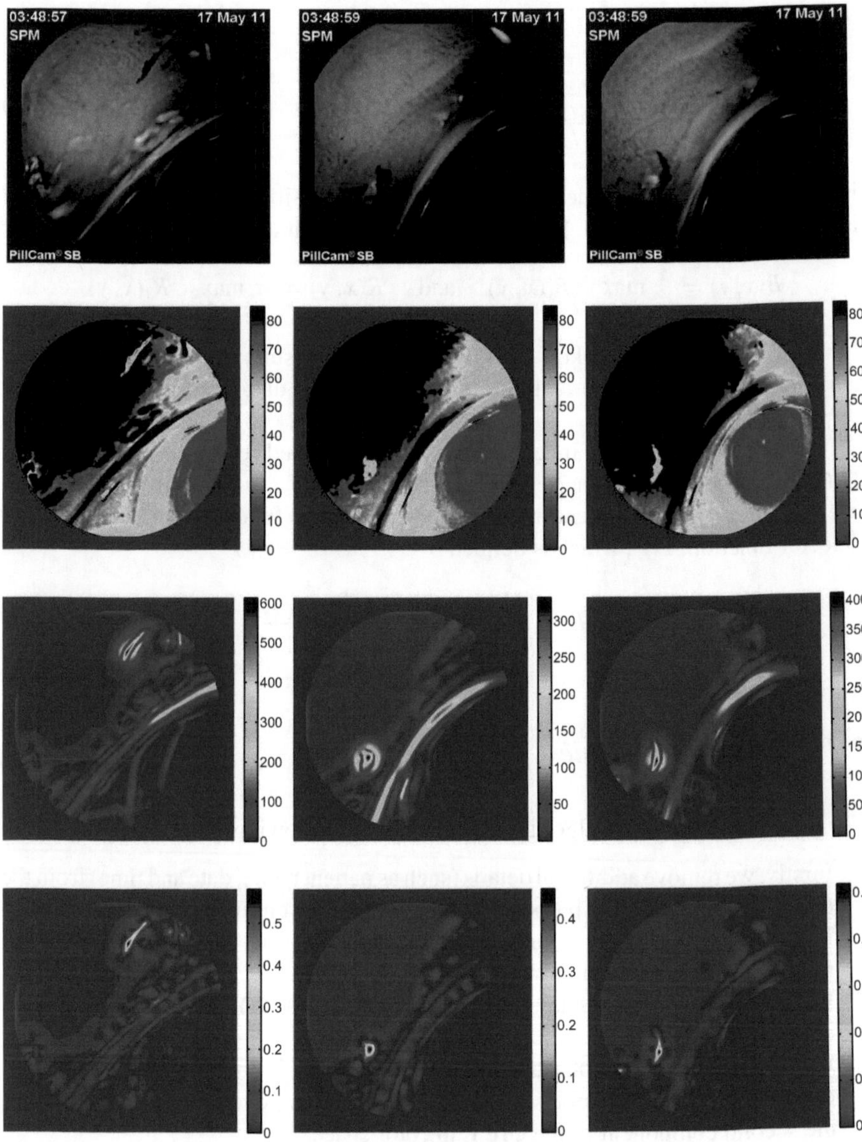

Fig. 3 *First row*: Original image with blood region. *Second row*: A_1 color channel. *Third row*: Function F. *Fourth row*: Function $B + R$

were collected from 4 patients video segments. The data set consists of 27 blood images and 663 normal images. We use standard performance measures: sensitivity, specificity and accuracy. These are defined as follows:

$$\text{Sensitivity} = \frac{\text{TP}}{\text{TP} + \text{FN}}, \quad \text{Specificity} = \frac{\text{TN}}{\text{TN} + \text{FP}},$$

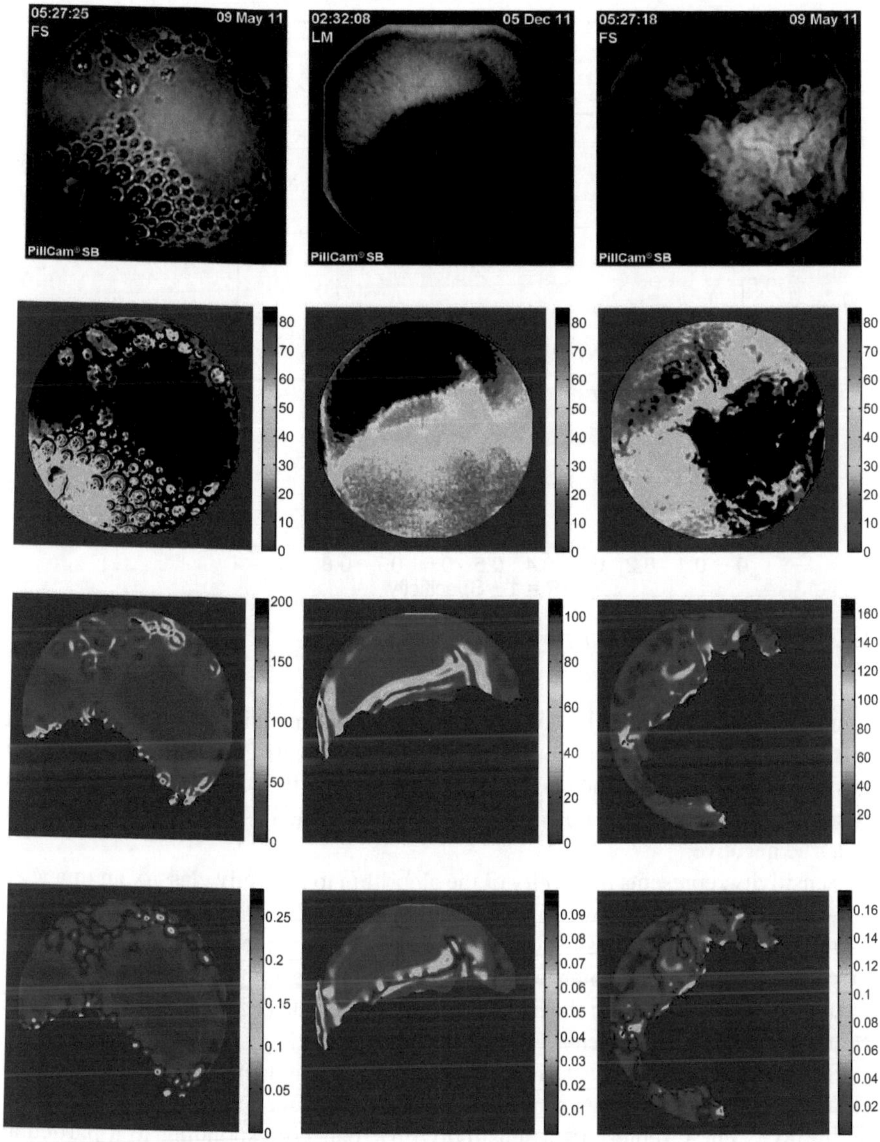

Fig. 4 *First row*: Original image without blood region. *Second row*: A_1 color channel. *Third row*: Function F. *Fourth row*: Function $B + R$

$$\text{Accuracy} = \frac{\text{TN} + \text{TP}}{\text{TN} + \text{FP} + \text{TP} + \text{FN}},$$

where TP, FN, FP and TN represent the number of true positives, false negatives, false positives and true negatives, respectively. For a particular decision threshold T, if for an image frame J, $DF > T$, it is a positive frame; if $DF \leq T$, it is a negative

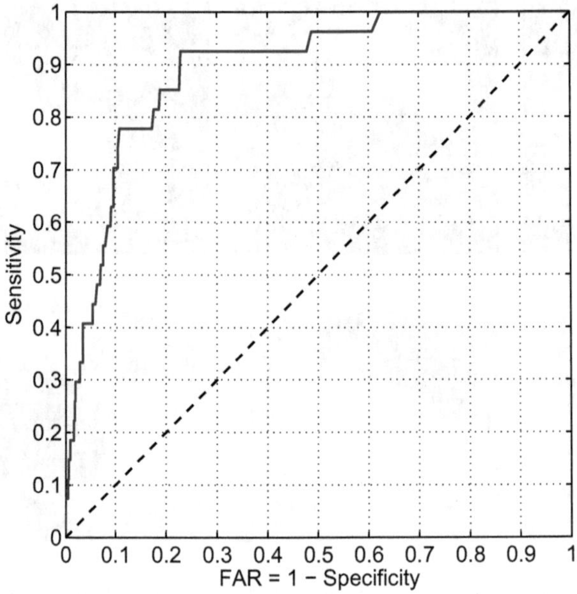

Fig. 5 ROC curve for function DF

frame. If J belongs to the class of blood image frames and it is classified as negative, it is counted as a false negative; if it is classified as positive, it is counted as a true positive. If J belongs to the class of non-blood image frames and it is classified as positive, it is counted as a false positive; if it is classified as negative, it is counted as a true negative.

Sensitivity represents the ability of the algorithm to correctly classify an image as a frame containing blood, while specificity represents the ability of the algorithm to correctly classify an image as a non-blood frame. The third measure, accuracy, is used to assess the overall performance of the algorithm. There is also another performance measure commonly used in the literature, false alarm rate (FAR). However, it can be computed from the specificity: FAR=1-Specificity.

Receiver operating characteristic (ROC) curve is a fundamental tool for detection evaluation. In a ROC curve sensitivity is plotted in function of FAR. Each point on the ROC curve represents a sensitivity/FAR pair corresponding to a particular decision threshold. It shows the tradeoff between sensitivity and specificity. Figure 5 represents the ROC curve with respect to the function DF. For FAR $\leq$ 10 %, the best sensitivity achieved is 70.37 %. In particular, the sensitivity, FAR and accuracy obtained are 70.37, 9.6 and 89.56 %, respectively, for the threshold $2.8928E + 007$. In summary, these results show that the presented algorithm is very promising for the detection of blood regions.

4 Speeding up the Segmentation and Detector Performance

In this section we describe general facts about the apparatus specifications. In particular, we detail the GPUs adopted and the underlying architectures. Finally, we address the parallelization of the algorithms proposed, namely by detailing the segmentation and blood detector parallelization procedures on the GPU, and reporting the results obtained for the current medical dataset.

The pipeline of the algorithm, described in Sect. 2, has been first implemented on a CPU Intel Core i7 950 CPU @ 3.07 GHz, with 12 GB of RAM, running a GNU/Linux kernel 3.8.0-31-generic. The C/C++ code was compiled using GCC-4.6.3.

In order to process more frames per second, the segmentation and blood detector steps have been paralellized, for executing on GPU NVidia C2050 and NVidia GTX 680, compiled using NVIDIA Compute Unified Device Architecture (CUDA) driver 5.5 [21].

4.1 *General Overview of the GPU Architecture*

The host system usually consists of a CPU that orchestrates the entire processing by sending data and launching parallel kernels on the GPU device. At the end of processing, it collects computed data from the device and terminates execution. The parallelization of segmentation and blood detection procedures is carried out using the CUDA parallel programming model, by exploiting the massive use of thread- and data-parallelism on the GPU. CUDA allows the programmer to write in a transparent way, scalable parallel C code [21] on GPUs.

As shown in Fig. 6, each thread processes one pixel and thus multiple elements can be processed at the same time. This introduces a significant reduction in the global processing time of the proposed algorithm. When the host launches a parallel kernel, the GPU device executes a grid of thread blocks, where each block has a predefined number of threads executing the same code segment. Organized in groups of 32 threads (a warp), they execute synchronously and are time-sliced among the stream processors of each multiprocessor.

Figure 7 depicts a simplified overview of the GPU architecture. It shows that several multiprocessors contain a large number of stream processors (the number of stream processors and multiprocessors depends on the model and architecture of the GPU). In the present case, the NVidia GTX 680 GPU, which contains eight multiprocessors with each multiprocessor containing 192 stream processors, performing a total of 1536 CUDA cores, executes the algorithm faster.

Before processing starts on the GPU, data is uploaded to device memory. This process is typically slow and consists in transferring the information from the host CPU memory to the GPU global memory (device). At the end of the processing, results are transferred from the GPU device global memory to the host CPU RAM memory.

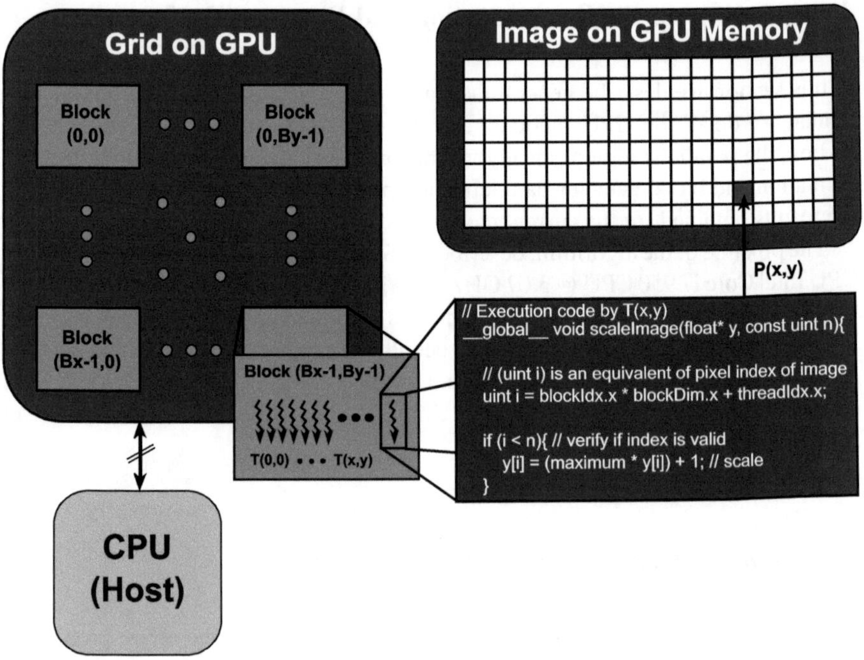

Fig. 6 Demonstration of the structure of a grid and thread blocks and how the same segment of code is executed by multiple threads. Each thread computes the result for one pixel

In the GPU, there are several memory types and they have different impacts on the throughput performance. We highlight two of them:

- Global memory accesses are time consuming operations with high latency and may represent a bottleneck in the desired system's performance. Instead, coalesced accesses should be performed whenever possible. They imply data in global memory to be contiguously aligned, so that all 32 threads within a warp can access the respective 32 data elements concurrently on the same clock cycle, with thread T(x,y) accessing pixel P(x,y), as depicted in Fig. 8.
- Also, modern GPUs have small and fast blocks of memory tightly coupled to the cores, which is shared by all threads within the same block. We can have several threads processing the same local data to optimize memory bandwidth (typically shared memory is faster than global memory when we need to share information among several threads), but shared memory is small in size. To maximize its use and performance, it is important to consider such size limitations. When large amounts of data have to be processed, data has to be partitioned in smaller blocks in order not to exceed the limits of shared memory. This action also represents penalties, since it increases the amount of data exchanges with global memory. Therefore, in the current work we use shared memory for calculating some procedures and global memory to perform the remaining functionalities, globally achieving an efficient memory usage as reported in later subsections.

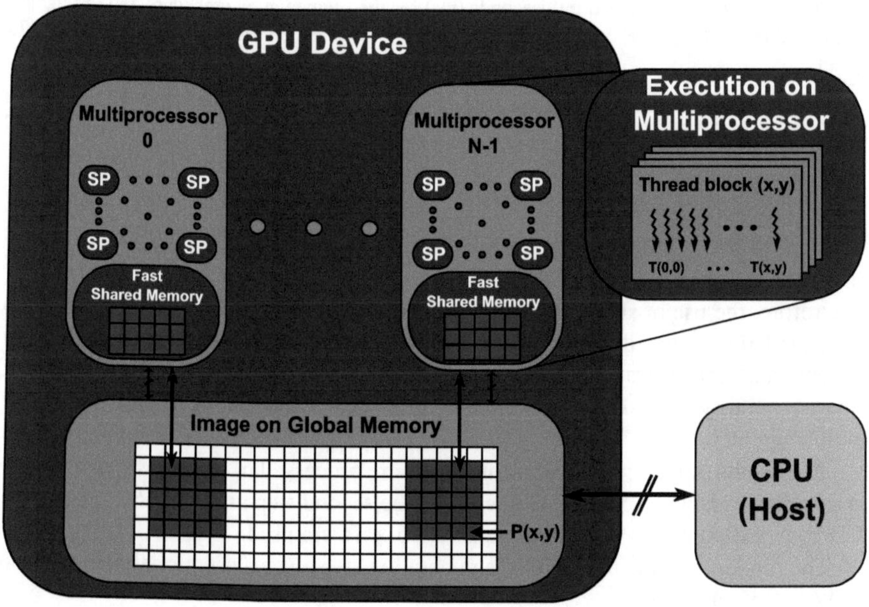

Fig. 7 Simplified GPU arquitecture. An example of how thread blocks are processed on GPU multiprocessors. A multiprocessor can execute more then one thread block concurrently

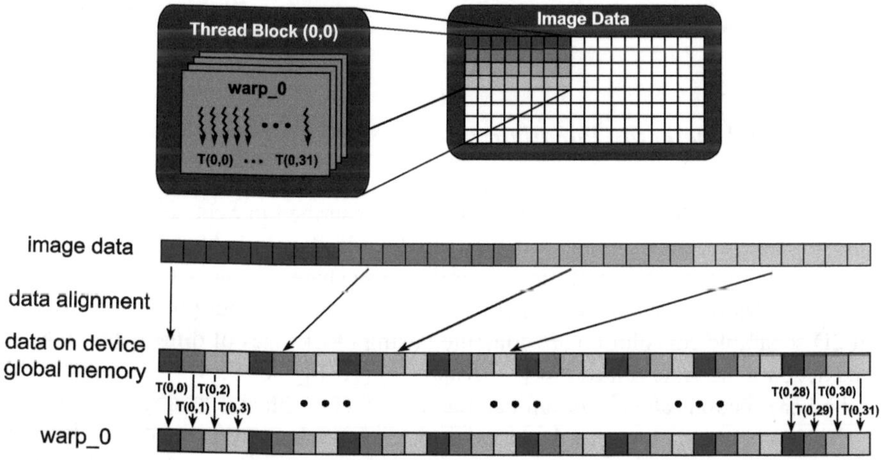

Fig. 8 Coalesced memory accesses illustrating a warp of 32 threads reading/writing the respective 32 data elements on a single clock cycle

4.2 Segmentation Parallelization

Some functions in the segmentation procedure, mentioned in Sect. 2.2, need to share image data between threads (e.g. neighboring pixels on the convolution procedure).

Table 1 Computation times in milliseconds (ms) for the segmentation procedure and throughput measured in frames per second (fps). The tests were performed on WCE images with 576×576 pixels

Processing Platform	Segmentation execution time (ms)	Segmentation (fps)
CPU Intel i7	240.0	4.2
GPU NVidia C2050	6.0	166.7
GPU NVidia GTX 680	4.8	208.3

Therefore, the use of shared memory is the best option to achieve a higher speedup (see [16] for a related work). These functions are: finding maximum and mean values, and 2D separable convolution [13]. All other functions perform slower if shared memory is used, because the total number of transactions to global memory will be greater.

The results of maximum and mean values are processed in two steps: the first step uses GPU grids with 256×256 block size; the second step uses 1×256 ; and in the 2D convolution, block sizes of dimension 16×16 are used.

The remaining functions in the segmentation step always use global memory and 1296×256 block sizes.

The computation times regarding the segmentation procedure are represented in Table 1, that shows the real speedups obtained using parallel computation on the GPU; as displayed, this procedure runs 40 times faster on GPU NVidia C2050 and 50 times faster on GPU NVidia GTX 680, when compared to an Intel i7 CPU.

4.3 *Blood Detector Parallelization*

For speeding up the blood detector procedure, described in Sect. 2.3, we only use one function that shares image data between threads: 2D separable convolution [13]. The remaining functions perform slower if we use shared memory because the total number of transactions to global memory would assume a higher impact. The results of 2D separable convolution are computed using block sizes of dimension 16×16 and 8×8 for the scale values $s = [8\ 10]$ and $s = [12\ 14]$ (see Sect. 2.3), respectively. All other functions always use global memory blocks with size 8×8.

The computation times of the blood detector procedure are presented in Table 2. We clearly see the speedup obtained using parallel computation on GPU. This algorithm runs 58.9 times faster on GPU NVidia C2050 and 59.5 times faster on GPU NVidia GTX 680, when compared to an Intel i7 CPU.

Table 2 Computation times in millisecons (ms) for the blood detector procedure and throughput measured in frames per second (fps). The tests were performed on WCE images with 576×576 pixels

Processing platform	Blood detector execution time (ms)	Blood detector (fps)
CPU Intel i7	529.9	1.9
GPU NVidia C2050	9.0	111.1
GPU NVidia GTX 680	8.9	112.4

Table 3 Throughput measured in fps and speedup archived to the complete algorithm (Segmentation and Blood Detector). Tests performed on WCE images with 576×576 pixels

Processing platform	Segmentation and blood detector (fps)	Speedup
CPU Intel i7	1.3	——
GPU NVidia C2050	66.7	51.3 times faster
GPU NVidia GTX 680	72.9	56.1 times faster

4.4 Speedup

Table 3 shows throughput measured in frames per second (fps) and the speedup of the full algorithm achieved. It can be seen that GPU NVidia GTX 680 is faster than NVidia C2050.

With the obtained speedup, the GPU NVidia GTX 680 shows to be able of processing 72 fps, which is equivalent to observe that the approximate total number of 56000 frames, generated by a complete WCE exam, can be computed in less than 13 min.

5 Conclusions

With the rapidly enhancing performances of graphics processors, improved programming support, and excellent price-to-performance ratio, GPUs have emerged as a competitive parallel computing platform for computationally expensive and demanding tasks in a wide range of medical image applications. We have proposed a GPU-based framework for blood detection in WCE images. The core of the algorithm lies in the definition of a good discriminator for blood and non-blood frames. This is accomplished by choosing a suitable color channel, image Hessian eigenvalue analysis and multiscale image analysis approach. Experimental results for our current dataset show that the proposed algorithm is effective, and achieves 89.56 % accuracy. Moreover, it is shown that the accelerated procedure is on average 50 times faster than the original one, and is able of processing 72 frames per second. This is achieved by parallelizing the two crucial steps, segmentation and blood detector functionalities in the algorithm, that were consuming most of the global processing time. To perform these steps more efficiently we now run parallel code on GPUs with an appropriate use of memory (shared and global). This novel approach allows processing multiple pixels of an image at the same time, thus sustaining the obtained throughput levels.

Acknowledgements This work was partially supported by the project PTDC/MATNAN/0593/2012, and also by CMUC and FCT (Portugal), through European program COMPETE/ FEDER and project PEst-C/MAT/UI0324/2011. The work of Gabriel Falcao was also partially supported by Instituto de Telecomunicações and by the project PEst-OE/EEI/LA0008/2013.

References

1. Bashar M, Kitasaka T, Suenaga Y, Mekada Y, Mori K (2010) Automatic detection of informative frames from wireless capsule endoscopy images. Med Image Anal 14:449–470
2. Bresson X, Esedoglu S, Vandergheynst P, Thiran JP, Osher S (2007) Fast global minimization of the active contour/snake model. J Math Imaging Vis 28:151–167
3. Chan TF, Vese LA (2001) Active contours without edges. IEEE Transac Image Process 10:266–277
4. Coimbra M, Cunha J (2006) MPEG-7 visual descriptors-contributions for automated feature extraction in capsule endoscopy. IEEE Transac Circuits Syst Video Technol 16:628–637
5. Cui L, Hu C, Zou Y, Meng MQH 2010) Bleeding detetction in wireless capsule endoscopy images by support vector classifier. In: Proceedings of the 2010 IEEE Conference on Information and Automation, pp. 1746–1751. Harbin, China, June 2010
6. Cunha JPS, Coimbra M, Campos P, Soares JM (2008) Automated topographic segmentation and transit time estimation in endoscopic capsule exams. IEEE Transac Med Imaging 27:19–27
7. Figueiredo IN, Kumar S, Figueiredo PN (2013) An intelligent system for polyp detection in wireless capsule endoscopy images. In: Computational Vision and Medical Image Processing IV: VIPIMAGE 2013, pp. 229–235. Madeira Island, Funchal, Portugal, 2013
8. Figueiredo IN, Kumar S, Leal C, Figueiredo PN (2013) An automatic blood detection algorithm for wireless capsule endoscopy images. In: Computational Vision and Medical Image Processing IV: VIPIMAGE 2013, pp. 237–241. Madeira Island, Funchal, Portugal, 2013
9. Figueiredo IN, Kumar S, Leal C, Figueiredo PN (2013) Computer-assisted bleeding detection in wireless capsule endoscopy images. Comput Meth Biomech Biomed Eng Imaging Visualization 1:198–210
10. Francis R (2004) Sensitivity and specificity of the red blood identification (RBIS) in video capsule endoscopy. In: 3rd international conference on capsule endoscopy. Miami, FL, USA, Feb 2004
11. Frangi AF, Niessen WJ, Vincken KL, Viergever MA (1998) Multiscale vessel enhancement filtering. In: Medical image computing and computer-assisted intervention, pp. 130–137. Cambridge, MA, USA, 1998
12. Idan G, Meron G, Glukhovsky A (2000) Wireless capsule endoscopy. Nature 405, 417–417
13. Lee H, Harris M, Young E, Podlozhnyuk V (2007) Image convolution with CUDA. NVIDIA Corporation
14. Li B, Q.-H-Meng M (2009) Computer-aided detection of bleeding regions for capsule endoscopy images. IEEE Transac Biomed Eng 56:1032–1039
15. Liedlgruber M, Uhl A (2011) Computer-aided decision support systems for endoscopy in the gastrointestinal tract: a review. IEEE Rev Biomed Eng 4:73–88
16. Martins M, Falcao G, Figueiredo IN (2013) Fast aberrant crypt foci segmentation on the GPU. In: ICASSP'13: Proceedings of the 36th IEEE International Conference on Acoustics, Speech and Signal Processing. IEEE

17. Ohta YI, Kanade T, Sakai T (1980) Color information for region segmentation. Comput Graphics Image Process 13:222–241
18. Pan G, Xu F, Chen J (2011) A novel algorithm for color similarity measurement and the application for bleeding detection in WCE. Int J Image Graphics Signal Process 5:1–7
19. Park SC, Chun HJ, Kim ES, Keum B, Seo YS, Kim YS, Jeen YT, Lee HS, Um SH, Kim CD, Ryu HS (2012) Sensitivity of the suspected blood indicator: an experimental study. World J Gastroenterol 18(31):4169–4174
20. Penna B, Tilloy T, Grangettoz M, Magli E, Olmo G (2009) A technique for blood detection in wireless capsule endoscopy images. In: 17th European signal processing conference (EUSIPCO 2009), pp. 1864–1868
21. Podlozhnyuk V, Harris M, Young E (2012) NVIDIA CUDA C programming guide. NVIDIA Corporation
22. Zheng Y, Yu J, Kang SB, Lin S, Kambhamettu C (2008) Single-image vignetting correction using radial gradient symmetry. In: Proceedings of the 26th IEEE conference on Computer Vision and Pattern Recognition (CVPR '08), pp. 1–8. Los Alamitos, California, USA, June 2008

Automated Image Mining in fMRI Reports: a Meta-research Study

N. Gonçalves, G. Vranou and R. Vigário

Abstract This chapter describes a method for meta-research, based on image mining from neuroscientific publications. It extends earlier investigation to the study of a large scale data set. Using a framework for extraction and characterisation of reported fMRI images, based on their coordinates and colour profiles, we propose that significant information can be harvested automatically. The coordinates of the brain activity regions, in relation to a standard reference templates are estimated. We focus on the analysis of scientific reports of the default mode network. Both the commonalities and the differences of brain activity between control, Alzheimer and schizophrenic patients are identified.

1 Introduction

1.1 Meta-Analysis in Neuroscience

There is an ever increasing number of scientific publications in many research fields in general, and in neuroscience in particular. Hundreds of articles are published every month, with a considerable amount devoted to functional magnetic resonance imaging (fMRI) ([7, 12]). When comparing results obtained with a particular experimental setup with those reported in the existing literature, one may validate, integrate or confront different theories. This analysis is usually performed in a rather human-intensive manner, through the use of dedicated curators, *e.g.* [14, 15]. The development of tools able to synthesise and aggregate such large-data can then be seen as crucial.

Meta-analysis of neuroscience research would clearly benefit from direct access to their original data sets. This is often not possible, due to the unavailability of such

N. Gonçalves (✉) · R. Vigário
Department of Information and Computer Science, Aalto University School of Science, 00076 Aalto, Finland
e-mail: nicolau.goncalves@aalto.fi

G. Vranou
Department of Informatics Technological Education Institute, Sindos 57400, Thessaloniki, Greece

J. M. R. S. Tavares, R. Natal Jorge (eds.), *Developments in Medical Image Processing and Computational Vision,* Lecture Notes in Computational Vision and Biomechanics 19, DOI 10.1007/978-3-319-13407-9_5

data. Yet, albeit of poorer quality, there is a plethora of summarising information, readily available in many published reports. Its analysis is the main topic of the current manuscript. That information is encoded both in text structures, as well as in image content, providing ample scope for mining information at various levels. The extraction of relevant information is not a simple task, and constitutes a major subject of information retrieval and data mining [11].

1.2 Previous Work

As stated above, previous approaches often used a considerable amount of curator work, with researchers reading from several sources, and extracting by hand the relevant information (*cf.*, [14]). This severely limits the range of possible analyses. It is, therefore, of significant importance that robust automated information retrieving approaches be added to the current attempts to build functional neuro-atlases. A recent, fully automated approach was proposed by [21]. Their framework combines text-mining, meta-analysis and machine-learning techniques, to generate probabilistic mappings between cognitive and neural states. One drawback of this method is that it addresses only text mining, and requires the presence of activation coordinates in the articles analysed. Those peak-coordinates and some text tags are the only representation of the activations, which results in the discarding of valuable information from the neural activity.

We see our approach as a complementary way to tackle the problem, when image information, rather than text, is automatically harvested from published data.

1.3 Default Mode Network

An open field of research with increasing interest in neuroscience is the resting state and default mode networks (RSN & DMN, respectively). These networks comprise areas such as the occipital, temporal and frontal areas of the brain. They are active when the individual is not performing any goal-oriented task, and suppressed during activity [6, 17]. In spite of the great attention to those networks, scientific research of brain's "resting state" still poses various conceptual and methodological difficulties [19]. A commonly topic of study consists in investigating the differences and commonalities in the activity of healthy brains when compared to, *e.g.*, Alzheimer or schizophrenic brains. Specifically, how different is the composition of RSN and DMN, in healthy and pathological brains, and how do these differences influence cognitive and functional performances.

1.4 Proposed Approach

In this chapter, we propose a complementary framework to text analysis, focusing instead on image information. It relies on the automatic extraction and characterisation of image information in fMRI literature. Such information often takes the form of activation/suppression of activity in the brain, in a variety of image settings, orientations and resolutions. This framework aims to open different means to building and improving functional atlases of the human brain, based solely on the large number of images published in neuroscientific articles.

We demonstrate the feasibility and results of our method in studies of the resting state and default mode networks, and highlight three outcomes of such research. The first is the identification of common neuronal activity across all subjects. Several regions are expected to participate in the DMN structures, in spite of possible existence of any of the aforementioned diseases. The second outcome focuses on differences between the activation patterns of healthy subjects and unhealthy ones, which can be explained with information already reported in articles within the data set used. Finally, we aim at identifying also variations in activity, not reported in the literature, and which could constitute evidence for proposing new research questions.

In the following sections, we will describe the procedure used for the extraction of reported fMRI images and subsequent mapping of functional activity patterns to a common brain template. Then we demonstrate the results obtained when mining information from a collection of articles related to the DMN. Using those results, we subsequently compare brain activity in healthy, Alzheimer and schizophrenic brains. We conclude the article with some remarks about the proposed approach, its limitations and possible future work.

2 Methodology

2.1 Data

The first step of our research consisted in the construction of a database of relevant publications. With this in mind, we searched for neuroscientific publications published online, in which the topic of discussion was related to the default mode network. This search was carried out using a keyword based search, with words such as DMN, Alzheimer, fMRI, cognitive impairment, Schizophrenia and resting state.

We gathered 183 articles in *pdf* format, from journals such as NeuroImage, Human Brain Mapping, Brain, Magnetic Resonance Imaging, PNAS and PLOS ONE. The time-frame for these articles ranged from early 2000 to June 2013. All papers were then separated according to the specificity of the analysis carried therein (see Table 1), distinguishing between studies on healthy brains (132), Alzheimer (29) and Schizophrenia (18) research.

Table 1 Number of articles used in this study, separated by type of study, as well as figures, images and blobs, obtained by our method

	Articles	Figures	Images	Blobs
Healthy	132	217	1200	5303
Alzheimer	29	44	184	573
Schizophrenia	18	23	103	307
	183	284	1487	6183

2.2 *fMRI Activity*

Consider typical images of fMRI activity, as shown in Fig. 1. In a brief glance, it is easy to identify several features of relevance, such as the kind of section of the image (axial in this case, as opposed to sagittal or coronal), various anatomical features of the section, as well as the functional activity regions or 'blobs' within the section. We do that by relating the image to an internal representation of our anatomical and physiological knowledge of the brain. This relation takes into account physical and geometrical properties of the underlying structural image, as well as of the superimposed blob. In addition to the activity location, other features, such as intensity, area, perimeter or shape can be used to fully characterise the activity, c.f. ([1, 18]). Other non-pictorial features, such as the text in the caption, could also be used to characterise said images.

In Fig. 1, one can also see the various reporting styles illustrated, including various underlying, gray-scale, structural images, colours and formats. The leftmost image shows a typical example where a slight increase of activity when compared to the reference corresponds to dark red while a big increase is depicted in bright yellow, which is typically called the *hot* colour scale. On the rightmost image, the decrease of activity when compared to the reference is shown in a gradation of blue, from dark to bright, corresponding to a small to big decrease. The image on the middle shows an example where the authors only chose to report the areas of difference in activation, without giving intensity information.

2.3 *Image Extraction Procedure*

In Fig. 2, we show a flowchart of our framework. We start by extracting figures from the PDF files of publications, using an open source command-line utility *pdfimages*, running in Linux.

For each journal publication there is a pre-defined, common reporting style, but, as shown before, different authors produce their figures with different styles. They have non-homogeneous content, such as multiple image frames per figure, other plots, annotations or captions. Since we desire a clear image in order to accurately isolate the fMRI activity of interest, it is necessary to morphologically process those figures.

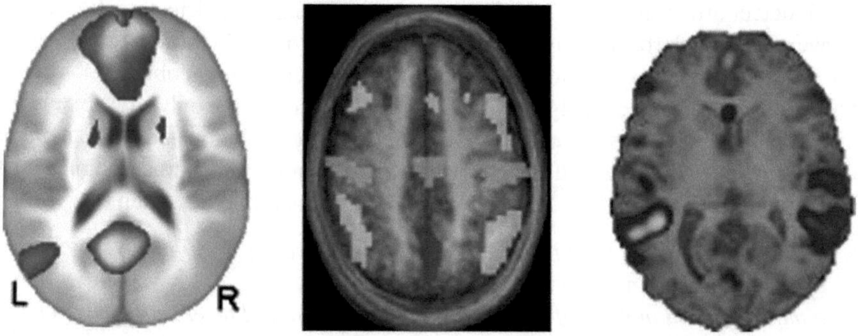

Fig. 1 Examples of images presented in fMRI reports. On the leftmost image (adapted from [13]), activity is present in the occipital, left temporal and frontal areas of the brain, and the activity is reported using the *hot* colour scale. The activity on the second image (adapted from [9]) is shown in three different uniform colours, while the third image (adapted from [22]) shows a combination of *hot* and *cold* colour scales, for increase and decrease of activity when compared to the reference

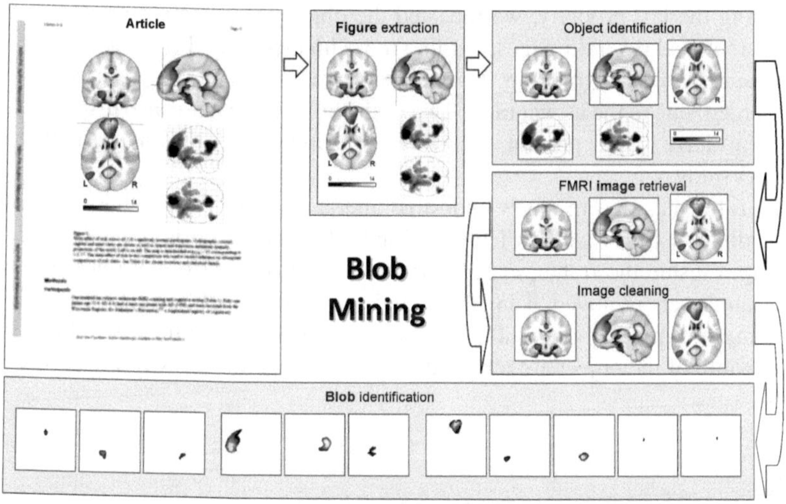

Fig. 2 Flowchart describing the blob mining procedure. First, figures are retrieved from articles (images adapted from Johnson et al.(2007)). This is then followed by the detection of possible objects containing fMRI activity reports. After processing and retrieval of these images, they are cleaned of artifacts, such as lines and text, allowing for a final stage of blob identification

The first stage is the object identification. Many figures have a simple background colour, like black or white, but others have different colours, *e.g.*, gray. Hence, the background colour needs to be detected, which is done through histogram and border analysis. The possible background colours are detected from the borders of the image, and the one with highest number of pixels is selected.

To detect different objects in a figure, and after background detection, figures are converted to black (background) and white (objects) colour. In those binary images, the white areas correspond to the smallest rectangle enclosing a object. Objects in the border of the respective figure, as well as those composed of only a few pixels are discarded. The next step is to analyse the images that are left inside the remaining objects. After extracting said images, we need to identify and extract the ones that correspond to fMRI reports. This is done using various properties, such as:

- *a minimum perimeter of the image, which we have set to 80 pixels*, to allow a sufficient processing resolution;
- *a minimum and maximum number of image/background pixel ratio, between 0.1 and 97.5*, to avoid non-brain images;
- *percentage of colour pixels in the image between 0 and 40 % of coloured pixels*, filtering out non-fMRI images or images with activity all over the brain;
- *image aspect ratio between 0.66 and 1.6*, typical of a brain image;
- *one image should occupy more than 50 % of the frame*, to eliminate multiple images in the same object frame.

Regarding the last property, we repeated the object identification procedure when objects included several images, until no more images could be found.

In the example shown in Fig. 2, the object frame containing the figure colour map is discarded, due to the aspect ratio. Two of the brain images are also discarded since they don't have colour present, therefore not being considered as originating from an fMRI study.

The following step removes undesired annotations. In Fig. 2, these correspond to coordinate axis as well as letters 'L' and 'R'. This stage is done by removing all images inside the frame, except for the biggest one. Also any lines in 0 or 90 degree angles are removed, using the Hough transform [8, 20] on each frame. Pixels belonging to vertical/horizontal lines that are present in more than two thirds of the height/width of the object are replaced with an average intensity of the surrounding pixels.

2.4 Volume and Section Identification

Once the activity images have been retrieved and cleaned, the type of template used in the images, *i.e.* volume type, and sections are identified, to estimate the three-dimensional coordinates of the activated regions. To represent the three dimensional changes in brain activity, views from three different planes are used to represent them in two dimensions. Thus we have axial sections, along the transversal plane that travels from the top of the brain to bottom; the sagittal section that travels along the median plane, from left to right; and the coronal section, along the frontal plane, that travels from front to back. To do a proper characterisation of the images, instead of focusing on the internal features of each section, the symmetry characteristics of the section shapes are used, as show in Fig. 3.

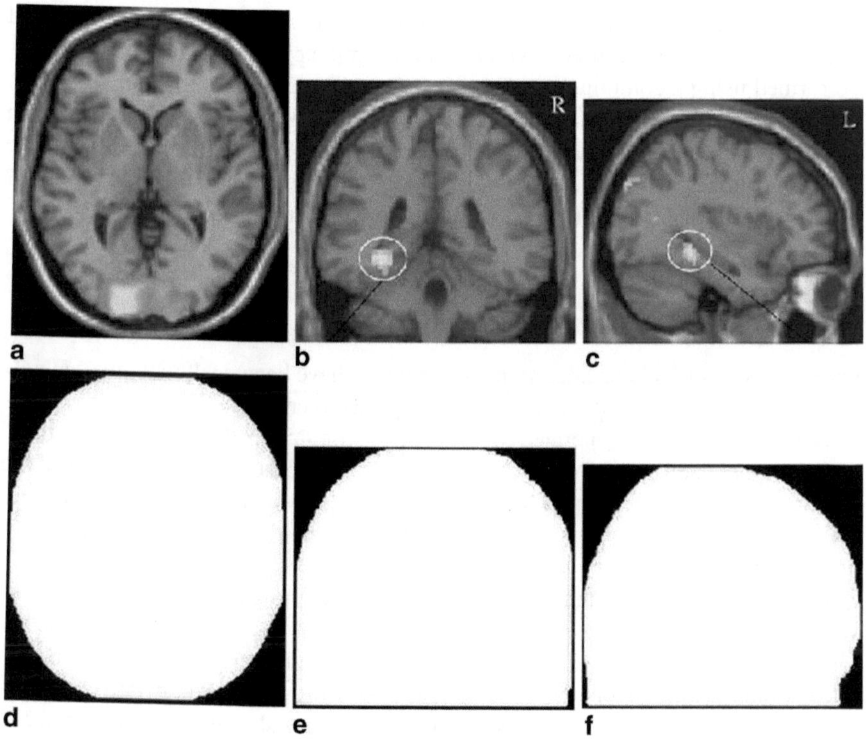

Fig. 3 Section identification—*Top column* contains example fMRI activity images (after conversion to *grey scale*) and below them their corresponding binary masks. From *left* to *right*, we have *axial*, coronal and sagittal sections

The images are again converted to binary images, thereby outlining the respective shape of the section. Simple symmetry allows for a suitable distinction between sections. One axial section is mostly symmetric about both the horizontal and vertical axis (Fig. 3a, d). The coronal section displays some symmetry only with respect to its vertical axis (Fig. 3b, e) while the sagittal section is asymmetric (Fig. 3c, f).

Most researchers map the activity changes found onto either SPM [10] or Colin [3] volume templates. Colin volumes contain higher resolution sections, when compared to SPM. Regarding the spatial separation between adjacent sections, SPM volume templates uses 2 mm, whereas that distance is 1mm for Colin templates.

To detect the volume type, one can use a complexity measure of the images. We used a *Canny* filter, [4], to detect the voxels corresponding to contrast edges. This is done for both template volumes, *i.e.* Colin and SPM, and for all the image slices from the section identified before. The volume template we select corresponds to the one with the minimal difference between the analysed image and the volume template images. This difference is calculated for the whole image and for a centred square with half the image size. We then average both values and use this as the difference measure.

To identify which slice of the template's volume corresponds to the extracted image, we compare that image with all of the template's slices. This comparison is performed using a combination of correlation and scale invariant feature transform (SIFT, [16, 20]). If there is a slice with a correlation of more than .9 with the extracted image, then that slice is selected. Otherwise, we select the slice which obtains the smallest distance of SIFT features as the correct mapping. Once this information is found, the complete coordinate set is identified for the reported image.

2.5 Blob Information Mapping

Once the geometrical considerations of the image have been dealt with, we can now characterise in the more detail the regions reported therein.

Activity regions are generated in response to stimulation. The properties of these regions largely define the fMRI activity and hence it is crucial that an analysis of the coloured blobs is carried out. Since we assume that only activations are color coded, these regions are easily segmented based on hue information (*cf.* 'blob identification' box in Fig. 2).

As mentioned before, the reporting style of different researchers can vary. This variety of reporting methods restricts the analysis that can be performed, since the same article can contain images with different colour scales. We tried to obtain intensity information from each fMRI image by using a colour map detection procedure, through histogram analysis. Since some images showed both increased and decreased activity, this step comprised from mild human intervention, aimed at fixing some wrongly detected colour maps. This was only applied to the rare cases where the automatic histogram analysis couldn't detect the correct colour scale, and was performed rather easily.

Using the Colin brain template as a reference to our own reporting, we mapped all blob intensity information to their respective coordinates. We sum all intensities found in the data, for each voxel. Then those intensities are normalised to a scale from 0 to 1, where one corresponds to the highest possible common activity.

This produces a three-dimensional intensity map, where each voxel displays the intensity corresponding to the average activity in the data, for the respective voxels. Since this intensity map was built using two-dimensional images, we also performed a 3D smoothing, using a Gaussian ellipsoid with dimensions corresponding to 5 % of the template size.

In our reporting, we decided to use the *jet* colour scale for the summarising intensity map. There, colours go from dark blue to dark red, covering also green and yellow. One big difference between our scale and typical fMRI reports is that we don't distinguish between increase or decrease of activity, when compared to a reference, but consider any coloured report as "interesting". Therefore the dark blue corresponds to locations with very low reporting of activity (positive or negative) while dark red is used for locations with many reports. To avoid showing all the brain in dark blue, we show only intensities for locations where the number of reported blobs is more than 10 % of the total.

By superimposing this intensity map over the template volume, we can obtain a visual summary of all the results found in the articles[1].

3 Results

3.1 *Extracted Information*

Table 1 shows how many articles, figures, images and blobs were found according to the publications analysed. Note that the number of samples for the unhealthy cases is quite small when compared to the healthy brains. This bias might affect the quality of the results, but the same problem would occur to any other meta-researcher, investigating brain activity in Alzheimer/Schizophrenia, due to the smaller sample of research dealing with these cases, when compared to the healthy controls.

Regarding the accuracy of the method, a simple visual inspection shows that once the volume and type of section are identified, the section coordinates were typically accurate within 1 voxel of distance. Also, the cleaning procedure of images mentioned in Sect. 2.3 doesn't remove all artifacts from images, *e.g.*, when the letters are inside the brain. Nonetheless we found that leftover artifacts rarely affected activity detection and subsequent mapping.

3.2 *Meta-Analysis*

After the compilation of all the results and the creation of the three-dimensional activity maps, one can perform analyses on the different types of brains studied.

3.2.1 Healthy Brain Activity

Figure 4 shows the brain activity reported for healthy subjects, displayed on axial section of the standard Colin reference. The highest areas of activity are the typical subsystems that compose the DMN: the posterior cingulate/precuneous, the medial pre-frontal cortex and the inferior parietal lobes. Note that, in the majority of the reports, including Alzheimer and Schizophrenia, most subjects presented the bulk of the activity in these major areas.

3.2.2 Alzheimer vs Healthy Brain Activity

We can now focus on the comparison between healthy, Alzheimer and Schizophrenia DMN activity, for example at axial height 114 of Colin's standard brain (see Fig. 5).

[1] The 2D projections of said summarising volumes were produced using the ITK-SNAP tool [23].

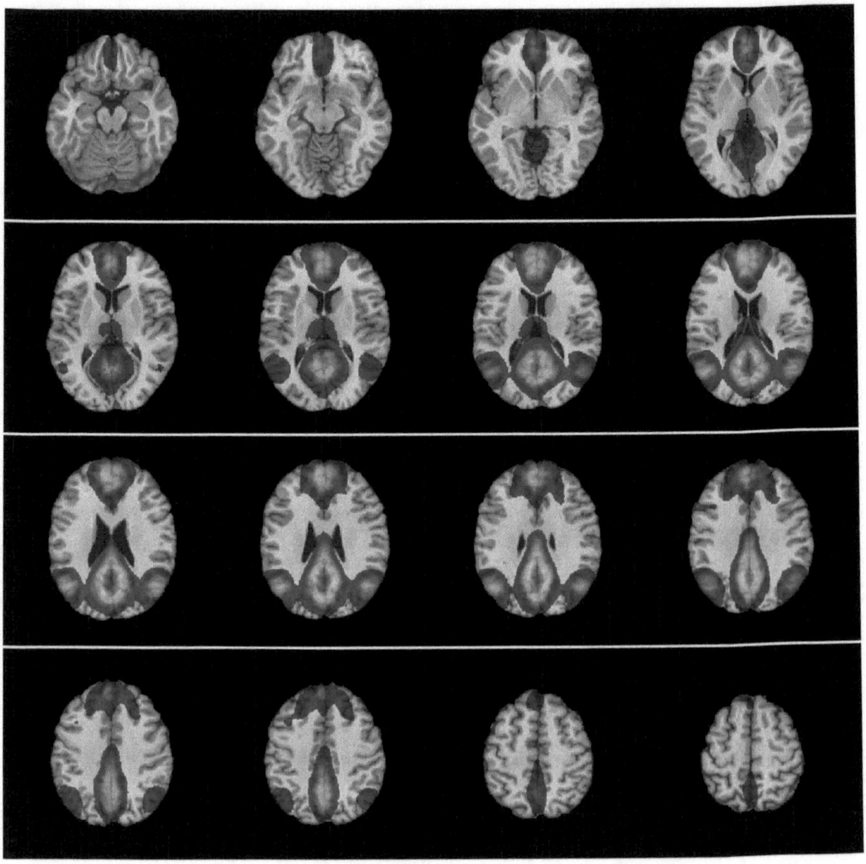

Fig. 4 Average brain activity reported in publications dealing with healthy brains, superimposed on a Colin-based brain template, shown at various axial heights. Most of the activity is reported on the occipital, temporal and frontal areas of the brain, which correspond to the typical default mode network areas

According to [2], one would expect that older brains have larger areas of activity than younger ones. We can see this in the posterior cingulate and in the inferior parietal lobes for Alzheimer when compared to the healthy brain image. On the other hand, the aged brain image shows somewhat less spread activity on the frontal lobe, when compared to the other areas of DMN. This seems counter-intuitive in light of the referred work. One may say that the lack of samples could cause this phenomenon, but our results seem rather consistent for the other areas. To find out a possible reason for this discrepancy, we can search for corroborating evidence in one of the articles analysed. In Fig. 1 of [5], there is a similar decrease in activity for aged brains, compared to healthier ones, confirming our own results.

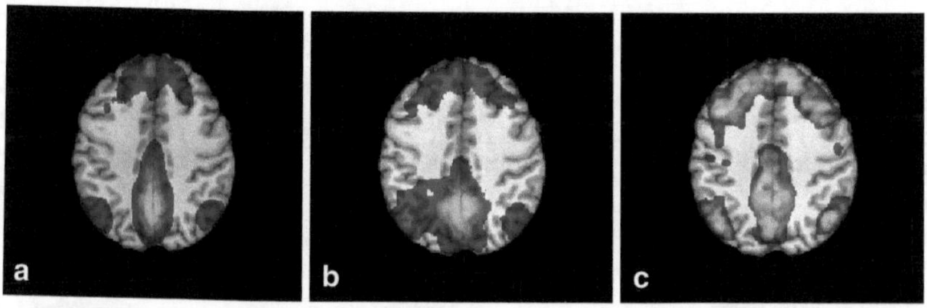

Fig. 5 Brain activity reported for healthy (**a**), Alzheimer (**b**) and schizophrenic (**c**) brains, at height 114 of the colin standard brain. The reports on brains affected by Alzheimer show a smaller intensity of activity in the pre-frontal cortex, when compared to the other DMN areas, unlike the reports for healthy and schizophrenic brains

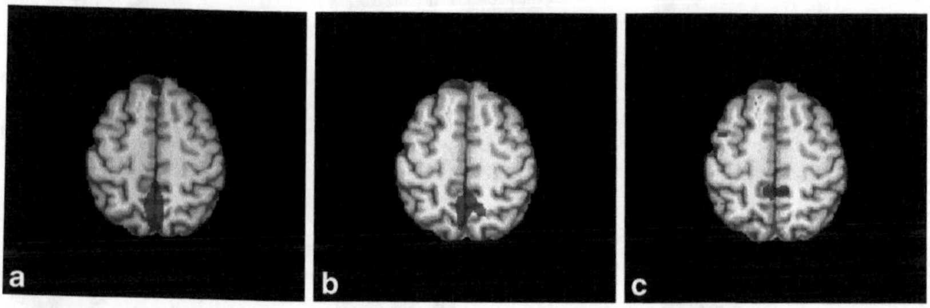

Fig. 6 Brain activity reported for healthy (**a**), Alzheimer (**b**) and schizophrenic (**c**) brains, at height 130 of the colin standard brain. (**a**) image shows wider activation in the posterior cingulate area, suggesting that both Schizophrenia and Alzheimer might play a big role in this area of the brain

3.2.3 Schizophrenia vs Healthy Brain Activity

Another analysis that can be performed with our method relates to finding areas of the brain with different activities between unhealthy brains and healthy ones. In Fig. 6, one can see images for axial height 130, where publications dealing with healthy brains report a bigger area of activity in the posterior cingulate area (PCC), when compared with brains suffering from Alzheimer, and even more so on schizophrenic brains.

3.2.4 Overall Comparison between Healthy, Alzheimer and Schizophrenia DMN Activity

To have a better overall perspective of the reported brain activations/deactivations, we can look at the 3D images of the intensity map, as depicted in Fig. 7. In this figure, we can clearly see that the areas reported on the healthy brains correspond exactly to the ones normally expected for studies of the DMN. On the brains suffering with Alzheimer, the intensity values decrease when compared to the healthy brain, as we suggested already in Fig. 5, although the areas reported are still the same as the

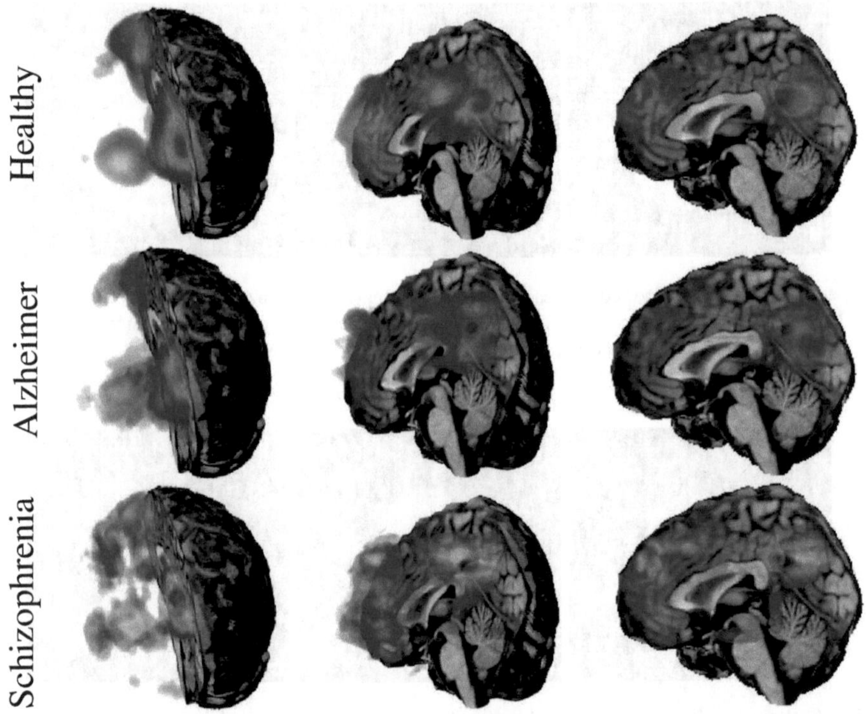

Fig. 7 Three dimensional images of brain activity reported for healthy (*top row*), Alzheimer (*middle row*) and schizophrenic (*bottom row*) brains. All reported images show the expected main DMN areas, although the reports on Alzheimer show a decreased intensity and the brains suffering with Schizophrenia report a more distributed activity pattern

from normal controls. Regarding the brains with Schizophrenia, we can see an area increase in the frontal region of the brain, while several smaller foci of activation appear, *e.g.*, near the cerebellum.

4 Discussion

We gathered more than 180 articles studying the default mode network, and analysed the images contained therein, in order to get a summarising overview of their results. Our main goal was to automatically map the results of studies reported by several researchers, onto a standard brain, and use this mapping to analyse the differences between healthy and unhealthy brains. This task would involve a tremendous amount of work and time if done by a human curator, whereas our method retrieves most information in a uniform and almost automatic manner.

The complete procedure is done in approximately 1 min per article (including human intervention if needed), while it takes 30–60 min when done by a curator, as in [15]. In that publication, the researchers went through 13 publications to obtain the information they desired. Using our method, not only it would save a considerable amount of manual work, it would enable them to find other fMRI studies related to the areas they are interested in.

Looking at the results, it seems clear that our method performs remarkably well, suggesting that it could be used to help creating a comprehensive functional brain atlas. Since we only performed a rough analysis of a particular research topic, we didn't aim at a complete report of all brain activities that might be studied.

There are some problems with our approach, that also occur in other automatic data-mining approaches. First, by using only image information we are giving the same weight to all publications, irrespectively of the number of subjects studied. Furthermore, statistical thresholds and analysis methods vary in every publication, hence we cannot claim to make a thorough statistical analysis. Also, the number of articles dealing with the unhealthy cases is quite small when compared to the healthy brains. All these problems will affect quantitatively our analysis, although we may still draw valuable information from the data. We also expect their influence to decrease with an increasing number of analysed publications.

We showed that with a clear topic in mind, it is possible to obtain results of high relevance. As an example, we have seen that most reports on DMN, regardless of the health condition of the subjects show activity on the posterior cingulate/precuneous, the medial pre-frontal cortex and the inferior parietal lobes. On the other hand, the pre-frontal activity of Alzheimer subjects is shown to be spatially restricted. Corroborating evidence for this finding can be traced back to the original published reports. Due to the reduced sample statistics for the unhealthy brains, we can't guarantee that there is a 'real' lack of activity, or just the absence of reports, but it suggests a possible area of investigation.

As stated before, there is a considerable variability in how each researcher displays their results. In the future, and to mitigate the lack of availability of original data, our method could be included in online submission systems for publication, after authors have uploaded their document. With minimal manual effort, the authors could validate the proposed summarising data, and hence improve the quality of the information gathered.

Lately there have been more and more efforts to increase data availability, either through common databases or by submitting the data at the same time as the article. Naturally, when available, this would allow for a much better analysis of the data, avoiding all the problems of detecting fMRI images or which colour scale they have. Nevertheless, these databases are still rather rare.

Despite the specificity of the method regarding fMRI images, we believe the principles behind it could be easily ported to other areas of investigation, such as weather reports or earthquake maps.

We hope to further refine our method by combining it with a text-mining approach, and test it in situations where there is either a clear agreement between different research reports, or a challenge between theories. The former is a key aspect to the construction of functional neuro-atlases, whereas the latter may lead to true findings in neuroscience.

5 Appendix–Articles Database

Healthy

1. A. Abou-Elseoud, *et al.*, *Human Brain Mapping* **31**, 1207 (2010).
2. E. A. Allen, *et al.*, *Front. Syst. Neurosci.* **5** (2011).
3. J. S. Anderson, M. A. Ferguson, M. Lopez-Larson, D. Yurgelun-Todd, *Brain Connectivity* **1**, 147157 (2011).
4. C. Aydin, O. Oktay, A. U. Gunebakan, R. K. Ciftci, A. Ademoglu, *35th International Conference on Telecommunications and Signal Processing (TSP)* (2012).
5. E. B. Beall, M. J. Lowe, *Journal of Neuroscience Methods* **191**, 263276 (2010).
6. L. Beason-Held, M. Kraut, S. Resnick, *Brain Imaging Behav* **3**, 123 (2009).
7. P. Bellec, *Intl. Workshop on Pattern Recognition in Neuroimaging* (2013).
8. C. Benjamin, *et al.*, *Frontiers in Human Neuroscience* **4** (2010).
9. H. M. de Bie, *et al.*, *Hum. Brain Mapp.* **33**, 11891201 (2012).
10. R. M. Birn, K. Murphy, P. A. Bandettini, *Hum. Brain Mapp.* **29**, 740750 (2008).
11. A. Botzung, *Frontiers in Human Neuroscience* (2010).
12. S. L. Bressler, V. Menon, *Trends in Cognitive Sciences* **14**, 277290 (2010).
13. J. A. Brewer, *et al.*, *Proceedings of the National Academy of Sciences* **108**, 2025420259 (2011).
14. R. L. Buckner, *NeuroImage* **62**, 11371145 (2012).
15. R. L. Buckner, J. L. Vincent, *NeuroImage* **37**, 10911096 (2007).
16. M. van Buuren, T. E. Gladwin, B. B. Zandbelt, R. S. Kahn, M. Vink, *Hum. Brain Mapp.* **31**, 11171127 (2010).
17. Z. Cai, J. Zhai, *International Conference on Multimedia Technology* (2011).
18. V. Calhoun, *IEEE International Symposium on Biomedical Imaging: From Nano to Macro* (2009).
19. V. Calhoun, T. Adali, *Proceedings of the 2004 14th IEEE Signal Processing Society Workshop Machine Learning for Signal Processing* (2004).
20. X. J. Chai, A. N. Castan, D. ngr, S. Whitfield-Gabrieli, *NeuroImage* **59**, 14201428 (2012).
21. C. Chang, J. P. Cunningham, G. H. Glover, *NeuroImage* **44**, 857869 (2009).
22. C. Chang, G. H. Glover, *NeuroImage* **50**, 8198 (2010).
23. C. Chang, G. H. Glover, *NeuroImage* **47**, 14481459 (2009).
24. Z. Chen, V. Calhoun, *Medical Imaging 2011: Biomedical Applications in Molecular, Structural, and Functional Imaging* (2011).
25. E. Congdon, *et al.*, *NeuroImage* **53**, 653663 (2010).
26. R. T. Constable, *et al.*, *NeuroImage* **64**, 371378 (2013).
27. S. M. Daselaar, *Frontiers in Human Neuroscience* **3** (2009).
28. J. A. De Havas, S. Parimal, C. S. Soon, M. W. Chee, *NeuroImage* **59**, 17451751 (2012).
29. M. De Luca, C. Beckmann, N. De Stefano, P. Matthews, S. Smith, *NeuroImage* **29**, 13591367 (2006).
30. F. De Martino, *et al.*, *NeuroImage* **57**, 10311044 (2011).
31. G. Derado, F. Bowman, T. Ely, C. Kilts, *Stat Interface* **3**, 45 (2010).
32. G. Deshpande, S. LaConte, S. Peltier, X. Hu, *Hum. Brain Mapp.* **30**, 1323 (2009).
33. G. Deshpande, K. Sathian, X. Hu, *IEEE Trans. Biomed. Eng.* **57**, 14461456 (2009).
34. L. Ekstrand, N. Karpinsky, Y. Wang, S. Zhang, *JoVE* (2013).
35. E. Erhardt, E. Allen, E. Damaraju, V. Calhoun, *Brain Connect* **1**, 1 (2011).
36. F. Esposito, *et al.*, *Magnetic Resonance Imaging* **26**, 905913 (2008).
37. F. Esposito, *et al.*, *Brain Research Bulletin* **70**, 263269 (2006).
38. L. Ferrarini, *et al.*, *NeuroImage* **56**, 14531462 (2011).
39. A. R. Franco, A. Pritchard, V. D. Calhoun, A. R. Mayer, *Hum. Brain Mapp.* **30**, 22932303 (2009).
40. W. FREEMAN, *International Journal of Psychophysiology* **73**, 4352 (2009).
41. W. Freeman, *IEEE Transactions on Circuits and Systems* **35**, 781783 (1988).
42. T. Gili, Time-frequency analysis of resting state networks recovery as a function of cognitive load., Master's thesis, University of Rome, La Sapienza, Department of Physics (2011).
43. M. Goldberg, *et al.*, *IEEE Conf. on Technologies for Homeland Security* (2008).
44. M. D. Greicius, V. Menon, *Journal of Cognitive Neuroscience* **16**, 14841492 (2004).
45. O. Grigg, C. L. Grady, *PLoS ONE* **5**, e13311 (2010).
46. B. Hahn, T. J. Ross, E. A. Stein, *Cerebral Cortex* **17**, 16641671 (2007).
47. T. Hedden, *et al.*, *Journal of Neuroscience* **29**, 1268612694 (2009).
48. M. van den Heuvel, R. Mandl, H. Hulshoff Pol, *PLoS ONE* **3**, e2001 (2008).
49. M. van den Heuvel, R. Mandl, J. Luigjes, H. Hulshoff Pol, *Journal of Neuroscience* **28**, 1084410851 (2008).
50. M. P. van den Heuvel, R. C. Mandl, R. S. Kahn, H. E. Hulshoff Pol, *Hum. Brain Mapp.* **30**, 31273141 (2009).
51. S. G. Horovitz, *et al.*, *Proceedings of the National Academy of Sciences* **106**, 1137611381 (2009).
52. G.-A. Hossein-Zadeh, B. Ardekani, H. Soltanian-Zadeh, *IEEE Trans. Med. Imaging* **22**, 795805 (2003).
53. J. H. Jang, *et al.*, *Neuroscience Letters* **487**, 358362 (2011).
54. S.-Y. Jeng, S.-C. Chen, P.-C. Lee, P.-S. Ho, R. Tsai, *9th International Conference on e-Health Networking, Application and Services* (2007).
55. H. Jin, *et al.*, *International Journal of Psychophysiology* **71**, 142148 (2009).
56. W. Jin-Jia, J. Ke-Mei, M. Chong-Xiao, *First International Conference on Pervasive Computing, Signal Processing and Applications* (2010).
57. H. J. Jo, Z. S. Saad, W. K. Simmons, L. A. Milbury, R. W. Cox, *NeuroImage* **52**, 571582 (2010).
58. R. E. Kelly, *et al.*, *Journal of Neuroscience Methods* **189**, 233245 (2010).
59. D.-Y. Kim, J.-H. Lee, *Neuroscience Letters* **498**, 5762 (2011).
60. V. Kiviniemi, *et al.*, *Hum. Brain Mapp.* **30**, 38653886 (2009).
61. V. Kiviniemi, *et al.*, *Brain Connectivity* **1**, 339347 (2011).
62. W. Koch, *et al.*, *NeuroImage* **51**, 280287 (2010).
63. N. A. Kochan, *et al.*, *PLoS ONE* **6**, e23960 (2011).
64. S. Kumar, A. Noor, B. K. Kaushik, B. Kumar, *International Conference on Devices and Communications (ICDeCom)* (2011).
65. A. R. Laird, *et al.*, *Journal of Neuroscience* **29**, 1449614505 (2009).
66. R. Leech, R. Braga, D. J. Sharp, *Journal of Neuroscience* **32**, 215222 (2012).
67. X. Lei, *et al.*, *PLoS ONE* **6**, e24642 (2011).
68. C.-S. R. Li, P. Yan, K. L. Bergquist, R. Sinha, *NeuroImage* **38**, 640648 (2007).
69. R. Li, *et al.*, *NeuroImage* **56**, 10351042 (2011).
70. R. Li, *et al.*, *Medical Imaging 2009: Biomedical Applications in Molecular, Structural, and Functional Imaging* (2009).
71. Littow, *Front. Syst. Neurosci.* (2010).
72. D. Liu, *Front. Syst. Neurosci.* (2010).
73. D. Lloyd, *Consciousness and Cognition* **21**, 695703 (2012).
74. X.-Y. Long, *et al.*, *Journal of Neuroscience Methods* **171**, 349355 (2008).
75. C. Madjar, *et al.* .
76. C. Malherbe, *et al.*, *IEEE International Symposium on Biomedical Imaging: From Nano to Macro* (2010).
77. S. H. Maramraju, *et al.*, *IEEE Nuclear Science Symposium Conference Record* (2008).
78. T. Meindl, *et al.*, *Hum. Brain Mapp.* p. NANA (2009).
79. M. Meinzer, *et al.*, *Neurobiology of Aging* **33**, 656669 (2012).
80. F. Musso, J. Brinkmeyer, A. Mobascher, T. Warbrick, G. Winterer, *NeuroImage* **52**, 11491161 (2010).
81. G. Northoff, *et al.*, *Nat Neurosci* **10**, 15151517 (2007).
82. E. van Oort, A. van Cappellen van Walsum, D. Norris, *NeuroImage* **90**, 381389 (2014).
83. H.-J. Park, B. Park, D.-J. Kim, *Annual Intl. Conf. of the IEEE Eng. in Medicine and Biology Society* (2009).
84. C. Parsons, K. Young, L. Murray, A. Stein, M. Kringelbach, *Progress in Neurobiology* **91**, 220241 (2010).
85. G. V. Pendse, D. Borsook, L. Becerra, *PLoS ONE* **6**, e27594 (2011).
86. V. Perlbarg, *et al.*, *5th IEEE International Symposium on Biomedical Imaging: From Nano to Macro* (2008).
87. P. L. Purdon, H. Millan, P. L. Fuller, G. Bonmassar, *Journal of Neuroscience Methods* **175**, 165186 (2008).
88. M. Pyka, *et al.*, *PLoS ONE* **4**, e7198 (2009).
89. P. Qin, G. Northoff, *NeuroImage* **57**, 12211233 (2011).
90. W. Qiu, *et al.*, *The 2011 IEEE/ICME International Conference on Complex Medical Engineering* (2011).
91. J. Rees, *Clinics in Dermatology* **31**, 806810 (2013).
92. J. J. Remes, *et al.*, *NeuroImage* **56**, 554569 (2011).
93. R. Sala-Llonch, *et al.*, *Cortex* **48**, 11871196 (2012).
94. P. G. Samann, *et al.*, *Cerebral Cortex* **21**, 20822093 (2011).
95. F. Sambataro, *et al.*, *Neurobiology of Aging* **31**, 839852 (2010).
96. S. Sargolzaei, A. S. Eddin, M. Cabrerizo, M. Adjouadi, *6th International IEEE/EMBS Conference on Neural Engineering (NER)* (2013).
97. A. Sarje, N. Thakor, *The 26th Annual Intl. Conference of the IEEE Engineering in Medicine and Biology Society* .
98. R. Scheeringa, *et al.*, *International Journal of Psychophysiology* **67**, 242251 (2008).
99. V. Schpf, *et al.*, *Journal of Neuroscience Methods* **192**, 207213 (2010).
100. M. L. Seghier, E. Fagan, C. J. Price, *Journal of Neuroscience* **30**, 1680916817 (2010).
101. K. Singh, I. Fawcett, *NeuroImage* **41**, 100112 (2008).
102. X. Song, X. Tang, *The 12th Annual Meeting of the Association for the Scientific Study of Consciousness (ASSC2008)* (2008).
103. X. Song, *et al.*, *Medical Imaging 2013: Biomedical Applications in Molecular, Structural, and Functional Imaging* (2013).
104. D. Sridharan, D. J. Levitin, V. Menon, *Proceedings of the National Academy of Sciences* **105**, 1256912574 (2008).

105. T. Starck, J. Remes, J. Nikkinen, O. Tervonen, V. Kiviniemi, *J Neurosci Methods* **186**, 179 (2010).
106. D. Stawarczyk, S. Majerus, P. Maquet, A. DArgembeau, *PLoS ONE* **6**, e16997 (2011).
107. K. Supekar, *et al.*, *NeuroImage* **52**, 290301 (2010).
108. S. J. Teipel, *et al.*, *NeuroImage* **49**, 20212032 (2010).
109. S. Teng, *et al.*, *35th Annual International Conference of the IEEE Engineering in Medicine and Biology Society (EMBC)* (2013).
110. M. Thomason, *Frontiers in Human Neuroscience* **3** (2009).
111. M. E. Thomason, *et al.*, *NeuroImage* **41**, 14931503 (2008).
112. M. E. Thomason, *et al.*, *NeuroImage* **55**, 165175 (2011).
113. P. Valsasina, *et al.*, *Proc. Intl. Soc. Mag. Reson. Med* (2009), vol. 17.
114. R. Veselis, *Best Pract Res Clin Anaesthesiol* **21**, 297 (2007).
115. H. Wang, Z. Lu, *Seventh International Conference on Natural Computation* (2011).
116. L. Wang, X. Guo, J. Sun, Z. Jin, S. Tong, *Annual International Conference of the IEEE Engineering in Medicine and Biology Society* (2012).
117. Z. Wang, J. Liu, N. Zhong, H. Zhou, Y. Qin, *The 2010 International Joint Conference on Neural Networks (IJCNN)* (2010).
118. I. Weissman-Fogel, M. Moayedi, K. S. Taylor, G. Pope, K. D. Davis, *Hum. Brain Mapp.* p. n/an/a (2010).
119. Y. D. van der Werf, E. J. Sanz-Arigita, S. Menning, O. A. van den Heuvel, *BMC Neuroscience* **11**, 145 (2010).
120. S Whitfield-Gabrieli, *et al.*, *NeuroImage* **55**, 225232 (2011).
121. L. B. Wilson, J. R. Tregellas, E. Slason, B. E. Pasko, D. C. Rojas, *NeuroImage* **55**, 724731 (2011).
122. M. Wirth, *et al.*, *NeuroImage* **54**, 30573066 (2011).
123. C. Wu, *et al.*, *Neuroimage* **45**, 694 (2009).
124. C. W. Wu, *et al.*, *NeuroImage* **59**, 30753084 (2012).
125. J.-T. Wu, *et al.*, *Neuroscience Letters* **504**, 6267 (2011).
126. L. Wu, T. Eichele, V. D. Calhoun, *NeuroImage* **52**, 12521260 (2010).
127. J. Yang, X. Weng, Y. Zang, M. Xu, X. Xu, *Cortex* **46**, 354366 (2010).
128. W. Zeng, A. Qiu, B. Chodkowski, J. J. Pekar, *NeuroImage* **46**, 10411054 (2009).
129. D. Zhang, A. Z. Snyder, J. S. Shimony, M. D. Fox, M. E. Raichle, *Cerebral Cortex* **20**, 11871194 (2010).
130. H. Zhang, *et al.*, *NeuroImage* **51**, 14141424 (2010).
131. S. Zhang, C.-s. R. Li, *Hum. Brain Mapp.* **33**, 89104 (2012).
132. Z. Zhou, *et al.*, *Magnetic Resonance Imaging* **29**, 418433 (2011).

Alzheimer

1. F. Bai, *et al.*, *Brain Research* **1302**, 167174 (2009).
2. V. Bonavita, C. Caltagirone, C. M. andAlessandro Padovani, E. Scarpini, S. Sorbi, *Journal of Alzheimer's Disease* **29**, 109 (2012).
3. J. S. Damoiseaux, K. E. Prater, B. L. Miller, M. D. Greicius, *Neurobiology of Aging* **33**, 828.e19828.e30 (2012).
4. N. Filippini, *et al.*, *Proceedings of the National Academy of Sciences* **106**, 72097214 (2009).
5. T. Gili, *et al.*, *Journal of Neurology, Neurosurgery & Psychiatry* **82**, 5866 (2011).
6. M. D. Greicius, G. Srivastava, A. L. Reiss, V. Menon, *Proceedings of the National Academy of Sciences* **101**, 46374642 (2004).
7. A. Hafkemeijer, J. van der Grond, S. A. Rombouts, *Biochimica et Biophysica Acta (BBA) - Molecular Basis of Disease* **1822**, 431441 (2012).
8. Y. Han, *et al.*, *NeuroImage* **55**, 287295 (2011).
9. S. C. Johnson, *et al.*, *Archives of General Psychiatry* **64**, 1163 (2007).
10. W. Koch, *et al.*, *Neurobiology of Aging* **33**, 466478 (2012).
11. N. A. Kochan, *et al.*, *Biological Psychiatry* **70**, 123130 (2011).
12. J. Lee, J. C. Ye, *IEEE International Conference on Systems, Man, and Cybernetics (SMC)* (2012).
13. K. Lee, J. C. Ye, *IEEE International Symposium on Biomedical Imaging: From Nano to Macro* (2010).
14. K. Li, *et al.*, *NeuroImage* **61**, 8297 (2012).
15. P. Liang, Z. Wang, Y. Yang, X. Jia, K. Li, *PLoS ONE* **6**, e22153 (2011).
16. A.-L. Lin, A. R. Laird, P. T. Fox, J.-H. Gao, *Neurology Research International* **2012**, 117 (2012).
17. Z. Liu, *et al.*, *NMR Biomed.* **25**, 13111320 (2012).
18. M. M. Lorenzi, *et al.*, *Drugs & aging* **28**, 205 (2011).
19. K. Mevel, G. Chtelat, F. Eustache, B. Desgranges, *International Journal of Alzheimers Disease* **2011**, 19 (2011).
20. J. Persson, *et al.*, *Neuropsychologia* **46**, 16791687 (2008).
21. J. R. Petrella, F. C. Sheldon, S. E. Prince, V. D. Calhoun, P. M. Doraiswamy, *Neurology* **76**, 511517 (2011).
22. Y.-w. Sun, *et al.*, *Behavioural Brain Research* **223**, 388394 (2011).
23. P. Toussaint, *et al.*, *IEEE International Symposium on Biomedical Imaging: From Nano to Macro* (2011).
24. P.-J. Toussaint, *et al.*, *NeuroImage* **63**, 936946 (2012).
25. F. Vogelaere, P. Santens, E. Achten, P. Boon, G. Vingerhoets, *Neuroradiology* **54**, 11951206 (2012).
26. X. Wu, *et al.*, *Hum. Brain Mapp.* **32**, 18681881 (2011).
27. H.-Y. Zhang, *et al.*, *Radiology* **256**, 598606 (2010).
28. J. Zhou, *et al.*, *Brain* **133**, 13521367 (2010).
29. Y. Zhou, *et al.*, *Alzheimers & Dementia* **4**, 265270 (2008).

Schizophrenia

1. C. Abbott, Decreased functional connectivity with aging and disease duration in schizophrenia, Master's thesis (2010). Master Thesis.
2. J.-C. Dreher, *et al.*, *Biological Psychiatry* **71**, 890897 (2012).
3. M. J. Escart, *et al.*, *Schizophrenia Research* **117**, 3141 (2010).
4. J. H. Jang, *et al.*, *Schizophrenia Research* **127**, 5865 (2011).
5. B. Jeong, M. Kubicki, *Psychiatry Research: Neuroimaging* **181**, 114120 (2010).
6. B. Nelson, *et al.*, *Neuroscience & Biobehavioral Reviews* **33**, 807817 (2009).
7. M. Nielsen, *et al.*, *IEEE SMC99 Conference Proceedings. 1999 IEEE International Conference on Systems, Man, and Cybernetics (Cat. No.99CH37028)*.
8. A. Rotarska-Jagiela, *et al.*, *Schizophrenia Research* **117**, 2130 (2010).
9. R. Salvador, *et al.*, *Hum. Brain Mapp.* **31**, 20032014 (2010).
10. F. C. Schneider, *et al.*, *Schizophrenia Research* **125**, 110117 (2011).
11. S. Teng, *et al.*, *2010 International Conference on Bioinformatics and Biomedical Technology*.
12. J. R. Tregellas, *et al.*, *Biological Psychiatry* **69**, 711 (2011).
13. D. Vargas-Vázquez, *Journal of Electronic Imaging* **14**, 013006 (2005).
14. L. Wang, P. D. Metzak, T. S. Woodward, *Schizophrenia Research* **125**, 136142 (2011).
15. S. Whitfield-Gabrieli, *et al.*, *Proceedings of the National Academy of Sciences* **106**, 12791284 (2009).
16. N. D. Woodward, B. Rogers, S. Heckers, *Schizophrenia Research* **130**, 8693 (2011).
17. Q. Yu, *et al.*, *Front. Syst. Neurosci.* **5** (2012).
18. D. ngr, *et al.*, *Psychiatry Research: Neuroimaging* **183**, 5968 (2010).

References

1. Bankman I (ed) (2000) Handbook of medical imaging. Academic, New York
2. Beason-Held LL (2011) Dementia and the default mode. Curr Alzheimer Res 8(4):361–365
3. Brett M, Johnsrude IS, Owen AM (2002) The problem of functional localization in the human brain. Nat Rev Neurosci 3(3):243–249
4. Canny J (1986) A computational approach to edge detection. Patt Anal Mach Intell IEEE Transac PAMI 8(6):679–698
5. De Vogelaere F, Santens P, Achten E, Boon P, Vingerhoets G (2012) Altered default-mode network activation in mild cognitive impairment compared with healthy aging. Neuroradiology 54(11):1195–1206

6. Deco G, Jirsa VK, McIntosh AR (2011) Emerging concepts for the dynamical organization of resting-state activity in the brain. Nat Rev Neurosci 12(1):43–56
7. Derrfuss J, Mar R (2009) Lost in localization: The need for a universal coordinate database. Neuroimage 48(1):1–7
8. Duda RO, Hart PE (1972) Use of the Hough transformation to detect lines and curves in pictures. Commun ACM 15(1):11–15
9. Esposito F, Pignataro G, Di Renzo G, Spinali A, Paccone A, Tedeschi G, Annunziato L (2010) Alcohol increases spontaneous BOLD signal fluctuations in the visual network. Neuroimage 53(2):534–43
10. FIL Methods Group: Statistical Parametric Mapping. http://www.fil.ion.ucl.ac.uk/spm/
11. Hand D, Mannila H, Smyth P (2001) Principles of data mining. MIT Press, Cambridge
12. Huettel SA, Song AW, McCarthy G (2008) Functional magnetic resonance imaging, 2nd ed. Sinauer, Sunderland
13. Johnson SC, Ries ML, Hess TM, Carlsson CM, Gleason CE, Alexander AL, Rowley HA, Asthana S, Sager MA (2007) Effect of Alzheimer disease risk on brain function during self-appraisal in healthy middle-aged adults. Arch Gen Psychiat 64(10):1163–1171
14. Laird AR, Lancaster JL, Fox PT (2009) Lost in localization? the focus is meta-analysis. Neuroimage 48(1):18–20
15. Levy DJ, Glimcher PW (2012) The root of all value: a neural common currency for choice. Curr Opin Neurobiol 22(6):1027–1038
16. Lowe DG (2004) Distinctive image features from scale-invariant keypoints. Int J Comput Vision 60:91–110
17. Raichle ME, MacLeod AM, Snyder AZ, Powers WJ, Gusnard DA, Shulman GL (2001) A default mode of brain function. Proc Natl Acad Sci USA 98(2):676–682
18. Rajasekharan J, Scharfenberger U, Gonçalves N, Vigário R (2010) Image approach towards document mining in neuroscientific publications. In: IDA, pp 147–158
19. Snyder AZ, Raichle ME (2012) A brief history of the resting state: the Washington University perspective. NeuroImage 62(2):902–910 http://www.sciencedirect.com/science/article/pii/S10538119120 00614
20. Szeliski R (2010) Computer vision: algorithms and applications, 1st edn. Springer, New York
21. Yarkoni T, Poldrack RA, Nichols TE, Van Essen DC, Wager TD (2011) Large-scale automated synthesis of human functional neuroimaging data. Nature Methods 8(8):665–670
22. Ylipaavalniemi J, Vigário R (2008) Analyzing consistency of independent components: an fMRI illustration. NeuroImage 39(1):169 – 180. http://dx.doi.org/10.1016/j.neuroimage.2007.08.027. http://www.sciencedirect.com/science/article/pii/S1053811907007288
23. Yushkevich PA, Piven J, Cody Hazlett H, Gimpel Smith R, Ho S, Gee JC, Gerig G (2006) User-guided 3D active contour segmentation of anatomical structures: significantly improved efficiency and reliability. Neuroimage 31(3):1116–1128

Visual Pattern Recognition Framework Based on the Best Rank Tensor Decomposition

B. Cyganek

Abstract In this paper a framework for visual patterns recognition of higher dimensionality is discussed. In the training stage, the input prototype patterns are used to construct a multidimensional array—a tensor—whose each dimension corresponds to a different dimension of the input data. This tensor is then decomposed into a lower-dimensional subspace based on the best rank tensor decomposition. Such decomposition allows extraction of the lower-dimensional features which well represent a given training class and exhibit high discriminative properties among different pattern classes. In the testing stage, a pattern is projected onto the computed tensor subspaces and a best fitted class is provided. The method presented in this paper, as well as the software platform, is an extension of our previous work. The conducted experiments on groups of visual patterns show high accuracy and fast response time.

1 Introduction

Recognition of patterns in different types of visual signals belongs to difficult computer tasks. Most problematic is high dimensionality of input data, as well as development of the methods of extraction of the features (a model) which well represent a given class of patterns and are sufficiently discriminative among the other. There are also some additional constraints superimposed on patter recognition methods, such as real-time operation or special platforms or conditions of operation. When analyzing different types of visual signals it becomes evident that a difficulty also comes from specific properties of different groups of images. For instance, the surveillance video may not be of well quality and the objects might be only partially seen and with high noise. On the other hand, medical images, such as radiograph images, may be of low contrast. All these scenarios cause research and engineering problems when designing pattern recognition systems. Frequently, additional expert knowledge is included into a design which results in highly specialized visual pattern recognition systems which are specialized in recognizing only specific types of objects. In this respect achievements in other disciplines frequently are of help.

B. Cyganek (✉)
AGH University of Science and Technology, Al. Mickiewicza 30, 30-059 Krakow, Poland
e-mail: cyganek@agh.edu.pl

J. M. R. S. Tavares, R. Natal Jorge (eds.), *Developments in Medical Image Processing and Computational Vision*, Lecture Notes in Computational Vision and Biomechanics 19,
DOI 10.1007/978-3-319-13407-9_6

In this paper a method of pattern recognition in visual data is discussed with special stress on medical and biometric images and videos. The presented method is based on the best rank tensor decomposition and extends its version presented in our previous publication [4]. In this group of method, object recognition is accomplished by comparing distances of the lower-dimensional features obtained by projecting a test pattern into the best rank tensor subspaces of different pattern classes [8]. The method was tested on the maxillary radiograph images and showed high accuracy and fast computation time. In this paper we follow this presentation and show additional aspects of the method. Specifically, the new pattern recognition framework was modified as compared to the method presented in [4]. In [4] it was proposed to select one of the best fitted prototypes for comparison. On the other hand, in this paper a modified version is proposed which account for impact of all prototype patterns which influence is averaged, as will be discussed. Also, the experimental results were extended onto the face recognition problem which builds into the biometric recognition framework.

The rest of this paper is organized as follows. In Sect. 2 the problem of pattern recognition with decompositions of pattern tensors is presented. Specifically, Sect. 2.1 presents an overview of pattern representation in the framework of best-rank prototype pattern decomposition, whereas in Sect. 2.2 pattern classification with the best rank tensor decomposition is discussed. Section 3 presents implementation details of the best rank tensor decomposition. In Sect. 4, the experimental results are presented and discussed. Finally, the paper ends with conclusions, presented in Sect. 5, as well as bibliography.

2 Pattern Recognition with the Pattern Tensor Decompositions

Recently, multidimensional arrays of data, called tensors, were proposed for pattern recognition. These, especially well fit into the problem of pattern recognition in visual signals due to a direct representation of each of the dimensions of the input signal.

Even more important are the methods of analyzing tensor content. In this respect a number of tensor decomposition methods were proposed [5, 10–12, 16]. In this respect the three decomposition methods are as follows.

1. The Higher-Order Singular Value Decomposition (HOSVD) [11].
2. The best rank-1 [12].
3. The best rank-(R_1, R_2, ..., R_K) approximations [12, 16].

First of the above, the HOSVD can be used to build the orthogonal space for pattern recognition [14]. Its variant operating on tensors obtained from the geometrically deformed prototype patterns is discussed in [5]. However, HOSVD is not well suitable for data reduction. Although there is a truncated version HOSVD, its results lead to excessive errors. Thus, usually a truncated HOSVD is treated only as a coarse approximation or it can serve as an initialization method for other decompositions.

In terms of dimensionality reduction, better results can be obtained with the best rank-1 decomposition [12]. However, the best rank-(R_1, R_2, ..., R_K) approximation offers much better behavior in terms of pattern representation in lower-dimensional subspaces, as shown by de Lathauwer [12], as well as other researchers, such as Wang and Ahuja [15, 16]. In this paper we follow this approach, discussing its properties and a method of pattern recognition, as well as providing an experimental and software framework for pattern recognition with the best rank tensor decomposition.

2.1 Pattern Representation in the Framework of Best-Rank Prototype Pattern Decomposition

As alluded to previously, the best-rank tensor prototype tensor decomposition allows best trade-off between data compression and recognition accuracy. The only control parameters of the method are requested new rank values for each of the dimensions of the prototype pattern tensor. These, in turn, can be determined experimentally or with one of the heuristic methods usually based on signal energy analysis [5, 13]. In this section, a brief introduction to multilinear analysis and best-rank tensor decomposition is presented. More information on tensors and different types of their decompositions can be found in literature [2, 3, 5, 10, 11].

For further discussion, a tensor $\mathcal{T} \in \Re^{N_1 \times N_2 \times \ldots N_K}$ can be seen as a K-dimensional cube of data, in which each dimension correspond to a different factor of the input data space. With this definition, the j-mode vector of the K-th order tensor is a vector obtained from elements of $\mathcal{T}$ by varying only one its index n_j while keeping all other indices fixed. Further, if from the tensor $\mathcal{T}$ the matrix $\mathbf{T}_{(j)}$ is created, where

$$\mathbf{T}_{(j)} \in \Re^{N_j \times (N_1 N_2 \ldots N_{j-1} N_{j+1} \ldots N_K)}, \tag{1}$$

then columns of $\mathbf{T}_{(j)}$ are *j-mode* vectors of $\mathcal{T}$. Also, $\mathbf{T}_{(j)}$ is a matrix representation of the tensor $\mathcal{T}$, called a j-mode tensor flattening. The j-th index becomes a row index of $\mathbf{T}_{(j)}$, whereas its column index is a product of all the rest K-1 indices. An analysis of sufficient computer representations of (1) are discussed in many publications, for instance in [5].

Further important concept is a p-mode product of a tensor $\mathcal{T} \in \Re^{N_1 \times N_2 \times \ldots N_K}$ with a matrix $\mathbf{M} \in \Re^{Q \times N_p}$. A result of this operation is the tensor $\mathcal{S} \in \Re^{N_1 \times N_2 \times \ldots N_{p-1} \times Q \times N_{p+1} \times \ldots N_K}$ whose elements are obtained based on the following scheme:

$$\mathcal{S}_{n_1 n_2 \ldots n_{p-1} q n_{p+1} \ldots n_K} = \left(\mathcal{T} \times_p \mathbf{M}\right)_{n_1 n_2 \ldots n_{p-1} q n_{p+1} \ldots n_K} = \sum_{n_p=1}^{N_p} t_{n_1 n_2 \ldots n_{p-1} n_p n_{p+1} \ldots n_K} m_{q n_p}. \tag{2}$$

As was shown, the *p-mode* product can be equivalently represented in terms of the flattened versions of the tensors $\mathbf{T}_{(p)}$ and $\mathbf{S}_{(p)}$. That is, if the following holds

$$\mathcal{S} = \mathcal{T} \times_p \mathbf{M}, \tag{3}$$

then we have the following

$$\mathbf{S}_{(p)} = \mathbf{M}\mathbf{T}_{(p)} \tag{4}$$

In some computations, it is more efficient to represent the tensor and matrix product given in (2) in an equivalent representation based on the p-mode tensor flattening and the Kronecker product. That is,

$$\mathcal{T} = \mathcal{Z}\times_1\mathbf{S}_1\times_2\mathbf{S}_2\ldots\times_K\mathbf{S}_K, \tag{5}$$

can be equivalently represented as follows

$$\mathbf{T}_{(n)} = \mathbf{S}_n\mathbf{Z}_{(n)}\left[\mathbf{S}_{n+1}\otimes\mathbf{S}_{n+2}\otimes\ldots\otimes\mathbf{S}_K\otimes\mathbf{S}_1\otimes\mathbf{S}_2\otimes\ldots\otimes\mathbf{S}_{n-1}\right]^T, \tag{6}$$

where $\otimes$ denotes the Kronecker product between the matrices.

Equipped with the above concepts, the best rank-(R_1, R_2, …, R_K) decomposition of a tensor $\mathcal{T} \in \Re^{N_1\times N_2\times\ldots N_K}$ can be defined as a problem of computying a tensor $\tilde{\mathcal{T}}$, which is characteristic of the ranks $rank_1\left(\tilde{\mathcal{T}}\right) = R_1$, $rank_2\left(\tilde{\mathcal{T}}\right) = R_2$, …, $rank_K\left(\tilde{\mathcal{T}}\right) = R_K$, and which as close as possible approximates to the input tensor $\mathcal{T}$ [11, 12], that is the following functional should be minimized:

$$E\left(\tilde{\mathcal{T}}\right) = \left\|\tilde{\mathcal{T}} - \mathcal{T}\right\|_F^2, \tag{7}$$

where $\|.\|_F$ denotes the Frobenius norm . It can be shown that the approximated tensor $\tilde{\mathcal{T}}$ conveys as much of the "energy", in the sense of the squared entries of a tensor, as the original tensor $\mathcal{T}$, under the requested rank constraints. A value of E is called the reconstruction error. Figure 1 depicts the best rank-(R_1, R_2, R_3) decomposition of a 3D tensor $\mathcal{T} \in \Re^{N_1\times N_2\times N_3}$. However, contrary to the rank definition of the matrices, there are different rank definitions for tensors. For more discussion see [5, 11].

It can be also easily observed that the assumed rank conditions mean that the approximation tensor $\tilde{\mathcal{T}}$ can be decomposed as follows

$$\tilde{\mathcal{T}} = \mathcal{Z}\times_1\mathbf{S}_1\times_2\mathbf{S}_2\ldots\times_K\mathbf{S}_K, \tag{8}$$

Each of the matrices $\mathbf{S}_1 \in \Re^{N_1\times R_1}$, $\mathbf{S}_2 \in \Re^{N_2\times R_2}$, …, and $\mathbf{S}_K \in \Re^{N_K\times R_K}$ in (8) has orthonormal columns. The number of columns for $\mathbf{S}_i$ is given by R_i.

The core tensor $\mathcal{Z} \in \Re^{R_1\times R_2\times\ldots\times R_K}$ is of dimensions R_1, R_2, …, R_K. It can be computed from the original tensor $\mathcal{T}$ as follows

$$\mathcal{Z} = \mathcal{T}\times_1\mathbf{S}_1^T\times_2\mathbf{S}_2^T\ldots\times_K\mathbf{S}_K^T. \tag{9}$$

Summarizing, to find the best rank-(R_1, R_2, …, R_K) approximation of $\mathcal{T}$ it is sufficient to determine only a set of $\mathbf{S}_i$ in (8), and then $\mathcal{Z}$ is computed from Eq. (9).

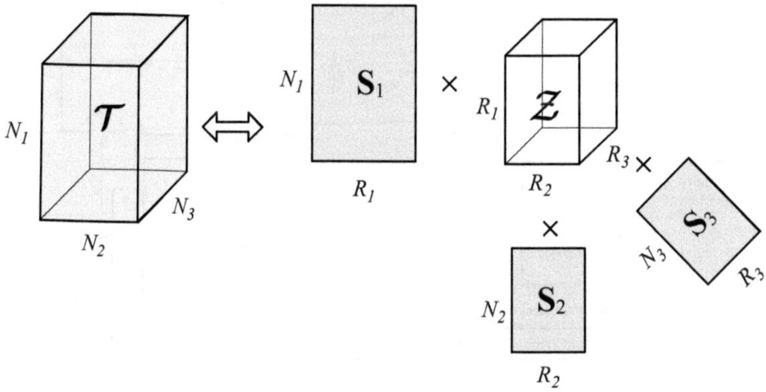

Fig. 1 Schematic representation of the best rank-(R_1, R_2, R_3) decomposition of a 3D tensor

Further analysis is constrained exclusively to 3D tensors, such as the one shown in Fig. 1. It can be seen that this decomposition leads to a significant data reduction. The compression C ratio can be expressed as follows:

$$C = (R_1 R_2 R_3 + N_1 R_1 + N_2 R_2 + N_3 R_3)/(N_1 N_2 N_3). \tag{10}$$

As alluded to previously, the only control parameters of the method are the ranks R_1, R_2, and R_3. A trade-off can be achieved between the compression ratio C in (10) with respect to the approximation error expressed in Eq. (7). This influences also pattern recognition accuracy, as will be discussed.

2.2 *Pattern Classification with the Best Rank Tensor Decomposition*

The already described, the subspace obtained after the best rank decomposition can be used to generate specific features of an image $\mathbf{X}$, which can be then used for pattern recognition [16]. The features are obtained by projecting the image $\mathbf{X}$ of dimensions $N_1 \times N_2$ into the space spanned by the two matrices $\mathbf{S}_1$ and $\mathbf{S}_2$ in accordance with (9). However, at first the pattern $\mathbf{X}$ needs to be represented in an equivalent tensor form $\mathcal{X}$ which is of dimensions $N_1 \times N_2 \times 1$. Then, the feature tensor $\mathcal{F}$ of dimensions $R_1 \times R_2 \times 1$ is obtained by projecting $\mathcal{X}$ onto the space spanned by $\mathbf{S}_1$ and $\mathbf{S}_2$, as follows

$$\mathcal{F}_{\mathbf{X}} = \mathcal{X} \times_1 \mathbf{S}_1^T \times_2 \mathbf{S}_2^T \tag{11}$$

Tensor $\mathcal{T}$ contains is constructed out of the available training patterns. However, the method can work depending on a number of available training patterns, starting from only one exemplar, as will be discussed. Hence, in our framework the following two scenarios were evaluated, depending on the available number of training patterns:

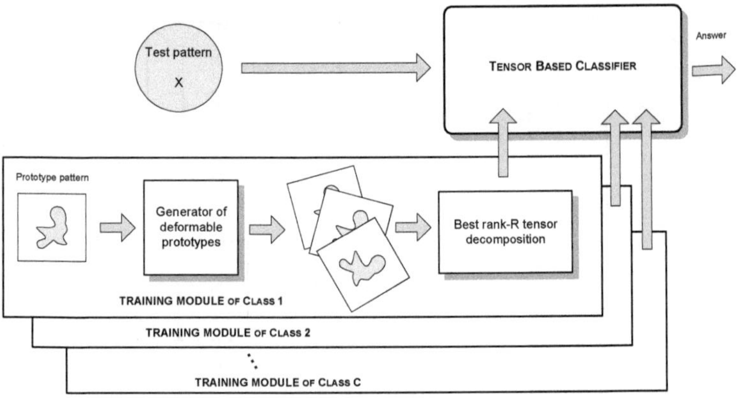

Fig. 2 The process of the 3D pattern tensor generation by geometrical warping of the prototype pattern

1. A set of prototype patterns $\mathbf{P}_i$ of the same object is available. These are used to form the input tensor $\mathcal{T}$.
2. If only one prototype $\mathbf{P}$ is available, its different appearances $\mathbf{P}_i$ are generated by geometrical warping of the available pattern. This process is visualized in Fig. 2.

As a result the patterns form a 3D tensor after the best-rank decomposition spans the space representing that class. In the case of multiple classes, a 3D tensor is built for each of the classes separately.

The next step after the best rank-(R_1, R_2, ..., R_K) decomposition consist of building features from each of the prototype patterns $\mathbf{P}_i$ from the tensor $\mathcal{T}$. These are computed as follows

$$\mathcal{F}_i = \mathcal{P}_i \times_1 \mathbf{S}_1^T \times_2 \mathbf{S}_2^T, \tag{12}$$

where $\mathcal{P}_i$denotes an $N_1 \times N_2 \times 1$ tensor representation of the pattern $\mathbf{P}_i$. In the same way features are computed for the tensor $\mathcal{P}_X$ created from the test pattern $\mathbf{P}_X$. It is interesting to notice that dimensions of the computed in this way features are much less than dimensions of the original patterns due to data compression expressed by (10). However, they represent the two-dimensional dominating spaces in each dimension independently. Thus, their discriminative properties are usually high despite low-dimensional representation.

Finally, a quantitative measure of the fitness of the test pattern $\mathbf{P}_X$ to the prototypes of a class c is computed based on the following formula

$$\rho_c = \frac{1}{N_3} \sum_{i=1}^{N_3} \left\| \mathcal{F}_{\mathbf{X}} - \mathcal{F}_i^{(c)} \right\|_F. \tag{13}$$

In a case of a multi-class classification scheme, a best fit class c^* is chosen which minimizes its fitness measure, as follows

$$c^* = \underset{1 \le c \le C}{\arg\min} \, (\rho_c). \tag{14}$$

Figure 3 depicts the described process of multi-class pattern recognition from the best-rank decomposition of the prototype pattern tensor.

As alluded to previously, the training parameters are the chosen rank values of R_1, R_2, and R_3 in (8). In our experiments these are usually determined experimentally, although they can be also chosen after analyzing signal energy level in the decomposed tensor. However, especially interesting is the case of $R_3 = 1$ which means that the third dimension of the pattern tensor, which reflects a number of training patterns, will be compressed to one the most prominent example. Such strategy frequently leads to superior results, as will be presented in the experimental part.

3 Implementation of the Best Rank Tensor Decomposition

Computation of the best rank-(R_1, R_2, ..., R_K) decomposition of tensors, given by Eqs. (8) and (9), can be done with the Alternating Least-Squares (ALS) method, as proposed by Lathauwer et al. [11, 12]. In each step of this method only one of the matrices $\mathbf{S}_k$ is optimized, whereas other are kept fixed [1, 5]. The main concept of this approach is to express the quadratic expression in the components of the unknown matrix $\mathbf{S}_k$ with orthogonal columns with other matrices kept fixed. That is, the following problem is solved

$$\max_{\mathbf{S}_i} \{\Psi(\mathbf{S}_i)\} = \max_{\mathbf{S}_i} \left\| \mathcal{T} \times_1 \mathbf{S}_1^T \times_2 \mathbf{S}_2^T \ldots \times_K \mathbf{S}_K^T \right\|^2. \quad (15)$$

Columns of $\mathbf{S}_i$ can be obtained finding the orthonormal basis of the dominating subspace of the column space of the approximating matrix $\hat{\mathbf{S}}_i$. As already mentioned, in each step only one matrix $\mathbf{S}_i$ is computed, while other are kept fixed. Such procedure—called the Higher-Order Orthogonal Iteration (HOOI)—is repeated until the stopping condition is fulfilled or a maximal number of iterations is reached [5, 12]. The pseudo-code of the algorithm is presented in Fig. 4.

In the above algorithm, the function $svds(\hat{\mathbf{S}}, R)$returns the R left leading singular vectors of a matrix $\hat{\mathbf{S}}$. These vectors are orthogonal. Frequently the matrix $\hat{\mathbf{S}}_k$has much more columns c than rows r. In such a case more efficient becomes computation of the *svds* from the product $\hat{\mathbf{S}}_k\hat{\mathbf{S}}_k^T$, instead of the matrix $\hat{\mathbf{S}}_k$using the fact that if a matrix $\mathbf{M} = \mathbf{SVD}^T$, then $\mathbf{MM}^T = \mathbf{SV}^2\mathbf{S}^T$.

Initialization of the matrices in the algorithm in Fig. 4 can be done with the prior HOSVD decomposition. Although such strategy does not guarantee the optimal solution, in practice usually it leads to good results [12]. However, HOSVD is computationally demanding, so for larger problems Wang and Ahuja propose to initialize $\mathbf{S}_k$, either with constant values, or with the uniformly distributed random numbers. These strategies when applied to image processing tasks gave almost the same results as initialization with the HOSVD [16]. Such an initialization method is also recommended in the paper by Chen and Saad [1]. In our software framework, accessible from [7], we also follow this way and initialize $\mathbf{S}_k$ with uniform random generator.

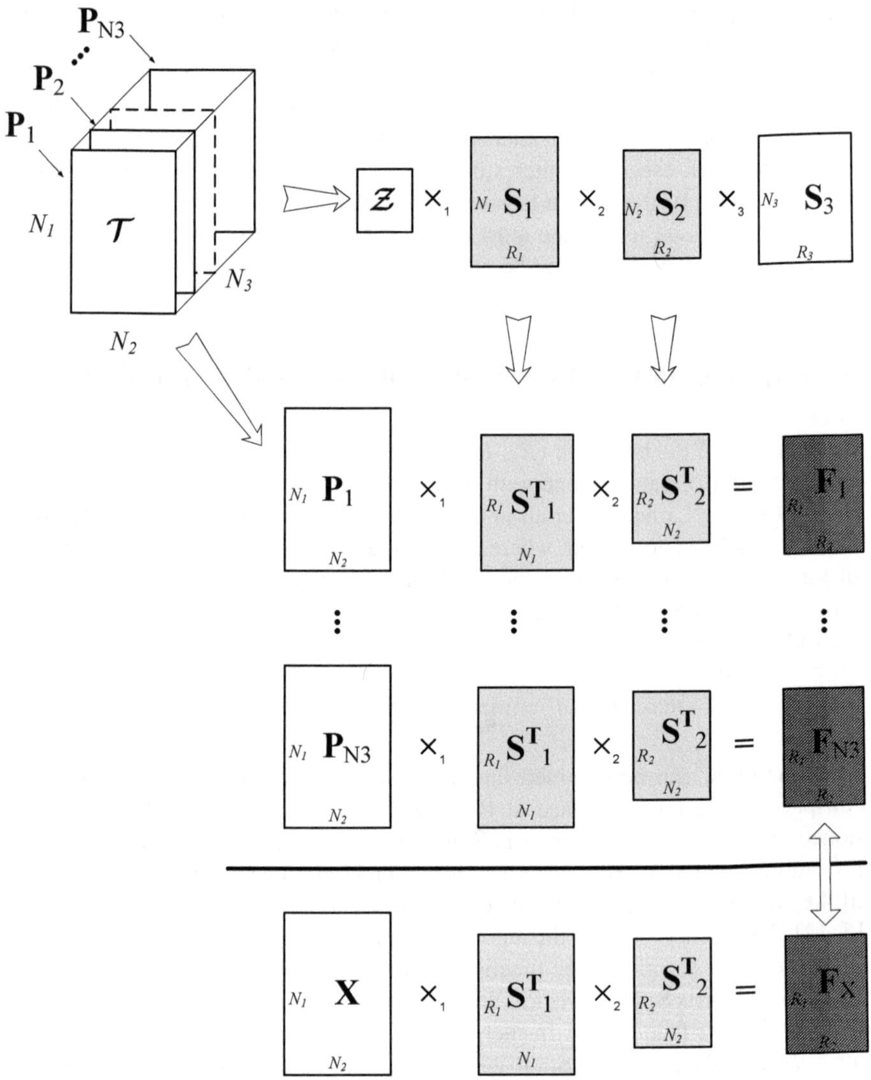

Fig. 3 Pattern recognition scheme with the best rank-(R_1, R_2, ..., R_K) decomposition of a tensor composed from the prototype patterns $\mathbf{P}_1$, $\mathbf{P}_2$, ..., $\mathbf{P}_{N3}$ of a single class. Decomposition of the pattern tensor provides the lower-dimensional subspaces given by the column orthogonal matrices $\mathbf{S}_1$, $\mathbf{S}_2$, and $\mathbf{S}_3$. Prototype features are obtained by projecting each prototype patterns onto the space spanned by the matrices $\mathbf{S}_1$ and $\mathbf{S}_2$. Features of the test pattern $\mathbf{X}$ are finally compared with the prototype features. The procedure is repeated for each class and the class with the best match of features is returned by the classifier

The above HOOI procedure has been implemented in our software framework, as described in [5]. The implementation utilizes C++ classes with basic data types defined as template parameters, as shown in Fig. 5. This allows time and memory

1. Set a number of ranks $R_1, R_2, \ldots, R_K$.
Set accuracy threshold e_{thresh}

2. Initialize the mode matrices with random values

$$\mathbf{S}_k^{(0)} \in \Re^{N_k \times R_k} \text{ for } 1 \leq k \leq K$$

$$t = 0$$

3. Do:

4. For each k in range ($1 \leq k \leq K$), do:

$$\hat{\mathbf{S}}_k^{(t+1)} = \mathbf{T}_{(k)} \left[\underbrace{\mathbf{S}_{k-1}^{(t)} \otimes \mathbf{S}_{k-2}^{(t)} \otimes \ldots \otimes \mathbf{S}_1^{(t)}}_{F_1} \otimes \underbrace{\mathbf{S}_P^{(t+1)} \otimes \ldots \otimes \mathbf{S}_{k+1}^{(t+1)}}_{F_2} \right]$$

$$\mathbf{S}_k^{(t+1)} = svds\left(\hat{\mathbf{S}}_k^{(t+1)}, R_k\right)$$

$$\mathcal{Z}_{t+1} = \mathcal{T} \times_1 \mathbf{S}_1^{(t+1)^T} \times_2 \mathbf{S}_2^{(t+1)^T} \ldots \times_P \mathbf{S}_P^{(t+1)^T}$$

$$e = \left| \left\| \mathcal{Z}_{t+1} \right\|^2 - \left\| \mathcal{Z}_t \right\|^2 \right|$$

while ($e > e_{thresh}$);

3. Output: a set of matrices $\mathbf{S}_k$.

Fig. 4 A procedure for computation of the best rank-($R_1, R_2, \ldots, R_K$) tensor decomposition

savings by using the fixed point representation of data instead of the floating point. In the presented experiments the 12.12 fixed point representation showed to be sufficient (each data is stored on 3 bytes instead of 8, needed in the case of the floating point representation).

The *Best_Rank_R_DecompFor*, shown in Fig. 5, is the main class for the best-rank tensor decomposition. It is derived from the *TensorAlgebraFor* class which implements all basic operations on tensors, such as the p-mode multiplications, discussed in the previous section. Tensors, are represented by objects of the class *TFlatTensorFor* which represents tensors in the flattened form. The *Best_Rank_R_DecompFor* class is accompanied by the *S_Matrix_Initializer* hierarchy. Its main role is to define the way of initial setup of the values of the $\mathbf{S}_i$ matrices for the HOOI process. In our case these were initialized with randomly generated values of uniform distribution [5, 7].

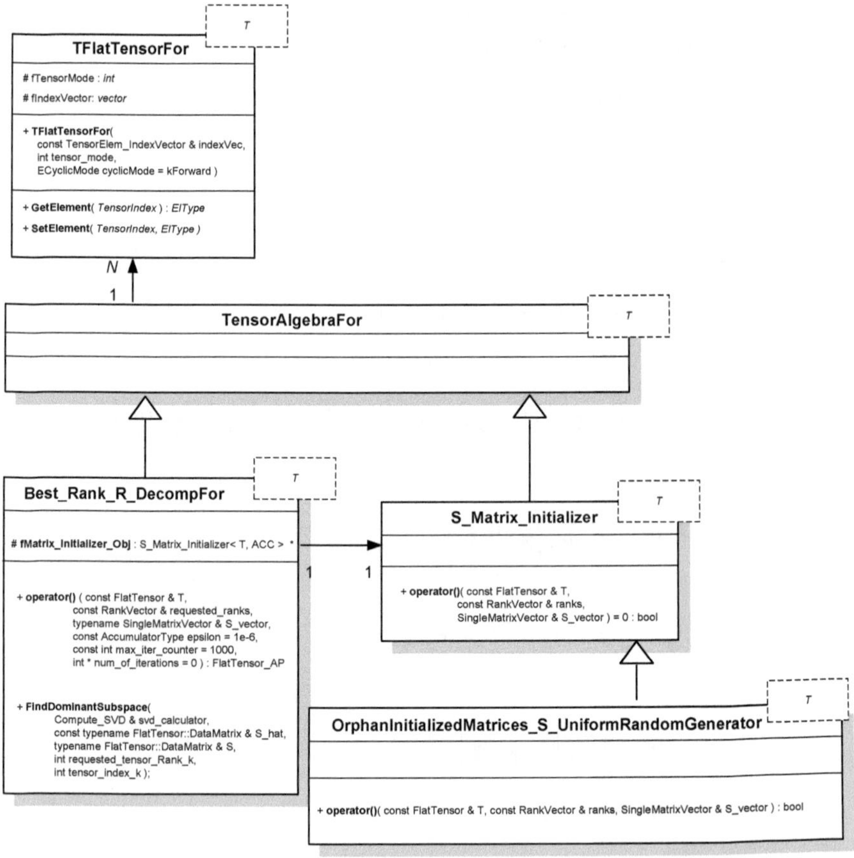

Fig. 5 Class hierarchy from the DeRecLib library implementing the best-rank tensor decomposition for tensors of any dimensions and any type of elements

4 Experimental Results

This paper is based on the previous version, presented in [4]. In this section we cite these results, augmented with results of the tests on face recognition. Figure 6 depicts a maxillary radiograph (left), as well as the implant pattern (right).

In the first task, the implants in the maxillary radiograph images are recognized with the proposed technique. At first, the places of implants are detected by exploiting their high contrast in the radiograph images [6]. These are detected as highly contrast areas, which after registration are fed to the tensor classifier described in the previous sections. Since only one example of the prototype image is usually available, its different appearances are generated by image warping, as described in the previous section. In the experiments an implant pattern is rotated in the range of $\pm 12^{\circ}$.

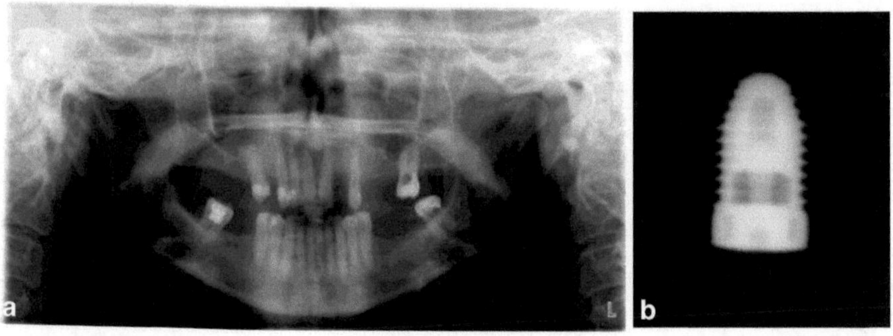

Fig. 6 An example of a maxillary radiograph image (**a**) and a dental implant to be recognized (**b**). (Based on [4])

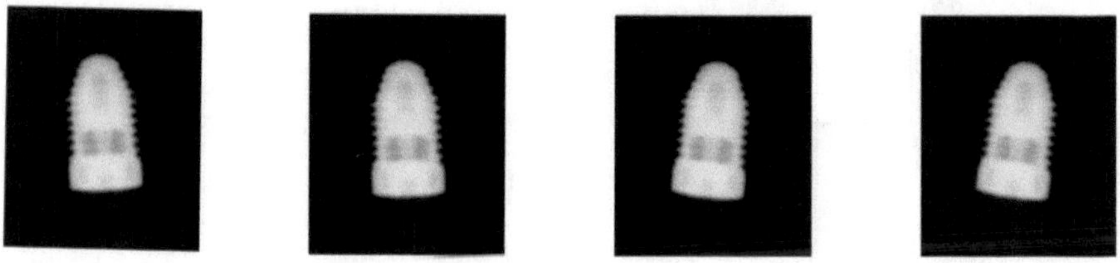

Fig. 7 Examples of the geometrically deformed versions of the prototype image of an implant. These are formed into a 3D tensor which after the best-rank approximation is used in object recognition. (From [4])

Additionally, a Gaussian noise is also added to increase robustness of the method. Examples of deformed versions of the prototype image of an implant are depicted in Fig. 7. These form a 3D tensor which, after the best-rank decomposition, is used in recognition process as already discussed.

Figure 8a shows a plot of the reconstruction error E, expressed in Eq. (7), in respect to the compression ratio C, given in Eq. (10).

In the presented experiments, size of the tensor $\mathcal{T}$ is $56 \times 56 \times 13$. Figure 8b depicts a plot showing accuracy of the pattern recognition, in respect to the compression ratio C. The accuracy with the best representing patter, presented in Fig. 3, allows accuracy at the level of 95–96 %. However, thanks to a different classification method, accuracy level was higher by 1–2 % in the presented experiments. The ranks were chosen 1/4 of the spatial resolution and 1/2 for the pattern dimension of the input tensors. In further research we plan to conduct more extensive comparison of different rank settings, as well as different pattern recognition strategy, in respect to the system accuracy.

In the second group of experiments, the method was tested in the tasks of face recognition. For this purpose the ATT Lab (formerly the ORL Database of Faces) face database were used, examples of which are depicted in Fig. 9. This database contains a set of face images taken in the laboratory conditions [9].

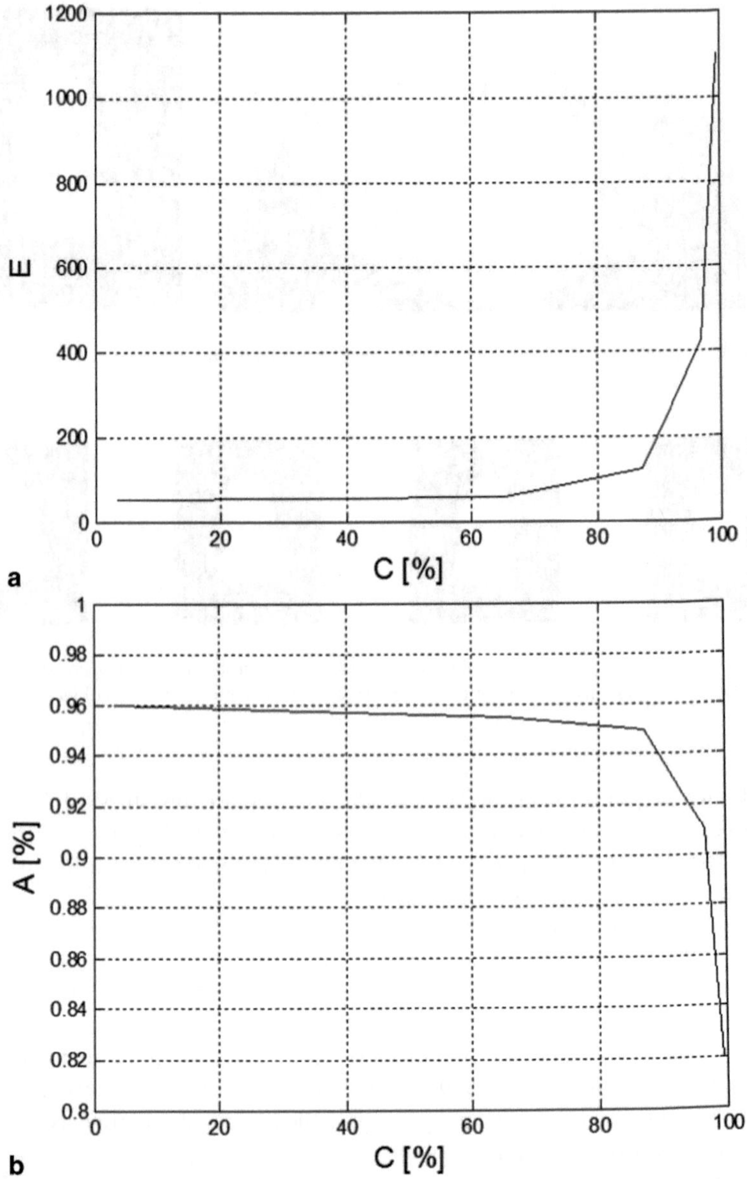

Fig. 8 Reconstruction error E in respect to the compression ratio C of the input patterns (**a**) Accuracy A of pattern recognition in respect to the compression ratio C of the input patterns (**b**). (From [4])

There are ten different images of each of 40 distinct persons. For few subjects, the images were taken at different times, at varying lighting conditions, as well as with different facial expressions (open/closed eyes, smiling/not smiling) and facial

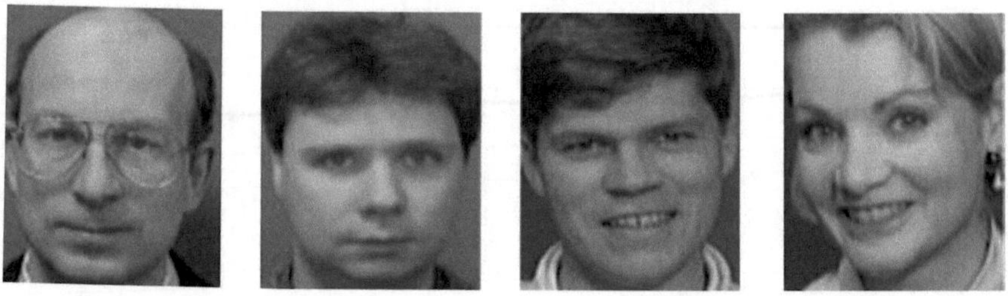

Fig. 9 Examples of the images from the Olivetti Research Lab (ORL)—now ATT Labs. There are 40 subjects, for each there are ten images from which a number were randomly selected for training and the remaining for testing

details (glasses/no glasses). All the images were taken against a dark homogeneous background with the subjects in an upright, frontal position (with tolerance for some side movement).

Figure 10 presents two accuracy plots obtained on the ATT face database with the presented method. In Fig. 10a accuracy is shown in respect to different rank assignments, which directly influence compression ratio, in accordance with formula (10). In this experiment nine images were used for training and the remaining one for testing. The procedure was repeated 10 times. The rank values in Fig. 10a are as follows: (20, 20, 1), (20, 20, 3), (40, 40, 1), (10, 10, 1), (20, 20.9). We notice, that different ranks lead to different accuracy and there is no simple formula joining the compression ration C with accuracy A. Nevertheless, high C leads to lowering A.

In Fig. 10b the same ranks (20, 20,1) are used and the accuracy is drawn in respect to different partitions of the database patterns into the training and testing groups respectively. These are as follows: 9 vs. 1, 7 vs. 3, 5 vs. 5, and 3 vs. 7. Although, a lowering number of training patterns with a higher number of test patterns leads to lower accuracy, the drop is by 0.1 (that is, by 10 %). For future research we plan further investigation, as well as we will try to develop the methods of automatic rank assignments based on signal properties.

The used database is demanding due to high diversity of face appearances within majority of single person. Despite this difficulty, the proposed method allows high accuracy and performs in real-time. Hence, the method can be used in many medical, as well as biometrical on other pattern recognition tasks.

5 Conclusions

The paper presents a framework for pattern recognition in the multi-dimensional image signals with help of the best rank decomposition of the prototype pattern tensors. The tensors are proposed to be formed from the patterns defining a class, either from the statistical group of prototype patterns, or from a series of patterns generated after geometrical transformations of a available single prototype. Pattern recognition

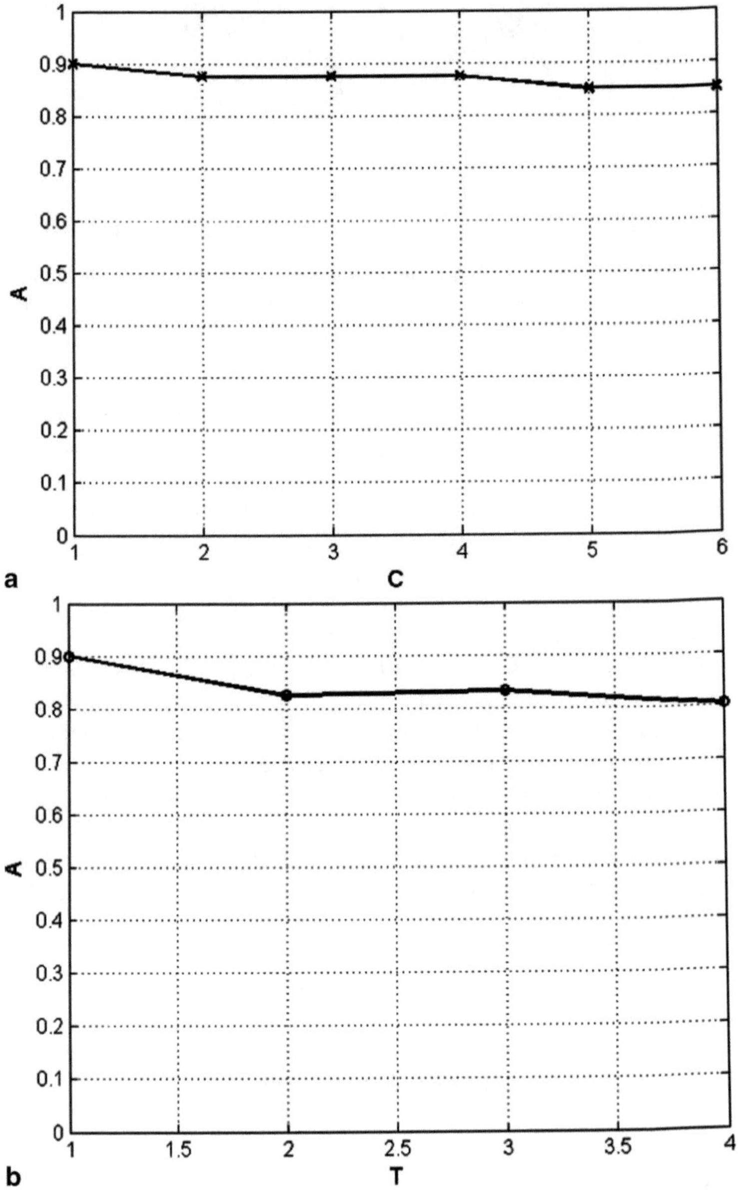

Fig. 10 Accuracy of face recognition in respect to different compression ratio C (**a**). Accuracy of face recognition for the same compression ratio (20, 20, 1) and different assignments T of training vs. testing images (**b**)

is accomplished by testing a distance of the features obtained by projection of the patterns into the best rank tensor subspace and comparing with features of all the projected prototypes. The method was tested on the number of image groups and showed high accuracy and fast response time. In the presented experiments with implant recognition in maxillary radiograph images, the reached accuracy is 97 %. The method was also tested on the problem of face recognition. In the task of face recognition from the face database the method achieves 90 % accuracy on average. Additionally, the object-oriented software platform was presented which, apart from training computations, allows real time response time. It was also indicated that the training process can be easily parallelized, since each class can be processed independently. The software for tensor decomposition is available from the webpage [7]. Our future research on this subject will concentrate on further analysis, measurement of different signal transformations, as well as on development of methods for best rank assignments.

Acknowledgements The financial support from the Polish National Science Centre NCN in the year 2014, contract no. DEC-2011/01/B/ST6/01994, is greatly acknowledged.

References

1. Chen J, Saad Y (2009) On the tensor svd and the optimal low rank orthogonal approximation of tensors. SIAM J Matrix Anal Appl 30(4):1709–1734
2. Cichocki A, Zdunek R, Amari S (2008) Nonnegative matrix and tensor factorization. IEEE Signal Process Mag 25(1):142–145
3. Cichocki A, Zdunek R, Phan AH, Amari S-I (2009) Nonnegative matrix and tensor factorizations. Applications to exploratory multi-way data analysis and blind source separation. Wiley, Chichester
4. Cyganek B (2013) Pattern recognition framework based on the best rank-($R_1, R_2, \ldots, R_K$) tensor approximation. In: Computational vision and medical image processing IV: proceedings of VipIMAGE 2013—IV ECCOMAS thematic conference on Computational vision and medical image processing, pp 301–306
5. Cyganek B (2013) Object detection and recognition in digital images: theory and practice. Wiley
6. Cyganek B, Malisz P (2010) Dental implant examination based on the log-polar matching of the maxillary radiograph images in the anisotropic scale space. IEEE Engineering in Medicine and Biology Conference, EMBC 2010, Buenos Aires, Argentina, pp 3093–3096
7. DeRecLib (2013) http://www.wiley.com/go/cyganekobject
8. Duda RO, Hart PE, Stork DG (2001) Pattern classification. Wiley, New York
9. https://www.cl.cam.ac.uk/research/dtg/attarchive/facedatabase.html
10. Tamara GK, Brett WB (2009) Tensor decompositions and applications. SIAM Rev 51(3): 455–500
11. Lathauwer de L (1997) Signal processing based on multilinear algebra. PhD dissertation, Katholieke Universiteit Leuven
12. Lathauwer de L, Moor de B, Vandewalle J (2000) On the best rank-1 and rank-($R_1, R_2, \ldots, R_N$) approximation of higher-order tensors. SIAM J Matrix Anal Appl 21(4):1324–1342
13. Muti D, Bourennane S (2007) Survey on tensor signal algebraic filtering. Signal Process 87:237–249
14. Savas B, Eldén L (2007) Handwritten digit classification using higher order singular value decomposition. Pattern Recognit 40(3):993–1003
15. Wang H, Ahuja N (2004) Compact representation of multidimensional data using tensro rank-one decomposition. In: Proceedings of the 17th international conference on pattern recognition, Vol 1, 4pp 4–47
16. Wang H, Ahuja N (2008) A tensor approximation approach to dimensionality reduction. Int J Comput Vision 76(3):217–229

Tracking Red Blood Cells Flowing through a Microchannel with a Hyperbolic Contraction: An Automatic Method

B. Taboada, F. C. Monteiro and R. Lima

Abstract The present chapter aims to assess the motion and deformation index of red blood cells (RBCs) flowing through a microchannel with a hyperbolic contraction using an image analysis based method. For this purpose, a microchannel containing a hyperbolic contraction was fabricated in polydimethylsiloxane by using a soft-lithography technique and the images were captured by a standard high-speed microscopy system. An automatic image processing and analyzing method has been developed in a MATLAB environment, not only to track both healthy and exposed RBCs motion but also to measure the deformation index along the microchannel. The keyhole model has proved to be a promising technique to track automatically healthy and exposed RBCs flowing in this kind of microchannels.

1 Introduction

Microfluidic devices have emerged as promising in vitro experimental technique to precisely control fluids with small volumes of blood cells and consequently to obtain more insight on the blood rheological properties at a micro-scale level, including red blood cell (RBC) deformability [8, 15]. One way to study blood flow behavior in detail is by measuring the displacements by tracking each RBC in a Lagrangian way [16]. This method is often referred as Particle Tracking Velocimetry (PTV) [16, 23]. Although this method is becoming indispensable in microcirculation [7, 10–14], most of these studies were performed with manual tracking methods. Recently, by

B. Taboada (✉) · R. Lima
ESTiG, IPB, C. Sta. Apolonia, 5301-857 Bragança, Portugal

CEFT, FEUP, R. Dr. Roberto Frias, 4200-465 Porto, Portugal
e-mail: brunataboada@ipb.pt

R. Lima
University of Minho, Mechanical Engineering Department, Campus de Azurém, 4800-058 Guimarães, Portugal
e-mail: ruimec@ipb.pt

F. C. Monteiro
ESTiG, IPB, C. Sta. Apolonia, 5301-857 Bragança, Portugal
e-mail: monteiro@ipb.pt

J. M. R. S. Tavares, R. Natal Jorge (eds.), *Developments in Medical Image Processing and Computational Vision,* Lecture Notes in Computational Vision and Biomechanics 19,
DOI 10.1007/978-3-319-13407-9_7

using manual methods several studies were able to measure motion [1, 7, 10–14] and dynamical deformation [6, 19, 22, 28] of RBCs flowing through microchannels.

However, the manual data collection is extremely time consuming and may introduce users' errors into the data. Hence, it is crucial to develop sophisticated computerized methods able to track automatically multiple cell trajectories and reduce possible errors by the users' evaluation. Several researchers have been developing different kinds of automatic particle tracking tools for Image J [18, 23, 24], Matlab [19, 24], LabVIEW [4, 18] and IDL [5]. A promising plugin for Image J is the "Particletracker" [23]. However, this plugin is still under development as the automatic tracking trajectories tend to overlap, especially at high concentration of particles and/or cells. Recently, Pinho et al. [20] have developed a Matlab module to track automatically individual RBCs flowing through a microchannel. However, this method did not measure the RBCs deformability. Hence, it is essential to develop an automatic method able to perform both tracking and deformability measurements of individual RBCs.

In this study, we propose an automatic image analysis technique based on the keyhole tracking algorithm that describes the probable movement of RBCs model [21]. First, a sequence of binary images containing segmented foreground objects were obtained by pre-processing videos, and then tracks were formed by linking the objects with common optical flow in contiguous frames. Finally, we measure the deformation of individual RBCs flowing through a microchannel having a hyperbolic contraction. In this geometry the RBCs mechanical properties are under the effect of a strong extensional flow.

Optical flow segmentation is usually defined as grouping of pixels of similar intensity that are associated with smooth and uniform motion information. However, this is a problem that is loosely defined and ambiguous in certain ways. Though the definition of motion segmentation says that regions with coherent motion are to be grouped, the resulting segments may not correspond to meaningful RBC regions in the image. To alleviate this issue the motion segmentation problem is placed at two levels namely low level and high level. Low level motion segmentation tries to group pixels with homogeneous motion vectors without taking any other information apart from intensity or image gradient. High level motion segmentation divides the image into regions that exhibit coherent motion and it also uses other image cues to produce image segments that correspond to projections of real RBCs.

It has been acknowledge by many authors that it is very difficult to determine the motion of pixels in areas of smooth intensity and that the motion in these areas must invariably be found by extrapolating from nearby features. These smooth areas of the image can be determined prior to any motion analysis by performing an initial segmentation based purely on intensity (or other spatial cues) to combine these smooth areas into individual atomic regions. The motion of these regions, rather than pixels, is then determined and these regions clustered together according to their motion.

Our method takes the spatial atomic regions produced by the watershed algorithm and a variational motion estimation method [2] and combines them into a complete algorithm producing a reliable motion segmentation framework which is used in the tracking step.

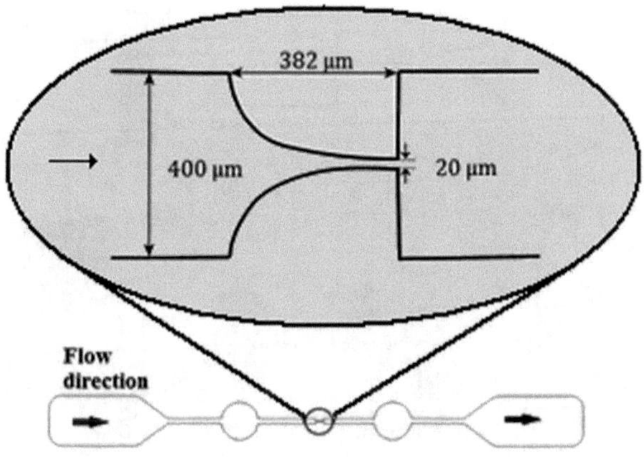

Fig. 1 Geometry of the hyperbolic microchannel used in this study

2 Materials and Methods

2.1 Working Fluids and Microchannel Geometry

The working fluid used in this study was Dextran 40 (Dx40) containing ~2 % of human RBCs (i.e., hematocrit, Hct ~2 %). The blood was collected from a healthy adult volunteer, and EDTA (ethylenediaminetetraacetic acid) was added to the samples to prevent coagulation. The blood samples were washed by centrifugation and then stored hermetically at 4° C until the experiments were performed at room temperature. For the RBCs exposed to chemicals, the cells were incubated for 10 mins at room temperature with 0.02 % diamide (Sigma-Aldrich). After the incubation time, RBCs exposed to chemicals were washed in physiological saline and re-suspended in Dextran 40 at 2 % Hct and then used immediately in our experiments.

The microchannels containing a hyperbolic contraction were produced in polydimethylsiloxane (PDMS) using a standard soft-lithography technique from a SU-8 photoresist mold. The molds were prepared in a clean room facility by photolithography using a high-resolution chrome mask. The geometry of the fabricated microchannel is shown in Fig. 1. The channel has a constant depth of 14 μm throughout the PDMS device and the width of the upstream and downstream channels is 400 μm. The minimum width in the hyperbolic contraction region is 20 μm.

2.2 Experimental Setup

For the microfluidic experiments, the device containing the microchannel was placed on the stage of an inverted microscope (IX71, Olympus). The flow rate of 0.5 μL/min was controlled using a syringe pump (PHD ULTRA). The images of the flowing RBCs were captured using a high speed camera (FASTCAM SA3, Photron) and transferred to the computer to be analyzed. An illustration of the experimental setup is shown in Fig. 2.

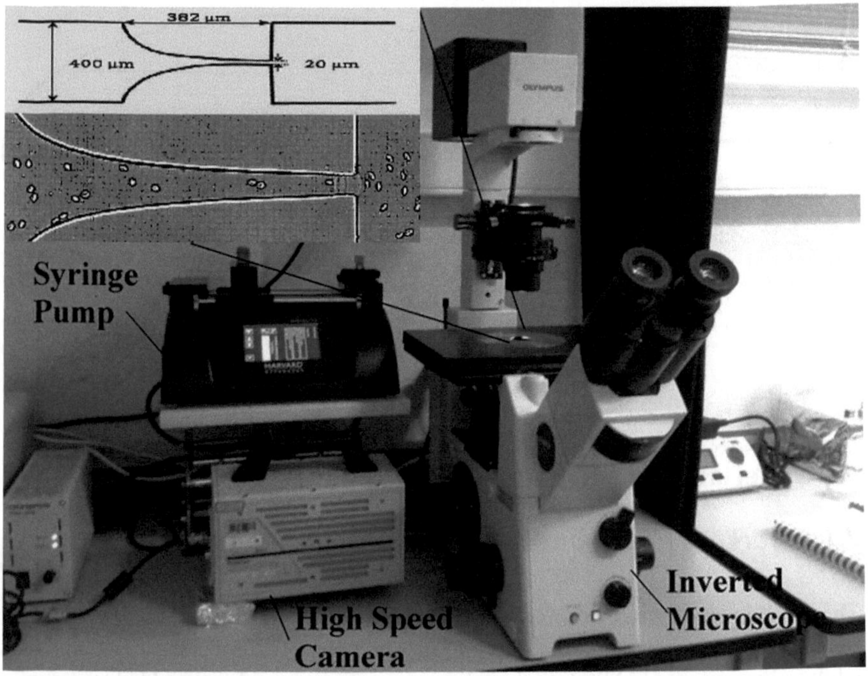

Fig. 2 Experimental setup: inverted microscope, high speed camera and syringe pump

2.3 Image Analysis Algorithm

The proposed methodology has five major stages. First, we remove background, noise and some artifacts of the original movie, as a pre-processing stage, obtaining an image only with the RBCs. Next, we create an over-segmented image, based on the initial magnitude gradient image, using the watershed transform. The optical flow information of these regions is obtained by using the variational method proposed by Brox et al. [2]. After that, the cell tracking links the atomic regions in contiguous frames, according to their motion, to form the tracks by means of a keyhole model proposed by Reyes-Aldasoro et al. [21]. Finally, we measure the deformation index of each RBC.

Optical flow is defined as the 2D vector field that matches a pixel in one image to the warped pixel in the other image. In other words, optical flow estimation tries to assign to each pixel of the current frame a two-component velocity vector indicating the position of the same pixel in the reference frame. The segmentation of an image sequence based on motion is a problem that is loosely defined and ambiguous in certain ways. Optical flow estimation algorithms often generate an inaccurate motion field mainly at the boundaries of moving objects, due to reasons such as noise, aperture problem, or occlusion. Therefore, segmentation based on motion alone results in segments with inaccurate boundaries.

A hybrid framework is proposed to integrate differential optical flow approach and region-based spatial segmentation approach to obtain accurate RBC motion. For the task at hand we adopt a high accuracy optical flow estimation based on a coarse-to-fine warping strategy [2] which can provide dense optical flow information. Using atomic regions implicitly resolves the problem which requires smoothing of the optical flow field since the spatial (static) segmentation process will group together neighbouring pixels of similar intensity, so that all the pixels in a area of smooth intensity grouped in the same region will be labelled with the same motion. We thereby presume two basic assumptions: (i) it is assumed that all pixels inside a region of homogeneous intensity follow the same motion model, and (ii) motion discontinuities coincide with the boundaries of those regions. To ensure that our assumptions are met, we apply a strong over-segmentation method to the image.

Our goal is to assign a unique motion vector to each region. While the atomic region motion vector is computed from the optical flows, it is necessary to consider the real situation that some of the optical flows might have been contaminated with noise, causing the computation of the region motion vector deviate from its genuine motion vector. For each optical flow, its contribution to the deviation depends both on its magnitude and on its direction. Thus, we want to detect and exclude those optical flows which tend to cause large errors to the computation of the region motion vector. We achieve these goals by obtaining the dominant motion of the atomic region from the mode of each optical flow component in the region.

2.3.1 Pre-Processing Stage

At this stage, the image background is removed by subtracting the average of all movie images from each image. To improve the identification of the RBCs the image contrast is adjusted by histogram expansion.

Images taken with digital cameras will pick up noise from a variety of sources. As the watershed algorithm is very sensitive to noise it is desirable to apply a noise reduction filter in the pre-processing step. Several filters have been proposed in the literature to reduce the spurious boundaries created due to noise. However, most of these filters tend to blur image edges while they suppress noise. To prevent this effect we use the non-linear bilateral filter [25].

The basic idea underlying the bilateral filter is to replace the intensity of a pixel by taking a weighted average of the pixels within a neighbourhood (in a circle) with the weights depending on both the spatial and intensity difference between the central pixel and its neighbours. In smooth regions, pixel values in a small neighbourhood are similar to each other and the bilateral filter acts essentially as a standard domain filter, averaging away the small, weakly correlated, differences between pixel values caused by noise. Bilateral filter preserves image structure by only smoothing over those neighbours which form part of the "same region" as the central pixel.

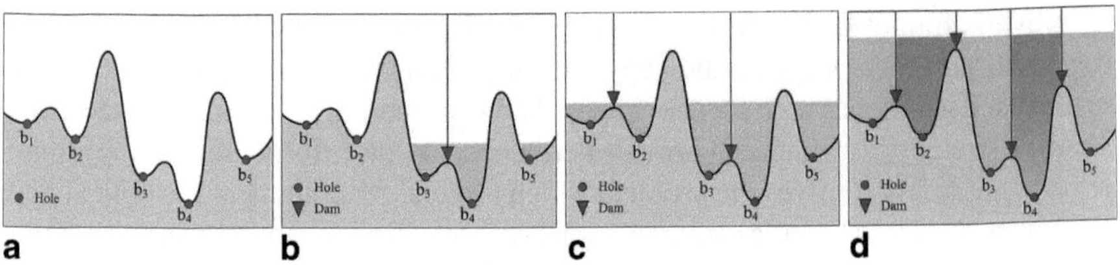

Fig. 3 Illustration of immersion watershed transform on a continuous 1D function interpreted as a landscape. The landscape is sequentially flooded from bottom to top. **a** Holes are pierced at each regional minimum. **b** At certain flooding height there are two regions with one dam between basin b_3 and basin b_4. **c** At intermediate flooding height there are three regions with two dams. **d** Final segmentation with five segments

2.3.2 Atomic Region Segmentation

An ideal over-segmentation should be easy and fast to obtain, and should not contain too many segmented regions and it should have its region boundaries as a superset of the true image region boundaries. In this section we present an algorithm step that groups pixels into "atomic regions". The motivations of this preliminary grouping stage resemble the perceptual grouping task: (1) abandoning pixels as the basic image elements, we instead use small image regions of coherent structure to define the optical flow patches. In fact, since the real world does not consist of pixels, it can be argued that this is even a more natural image representation than pixels as those are merely a consequence of the digital image discretization.

Watershed transform is a classical and effective method for image segmentation in grey scale mathematical morphology. For images the idea of the watershed construction is quite simple. An image is considered as a topographic relief where for every pixel in position (x, y), its brightness level plays the role of the z-coordinate in the landscape. Local maxima of the activity image can be thought of as mountain tops, and minima can be considered as valleys.

In the flooding or immersion approach [26], single pixel holes are pierced at each regional minimum of the activity image which is regarded as topographic landscape. When sinking the whole surface slowly into a lake water leaks through the holes, rising uniformly and globally across the image, and proceeds to fill each catchment basin. Then, in order to avoid water coming from different holes merge, virtual dams are built at places where the water coming from two different minima would merge.

Figure 3 illustrates the immersion simulation approach. Fig. 3a shows a 1D function with five minima. Water rises in and fills the corresponding catchment basins, as in Figs. 3b–c. When water in basins b_3 and b_4 begin to merge a dam is built to prevent this overflow of water. Similarly, the other watershed lines are constructed. When the image surface is completely flooded the virtual dams or watershed lines separate the catchment basins from one another and correspond to the boundaries of the regions as shown in Fig. 3d.

2.3.3 Optical Flow

In many differential methods, the estimation of optical flow relies on the assumption that objects in an image sequence may change position but their appearance remains the same or nearly the same (brightness constancy assumption) [17] from time t to time $t+1$. Brox et al. [2] proposed a variational method that combines a brightness constancy assumption, a gradient constancy assumption and a discontinuity-preserving spatio-temporal smoothness constraint.

Estimating optical flow involves the solution of a correspondence problem. That is, what pixel in one frame corresponds to what pixel in the other frame. In order to find these correspondences one needs to define some assumptions that are not affected by the displacement. The combined variational approach [2] differs from usual variational approaches by the use of a gradient constancy assumption. This assumption provides the method with the capability to yield good estimation results even in the presence of small local or global variations of illumination.

Constancy Assumptions on Data Given two successive images of a sequence $I(x,y,t)$ and $I(x+u,y+v,t+1)$ we seek at each pixel $\mathbf{x} := (x,y,t)^{\mathrm{T}}$ the optical flow vector $\mathbf{v}(\mathbf{x}) := (u,v,1)^{\mathrm{T}}$ that describes the motion of the pixel at $\mathbf{x}$ to its new location $(x+u,y+v,t+1)$ in the next frame.

- **Brightness constancy assumption**
  The common assumption is that the grey value of the pixel does not change as it undergoes motion:

$$I(x,y,t) = I(x+u,y+v,t+1) \tag{1}$$

  However, this constancy assumption cannot only deal with image sequences with either local or global change in illumination. In this case other assumptions that are invariant against brightness changes must be applied. Invariance can be ensured by considering spatial derivatives. Horn and Schunck [9] add a smoothness assumption to regularize the flow, and Lucas and Kanade [17] assume constant motion in small windows.
- **Gradient constancy assumption**
  A global change in illumination both shifts and/or scales the grey values of an image sequence. Shifting the grey values will not affect the gradient. Although scaling the grey values changes the length of the gradient vector it does not affect its direction. Thus, we assume that the spatial gradients of an image sequence can be considered as constant during motion:

$$\nabla I(x,y,t) = \nabla I(x+u,y+v,t+1) \tag{2}$$

  where $\nabla = (\partial x, \partial y)$ denotes spatial gradient. Although the gradient can slightly change due to changes in the grey value too, it is much less dependent on the illumination than on the brightness assumption.

Finding the flow field by minimizing the data term alone is an ill-posed problem since the optimum solution, especially in homogeneous areas, might be attained by many dissimilar displacement fields. This is the aperture problem: the motion of a homogeneous contour is locally ambiguous. In order to solve this problem some regularisation is required. The most suitable regularisation assumption is *piecewise smoothness* [2], that arises in the common case of a scene that consists of semi-rigid objects.

The data term $E_D(u,v)$ incorporates the brightness constancy assumption, as well as the gradient constancy assumption. While the first data term models the assumption that the grey-level of objects is constant and does not change over time, the second one accommodates for slight changes in the illumination. This is achieved by assuming constancy of the spatial image gradient:

$$E_D(u,v) = \int_{\Omega} \psi\left(|I(\mathbf{x}+\mathbf{v}) - I(\mathbf{x})|^2 + \gamma\,|\nabla I(\mathbf{x}+\mathbf{v}) - \nabla I(\mathbf{x})|^2\right) \mathrm{d}\mathbf{x} \tag{3}$$

where Ω is the region of interest (the image) over which the minimization is done. The parameter γ relates the weight of the two constancy assumptions, and $\psi\left(s^2\right) = \sqrt{s^2+\varepsilon^2}$ is a non-quadratic (convex) penaliser applied to both the data and the smoothness term which represents a smooth approximation of the L_1 norm, $L_1(s) = |s|$. Using the L_1 norm rather than the common L_2 norm reduces the influence of outliers and makes estimation robust. Due to the small positive constant ε, $\psi\left(s^2\right)$ is still convex which offers advantages in the minimization process. The incorporation of the constant ε makes the approximation differentiable at $s = 0$; the value of ε sets the level of approximation which we choose to be 0.001.

Applying a non-quadratic function to the data term addresses problems at the boundaries of the image sequence, where occlusions occur and therefore outliers in the data compromise the correct estimation of the flow field.

Smoothness Assumption The smoothness assumption [2, 9, 27] is motivated by the observation that it is reasonable to introduce a certain dependency between neighbouring pixels in order to deal with outliers caused by noise, occlusions or other local violations of the constancy assumption. This assumption states that disparity varies smoothly almost everywhere (except at depth boundaries). That means we can expect that the optical flow map is piecewise smooth and it follows some spatial coherency. This is achieved by penalising the total variation of the flow field. Smoothness is assumed by almost every correspondence algorithm. This assumption fails if there are thin fine-structured shapes (e.g. branches of a tree, hairs) in the scene.

Horn and Schunck proposed in their model the following smoothness (homogeneous) term [9]:

$$E_{S_{HS}}(u,v) = \int_{\Omega} |\nabla u|^2 + |\nabla v|^2 \mathrm{d}\mathbf{x} \tag{4}$$

However, such a smoothness assumption does not respect discontinuities in the flow field. In order to be able to capture also locally non-smooth motion it is necessary to allow outliers in the smoothness assumption. This can be achieved by the non-quadratic penaliser ψ also used in the data term. Thus, the smoothness term $E_S(u,v)$ becomes:

$$E_S(u,v) = \int_{\Omega} \psi\left(|\nabla u|^2 + |\nabla v|^2\right) \mathrm{d}\mathbf{x} \tag{5}$$

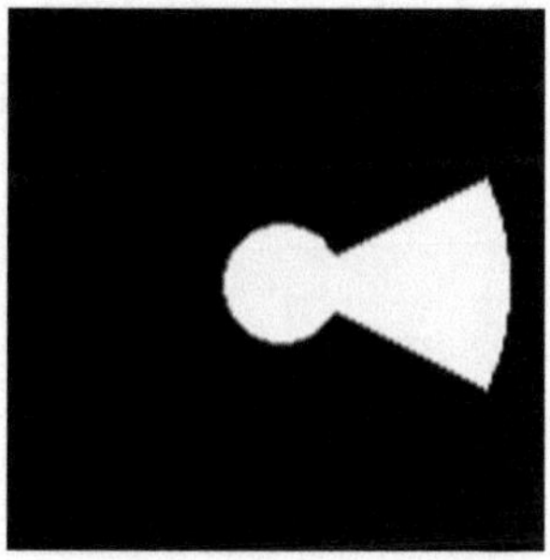

Fig. 4 Mask for the keyhole model

The smoothness term gives a penalty to adjacent segments which have different motion parameters.

Energy Functional Applying non-quadratic penaliser functions to both the data and the smoothness term and also integrating the gradient constancy assumption, results in the optical flow model described by the following energy functional:

$$E(u,v) = E_D(u,v) + \alpha E_S(u,v) \tag{6}$$

where α is some positive regularisation parameter which balances the data term E_d with the smoothness term E_s: Larger values for α result in a stronger penalisation of large flow gradients and lead to smoother flow fields.

The minimization of $E(u,v)$ is an iterative process, with external and internal iterations. The reader is referred to Brox et al. [2] for a solution to minimize this functional.

2.3.4 Tracking

The cell tracking is performed following the keyhole model proposed by Reyes-Aldasoro et al. [21] which predicted the most probable position of a RBC at time $t+1$ from the position in times $t-1$ and t. Assuming that child RBC (cell at frame t) moves in the same direction and velocity as its parent (cell at frame $t-1$) it is possible to predict the position of the cell in the next frame $t+1$. Of course, this would not cover major changes in speed or turns. Two regions of probability where the RBC is most probable to be were therefore defined: a narrow wedge (60° wide) oriented towards the predicted position, and a truncated circle (300°) that complements the wedge; together they resemble a keyhole. This model was designed in a mask of 141×141 pixels, as shown in Fig. 4, where the keyhole has a wedge length of 60 pixels and the circle has a radius of 15 pixels. This design allows the keyhole model to rotate 180° within the mask.

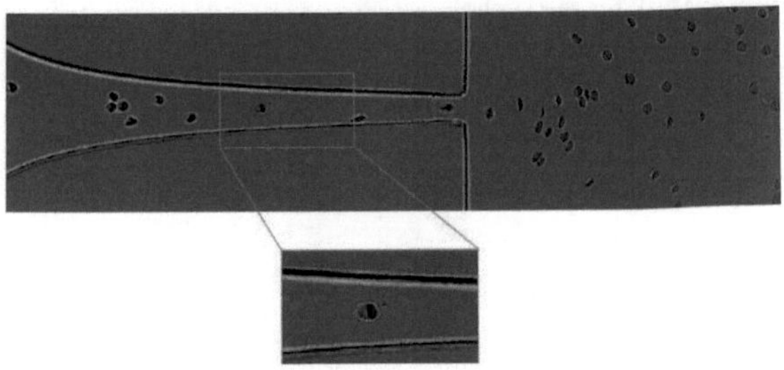

Fig. 5 Selected healthy RBC flowing through a microchannel having a hyperbolic contraction shape

2.3.5 Deformation Index Measure

Deformation Index (DI) is a well-used dimensionless value for expressing the degree of RBCs deformation and is defined as:

$$DI = \frac{L_{major} - L_{minor}}{L_{major} + L_{minor}} \tag{7}$$

where L_{major} and L_{minor} are the major and minor axis lengths of a RBC. The DI value is between 0 and 1, i. e., 0 means a RBC with a shape close to a circle and the higher value means a more deformed shape such an elongated ellipse.

3 Results and Discussion

For the selected RBC (see Fig. 5), the proposed method was able to track automatically the cell through the hyperbolic microchannel. Figure 6 shows the RBC trajectory obtained by the proposed method. The RBC trajectory has a linear behavior mainly due to its location in the middle of hyperbolic microchannel.

By using the proposed image analysis method we have also calculated automatically the deformation index (DI) of the selected RBC flowing along the microchannel. Detailed information about the DI calculation can be found elsewhere [28].

From Fig. 7 it is possible to observe that the proposed method is able to calculate automatically the DI of the selected RBC. Although the DI results are extremely oscillatory, overall the results show that the DI tends to decrease as the RBC leaves the hyperbolic contraction. This result corroborates recent studies performed by Yaginuma et al. [28] and Faustino et al. [6] where they have used a manual method to calculate the DI. Additionally, the proposed method was tested to track a RBC treated with diamide (0.02 %) throughout a microchannel with a hyperbolic contraction (see Fig. 8).

For this particular case the selected RBC (see Fig. 9) is located near the wall of the hyperbolic contraction and consequently its trajectory has a tendency flowing along the wall of the contraction region. After the contraction this RBC has a tendency to flow towards the wall of the sudden expansion region of the microchannel. This is an expected behavior under a laminar regime.

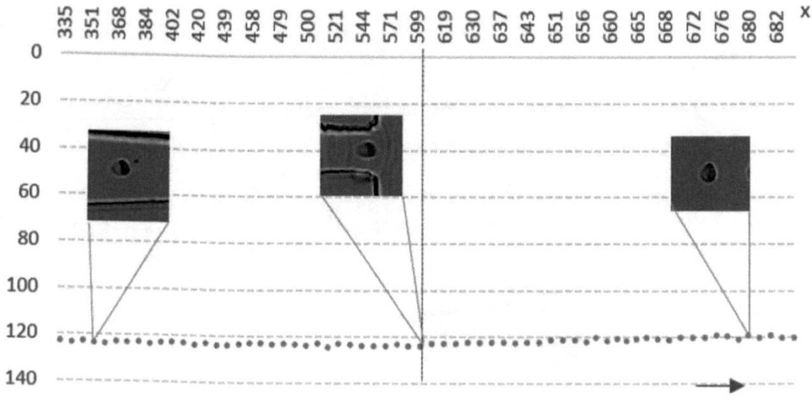

Fig. 6 Trajectory of a selected RBC tracked by the proposed image analysis method. The vertical red line represents the exit of the hyperbolic contraction

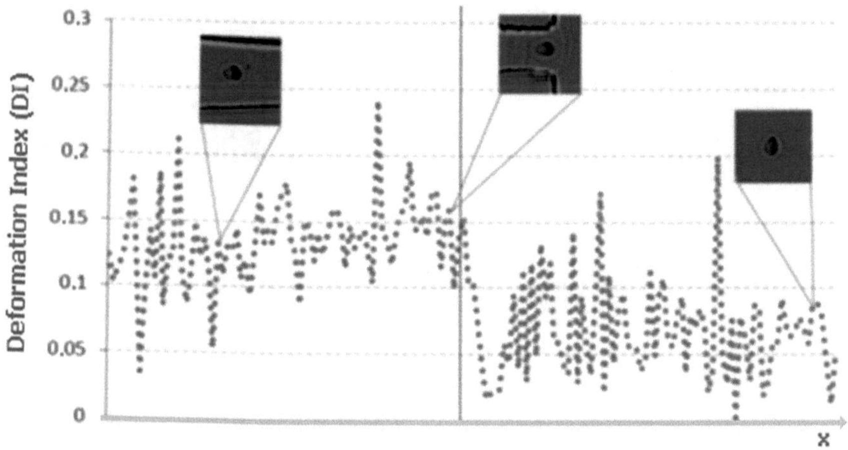

Fig. 7 Deformation index (DI) of a selected RBC by using the keyhole model. The vertical red line represents the exit of the hyperbolic contraction

Figure 10 shows the DI for a RBC exposed to 0.02 % diamide flowing through a hyperbolic microchannel. For this particular case the RBC DI tends to increase until the exit of the hyperbolic contraction. As soon as the RBC enters the sudden expansion region, the RBC DI decreases.

Figure 11 shows clearly that for both RBCs the DI tends to reduce when the RBCs enter the expansion region, which is consistent with other past results [6, 22, 28]. The results from Fig. 11 also show that the DI of a RBC exposed to 0.02 % diamide is higher than the DI of the selected healthy RBC. This latter result needs to be analysed with some caution as the exposed RBC is flowing close to the wall where the shear rate is extremely high and may play a key role on the increase of the RBC DI. Further studies are needed to clarify this phenomenon.

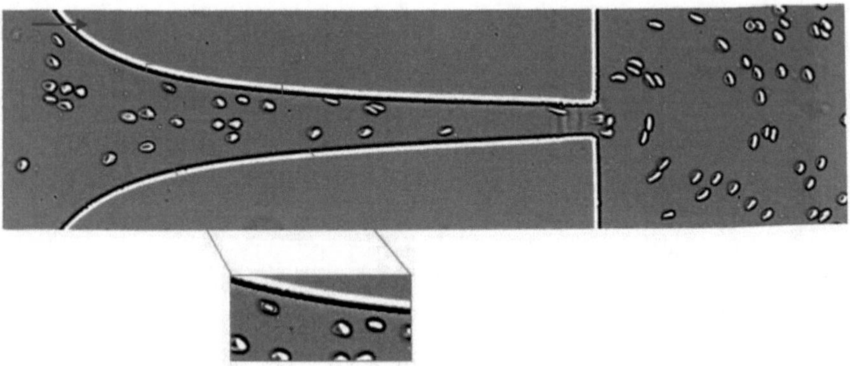

Fig. 8 RBCs exposed to 0.02 % diamide flowing through a microchannel having a hyperbolic contraction

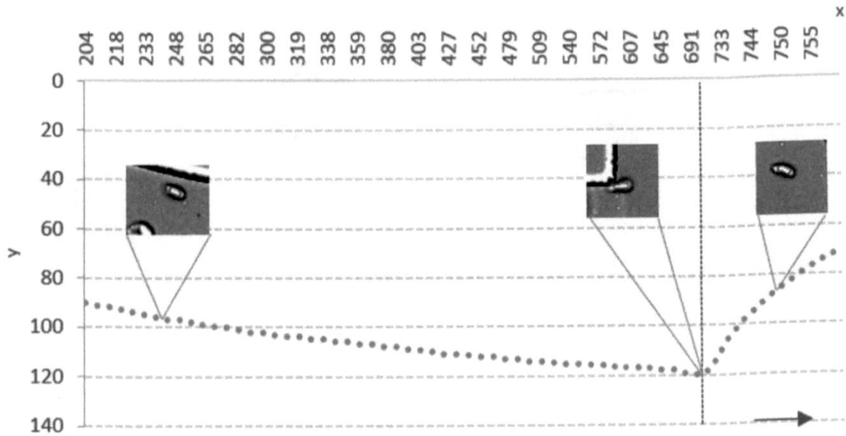

Fig. 9 Trajectory of a selected RBC exposed to 0.02 % diamide flowing through a hyperbolic microchannel. The vertical red line represents the exit of the hyperbolic contraction

4 Conclusion and Future Directions

The present study has tested an image analysis technique to track RBCs flowing through a microchannel with a hyperbolic contraction. The proposed automatic method is based on a keyhole model and its main purpose is to provide a rapid and accurate way to obtain automatically multiple RBC trajectories and deformability data. The results have shown that the proposed automatic method was able not only to track both healthy and exposed RBCs motion but also to measure RBCs DI along the microchannel. The DI data have shown clearly that for both RBCs the DI tends to reduce when the RBCs enter the microchannel expansion region. Hence, the results have shown that the proposed method can be successfully integrated with a

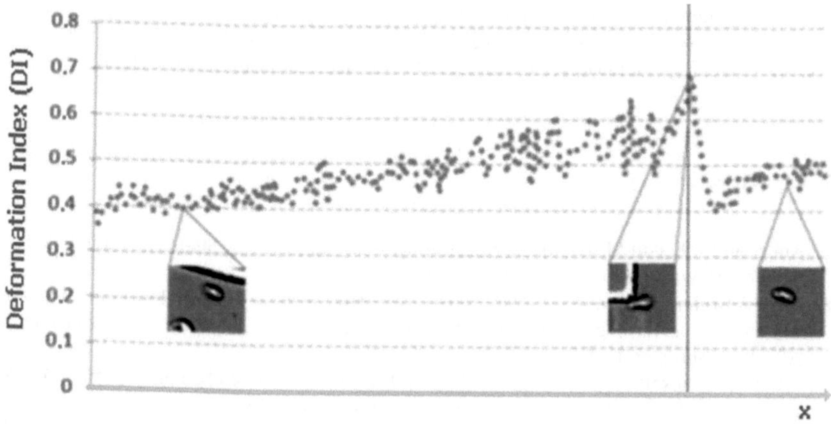

Fig. 10 DI of a selected RBC exposed to 0.02 % diamide flowing through a hyperbolic microchannel tracked by the keyhole model. The vertical red line represents the exit of the hyperbolic contraction

Fig. 11 Average DI for two different RBCs: healthy RBC and RBC exposed to 0.02% diamide

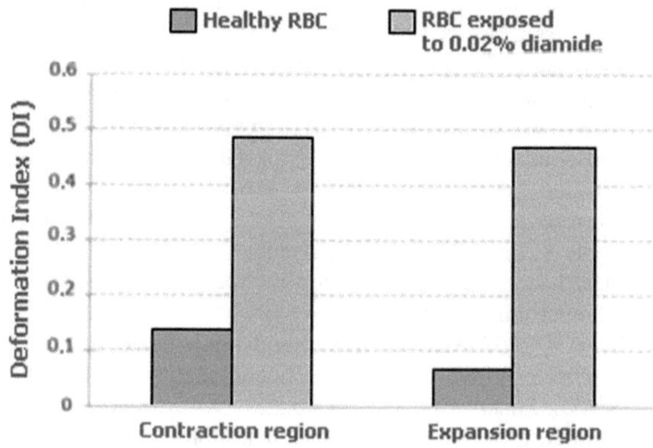

high-speed microscopy system and used as a fast way to obtain RBC measurements. Additionally, by reducing the time consuming tasks and errors from the users, this method will provide a powerful way to obtain automatically multiple RBC trajectories and DIs specially when compared with the manual tracking methods often used in blood microflow studies.

The algorithm takes advantage of spatial information to overcome inherent problems of conventional optical flow algorithms, which are the handling of untextured regions and the estimation of correct flow vectors near motion discontinuities. The assignment of motion to regions allows the elimination of optical flow errors originated by noise. Detailed studies with different optical conditions need to be performed in the near future as the optics and illumination source strongly affects the quality of the images. Moreover, the application of the proposed method to other more complex flows are also worth studying in the near future.

Acknowledgements The authors acknowledge the financial support provided by PTDC/SAU-BEB/105650/2008, PTDC/SAU-ENB/116929/2010, EXPL/EMS-SIS/2215/2013 from FCT (Science and Technology Foundation), COMPETE, QREN and European Union (FEDER).

References

1. Abkarian M, Faivre M, Horton R, Smistrup K, Best-Popescu CA, Stone HA (2008) Cellular-scale hydrodynamics. Biomed Mater 3(3):034011
2. Brox T, Bruhn A, Papenberg N, Weickert J (2004) High accuracy optical flow estimation based on a theory for warping. In: PajdlaT, Matas J (eds) European conference on computer vision, vol. 3024. Springer, LNCS, pp 25–36
3. Bruhn A, Weickert J, Schnörr C (2005) Luca/Kanade meets Horn/Schunck: combining local and global optic flow methods. Int J Comput Vision 61(3):1–21
4. Carter BC, Shubeita GT, Gross SP (2005) Tracking single particles: a user-friendly quantitative evaluation. Phys Biol 2:60–72
5. Crocker JC, Grier DG (1996) Methods of digital video microscopy for colloidal studies. J Colloid Interface Sci 179(1):298–310
6. Faustino V, Pinho D, Yaginuma T, Calhelha R, Ferreira I, Lima R (2014) Ex-tensional flow-based microfluidic device: deformability assessment of red blood cells in contact with tumor cells. BioChip J 8:42–47
7. Fujiwara H, Ishikawa T et al (2009) Red blood cell motions in high-hematocrit blood flowing through a stenosed microchannel. J Biomech 42:838–843
8. Garcia V, Dias R, Lima R (2012) In vitro blood flow behaviour in microchannels with simple and complex geometries. In: Naik GR (ed) Applied biological engineering–principles and practice. InTech, Rijeka, pp 393–416
9. Horn BKP, Schunck BG (1981) Determining optical flow. Artif Intell 17(1–3):185–203
10. Leble V, Lima R, Dias R, Fernandes C, Ishikawa T, Imai Y, Yamaguchi T (2011) Asymmetry of red blood cell motions in a microchannel with a diverging and converging bifurcation. Biomicrofluidics 5:044120
11. Lima R (2007) Analysis of the blood flow behavior through microchannels by a confocal micro-PIV/PTV system. PhD (Eng), Bioengineering and Robotics Department, Tohoku University, Sendai, Japan
12. Lima R, Ishikawa T et al (2009) Measurement of individual red blood cell motions under high hematocrit conditions using a confocal micro-PTV system. Ann Biomed Eng 37:1546–1559
13. Lima R, Ishikawa T, Imai Y, Takeda M, Wada S, Yamaguchi T (2008) Radial dispersion of red blood cells in blood flowing through glass capillaries: role of heamatocrit and geometry. J Biomech 44:2188–2196
14. Lima R, Oliveira MSN, Ishikawa T, Kaji H, Tanaka S, Nishizawa, M, Yamaguchi T (2009) Axisymmetric PDMS microchannels for in vitro haemodynamics studies. Biofabrication 1(3):035005
15. Lima R, Ishikawa T, Imai Y, Yamaguchi T (2012) Blood flow behavior in microchannels: advances and future trends. In: Dias R et al (eds) Single and two-phase flows on chemical and biomedical engineering. Bentham Science, Sharjah, pp 513–547
16. Lima R, Ishikawa T, Imai Y, Yamaguchi T (2013) Confocal micro-PIV/PTV measurements of the blood flow in micro-channels. In: Collins MW, König CS (eds) Nano and micro flow systems for bioanalysis, vol. 2. Springer, New York, pp 131–151
17. Lucas BD, Kanade T (1981) An iterative image registration technique with an application to stereo vision. Proceedings of Imaging Understanding Workshop, pp 121–130
18. Meijering E, Dzyubachyk O, Smal I (2012) Methods for cell and particle tracking. In: Conn PM (ed) Imaging and spectroscopic analysis of living cells. Methods in enzymology, vol. 504. Elsevier, Amsterdam, pp 183–200

19. Pinho D, Yaginuma T, Lima R (2013) A microfluidic device for partial cell separation and deformability assessment. BioChip J 7:367–374
20. Pinho D, Gayubo F, Pereira AI, Lima R (2013) A comparison between a manual and automatic method to characterize red blood cell trajectories. Int J Numer Meth Biomed Eng 29(9):977–987
21. Reyes-Aldasoro CC, Akerman S, Tozer G (2008) Measuring the velocity of fluorescently labelled red blood cells with a keyhole tracking algorithm. J Microsc 229(1):162–173
22. Rodrigues R, Faustino V, Pinto E, Pinho D, Lima R (2014) Red blood cells deformability index assessment in a hyperbolic microchannel: the diamide and glutaraldehyde effect. WebmedCentralplus Biomedical Engineering. 1: WMCPLS00253
23. Sbalzarini IF, Koumoutsakos P (2005) Feature point tracking and trajectory analysis for video imaging in cell biology. J Struct Bio 151(2):182–195
24. Smith MB, Karatekin E, Gohlke A, Mizuno H, Watanabe N, Vavylonis D (2011) Interactive, computer-assisted tracking of speckle trajectories in fluorescence microscopy: application to actin polymerization and membrane fusion. Biophys J 101:1794–1804
25. Tomasi C, Manduchi R (1998) Bilateral filtering for gray and color images. International Conference on Computer Vision, pp 839–846
26. Vincent L, Soille P (1991) Watersheds in digital spaces: an efficient algorithm based on immersion simulations. IEEE PAMI 13(6):583–598
27. Weiss Y (1997) Smoothness in layers: motion segmentation using nonparametric mixture estimation. Watersheds in digital spaces: An efficient algorithm based on immersion simulations, Int Conf on Computer Vision and Pattern Recognition, pp 520–527
28. Yaginuma T, Oliveira MS, Lima R, Ishikawa T, Yamaguchi T (2013) Human red blood cell behavior under homogeneous extensional flow in a hyperbolic-shaped microchannel. Biomicrofluidics 7:54110

[illegible]

A 3D Computed Tomography Based Tool for Orthopedic Surgery Planning

João Ribeiro, Victor Alves, Sara Silva and Jaime Campos

Abstract The preparation of a plan is essential for a surgery to take place in the best way possible and also for shortening patient's recovery times. In the orthopedic case, planning has an accentuated significance due to the close relation between the degree of success of the surgery and the patient recovering time. It is important that surgeons are provided with tools that help them in the planning task, in order to make it more reliable and less time consuming. In this paper, we present a 3D Computed Tomography based solution and its implementation as an OsiriX plugin for orthopedic surgery planning. With the developed plugin, the surgeon is able to manipulate a three-dimensional isosurface rendered from the selected imaging study (a CT scan). It is possible to add digital representations of physical implants (surgical templates), in order to evaluate the feasibility of a plan. These templates are STL files generated from CAD models. There is also the feature to extract new isosurfaces of different voxel values and slice the final 3D model according to a predefined plane, enabling a 2D analysis of the planned solution. Finally, we discuss how the proposed application assists the surgeon in the planning process in an alternative way, where it is possible to three-dimensionally analyze the impact of a surgical intervention on the patient.

1 Introduction

The surgery's success is intimately related with its planning. The pre-operative planning consists in an evaluation supported by the clinical information and the patient's studies to establish a surgical procedure suitable to it. During the planning process, a

J. Ribeiro (✉) · V. Alves · S. Silva · J. Campos
CCTC-Computer Science and Technology Center, University of Minho, Braga, Portugal
e-mail: joaopedroribeiro@me.com

V. Alves
e-mail: valves@di.uminho.pt

S. Silva
e-mail: sara.isa.silva@gmail.com

J. Campos
e-mail: jaimefbc@gmail.com

J. M. R. S. Tavares, R. Natal Jorge (eds.), *Developments in Medical Image Processing and Computational Vision*, Lecture Notes in Computational Vision and Biomechanics 19,
DOI 10.1007/978-3-319-13407-9_8

group of steps are defined that increase the chances of a successful surgery, improving the communication between the surgeon and the other members of the surgery, e. g., nurses, and anesthetist [21].

One of the difficulties that a surgeon faces is the need of visually precept the impact that his planned surgery will have on the patient. In the case of orthopedic surgery, this is even more important, since the analysis of implant's placement (when necessary) is only possible in real time (surgery). Moreover, it is important to annotate the location / actual position of a pre-surgical implant, thereby reducing the risk inherent to any surgical intervention. Allowing the patient situation to be previously analyzed in detail and with greater time interval, the task of the orthopedic surgeon is facilitated, because the pressure of the decision making during surgery is reduced. A surgeon tends to become less formal when planning only based on his previous professional experience. However, there is a need to become more effective and rigorous in the planning of more complex surgeries [10, 20, 21]. Surgeons are continuously searching to improve their performance, increasing their accuracy levels.

One of the current trends are the three dimension reconstructions which are used in several sectors of activity, namely in healthcare, particularly in diagnostics [5, 19]. Currently, there are several companies that offer computer-assisted orthopedic surgery (CAOS) solutions to help surgeons plan the surgical intervention. However, some of them are still based on orthogonal X-ray views, which remove the three dimensionality of the tissues (e.g. organs, bones). Although others use Computed Tomography (CT) scans, it is not possible for the surgeon to add templates that represent the implants that will be used in surgery, not allowing a global view of the planned solution. Some of these tools are Orthoview, TraumaCad, SurgiCase, HipOp [16].

The Orthoview solution can be integrated with DICOM Picture Archiving and Communication Systems (PACS) and uses two orthogonal X-ray images. After importing these images, the user is able to add vector lines (always in 2D) representing real physical implants [4]. Nonetheless, the surgeon is unable to visualize the resultant model in a 3D space. Due to the impossibility to convert a 3D structure into 2D without losing details, it is impossible to analyze the fracture (if there is one) with detail [3]. After these steps the surgeon can generate a report to use at the surgery.

Another application called TraumaCad is available from VoyantHealth. This application is fairly similar to Orthoview, although it uses CT scans instead of X-rays. However, both applications use 2D implants models (templates). In the surgeon's perspective, these models are represented through vector lines which decrease the perception of the trauma. In TraumaCad, the 3D visualization only allows the analysis of the study in other angles. The surgeon can add surgical templates to the CT scan and position them by using a multi view approach for guidance. For this to be accomplished, the software reslices the CT scan by using a multi-planar algorithm, therefore enabling the user to analyze the same image in four different angles (Axial, Coronal, Sagittal and Oblique). Although not being a real 3D model representation, it is a major step when compared with the previously mentioned application [18].

SurgiCase is available from the Belgian company Materialise. It allows the pre-operative planning with the help of an engineer, where the surgeon can create a 3D model of the planned resolution but this is achieved with a remote assistant's help. This assistant is an engineer from Materialise that will work with him in a cooperative way, in order to develop a plan for the surgery. So, the surgeon has little autonomy since he cannot add templates or test other procedures. Consequently, if he wants to change anything in the plan, he must contact the assistant [1].

There is a free software application for pre-operative planning developed by Istituti Ortopedici Rizzoli and CINECA, named HipOp. This application was conceived for the total hip replacement. The system imports a CT scan which defines a 3D anatomical space. The anatomical objects are represented through multiple views. The implants can be loaded by the surgeon and they are represented by their 3D model in the same space. However, it is not possible to move both components at the same time independently [8].

Steen and Widegren [17] in association with Sectra Medical Systems AB in Sweden presented a prototype to analyze the fit of implants. The application shades the implants depending on the distance between them and the bone. Aiming for the total hip replacement, it offers the possibility to measure its critical distances. There are some limitations towards its 3D environment. The 3D implant model and the 3D volume reconstruction of the CT study are rendered independently which causes failures in the transparency. Beyond that, it is not possible to intersect both components, in this case the implant model is always totally in front or behind the 3D CT volume. Thus, it is difficult to predict surgery outcome for the patient.

Some other planning solutions use professional image editing tools, such as Adobe Photoshop. By using tools typically design for digital image processing, the surgeons create an image of the final result [15]. Some publications point out that the success of the surgery increases using virtual reality techniques where surgeons can practice their surgeries. This kind of technology is normally associated with the training carried out by pilots and astronauts [10].

The main reason for the lack of software that merge a CT scan and templates representing the implants to be used in surgery is due to the difficulty of dealing with two different major graphic types representations: 3D bitmaps (voxels) and vector images. On one hand, the CT scan, which is a series of volume based images with same thickness and equally spaced (i.e. matrix of voxels). On the other hand, we have a template provided by an orthopedic implants manufacturer, which is vector type. This template is a virtual representation of a physical support and its structure is a set of arranged triangles. Due to these structurally different image types, the development of a solution that aggregates these two types together on a same plane is somewhat challenging. In order to visualize and analyze all the angles of the fracture, a surgeon needs to freely manipulate the templates on the patient's imaging studies. This can only be satisfactorily achieved with a 3D model. Since a CT scan is a series of images with the same thickness and equally spaced, it allows us to create the corresponding 3D model. This model, allows a greater viewing and understanding of the fracture extent (in the case of bone tissue) [5, 19].

The three main rendering techniques that enable the creation of a CT scan 3D model are Multi-planar Rendering (MPR), Volume Rendering (VR) and Surface Rendering (SR). The MPR is usually used when only weak computational resources are available because the processing required is lower. It is widely used whenever the goal is to visualize the imaging study through different planes simultaneously (e.g. Axial, Coronal, Sagittal and Oblique). The VR technique is used when the purpose is to visualize the entire volume. Images are created by projecting rays in the volume from a viewpoint (Ray Casting method) [14]. For each ray that intersects the volume (one or more voxels), color and opacity values are calculated and then represented as a pixel. This technique requires a huge amount of runtime calculations, which implies more powerful machines. SR is the technique that was used in this work. It is, by definition, the visualization of a 3D object from a set of isosurfaces. They are only made by points with the same intensity which in this case refers to the attenuation value for radiation using the Hounsfield's scale. It is widely used whenever the goal is to visualize structures close to each other (e.g. visualize the skull on a brain CT scan) [22]. These isosurfaces can be constructed by contours that are extracted from each slice in order to create a surface based on the volume's contour or by voxels where the isosurfaces are generated directly from voxels with a predefined value from the Hounsfield's scale. One of the algorithms used in this reconstruction is the Marching Cubes (MC) [2, 9].

The surgeon using any of these techniques can extract more information about the study because he is given the capability to analyze it in all possible angles. Yet, he is unable to add templates to elaborate a plan for the surgery. In this study, we present a solution for the problem of structural differences between images. With the proposed solution, the surgeon can import a CT scan, generate a 3D surface from it and add 3D surgical templates on top of it. This means that 3D vector graphics can be merged with a 3D matrix (generated) surface. The present article is structured as follows: first, 3D Modeling principles are introduced, then it is presented the features and the operation of the proposed solution, finishing with conclusions and the future steps to improve the application.

2 3D Modeling and Visualization

Each CT scan produces a volume of data that can be manipulated. In order to extract the isosurfaces from the CT scan, the MC algorithm was chosen [9]. These isosurfaces are constituted by a polygonal mesh which was computed from a scalar field, i.e., set of voxels. The process starts with a given predefined Hounsfield Unit (HU) value from the original imaging study. The voxels that meet this threshold requirement are then used by the MC algorithm to construct the isosurface by marching iteratively with an imaginary cube through the 3D grid where the voxels are projected. Constructing the 3D model entails proceeding with the scalar field and evaluating each vertices of the cube in order to use the best polygons to represent the original surface. These vertices are then aggregated to form the final isosurface of a polygon mesh. A lookup table (Fig. 1) is used by the MC algorithm in order to decide how to fuse the vertices and resolve ambiguity when choosing the points which belong to the polygon mesh

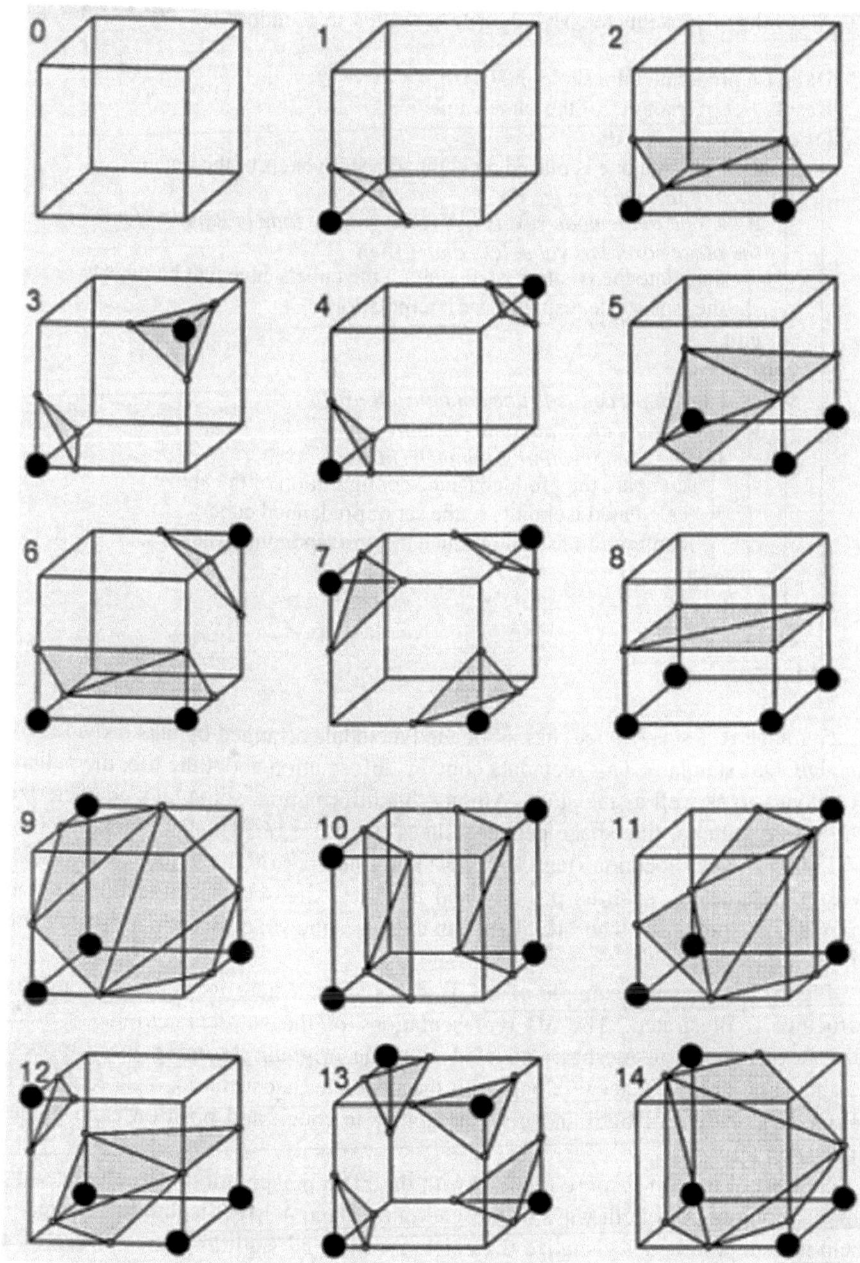

Fig. 1 The original published lookup table

surface. Since the first algorithm implementation, this table has been refined over the years to provide better results.

Algorithm 1 presents the MC algorithm written in pseudocode.

Data: t-a predefined threshold in HU
Result: Set of triangles of the same value
for *each image voxel* **do**
  a cube of length one is placed on eight adjacent voxels of the image;
  for *each of the cube's edge* **do**
    if *the one of the node voxels has value greater than or equal to t* ***and*** *the other voxel has value less than t* **then**
      calculate the position of a point on the cube's edge that belongs to the isosurface, using linear interpolation;
    end
  end
  for *each of the predefined cube configurations* **do**
    for *each of the eight possible rotations* **do**
      for *the configuration's complement* **do**
        compare the produced cube configuration of the above calculated isopoints to the set of predefined cube configurations and produce the corresponding triangles;
      end
    end
  end
end

Each image (CT scan's slice) has associated metadata arranged by tags provided by the DICOM standard. This metadata contains information about the file, the patient it belongs to as well as the study. Among this information, some tags characterize the whole volume, like space between slices (tag 0018,0088), slice thickness (tag 0018,0050), slice location (tag 0020,1041) and number of slices (tag 0054,0081). Voxels parameters, such as position and thickness are set using the information provided by these tags. The MC algorithm then uses the voxels information to create the 3D models.

Figure 2 shows an example of a CT scan's slice, where its volumetric matrix structure is illustrated. The 3D representations of the surgical template's models are also polygon meshes, modeled after the original. Merging these models in the same graphic's scene along with the generated isosurfaces, will enable the visual intersection of both and give the ability to rotate and position each model independently.

Since the surgeon is more familiar with the 2D representation of each slice, the application provides both ways of presenting the data. A MPR technique is used to help the surgeon better visualize the axial, coronal and sagittal planes of each CT scan's slice (Fig. 3). When rendering in conjunction with the 3D generated model in the same scene, the surgeon is able to pan each 2D plane and visualize each slice representation independently in another viewer.

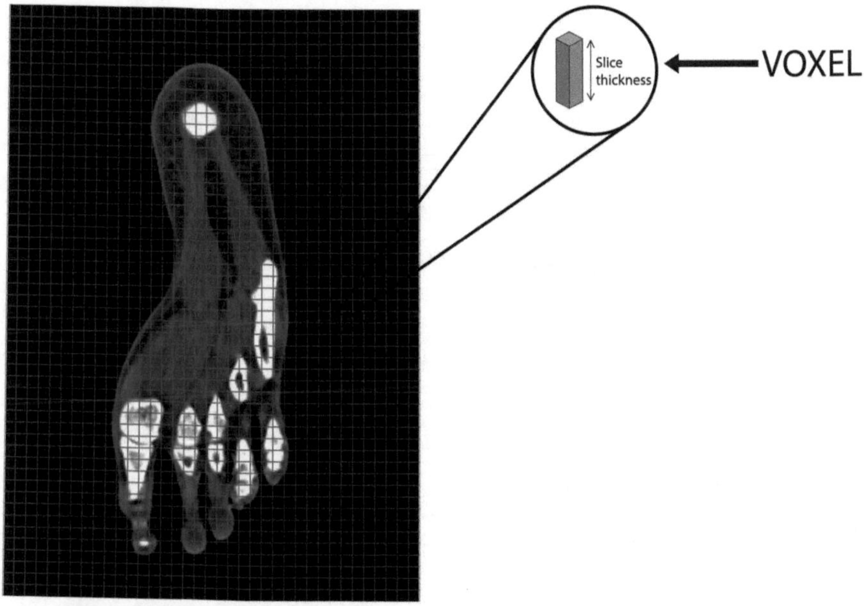

Fig. 2 Example of a CT scan's slice

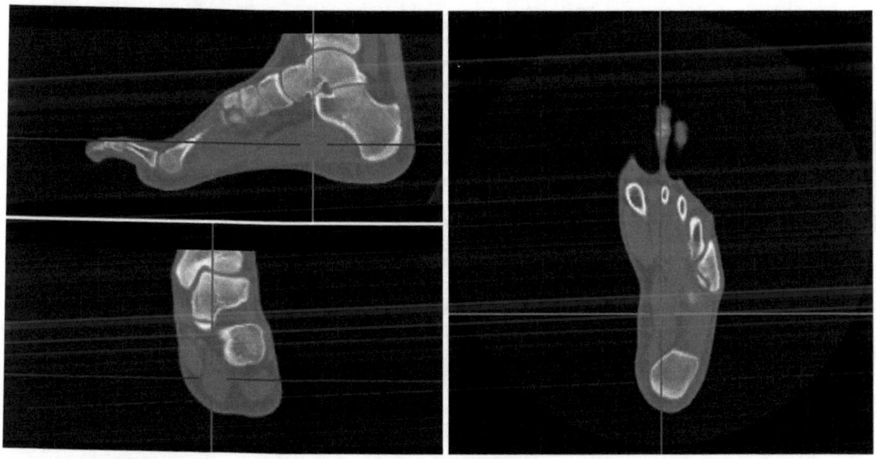

Fig. 3 OrthoMED Multi-planar Rendering visualization

3 The OrthoMED Plugin

The proposed solution, which we named OrthoMED, was developed in C++ and Objective-C as a plugin for OsiriX [12, 13] using a set of open source libraries written in the same programming language. They are OsiriX DCM Framework, used

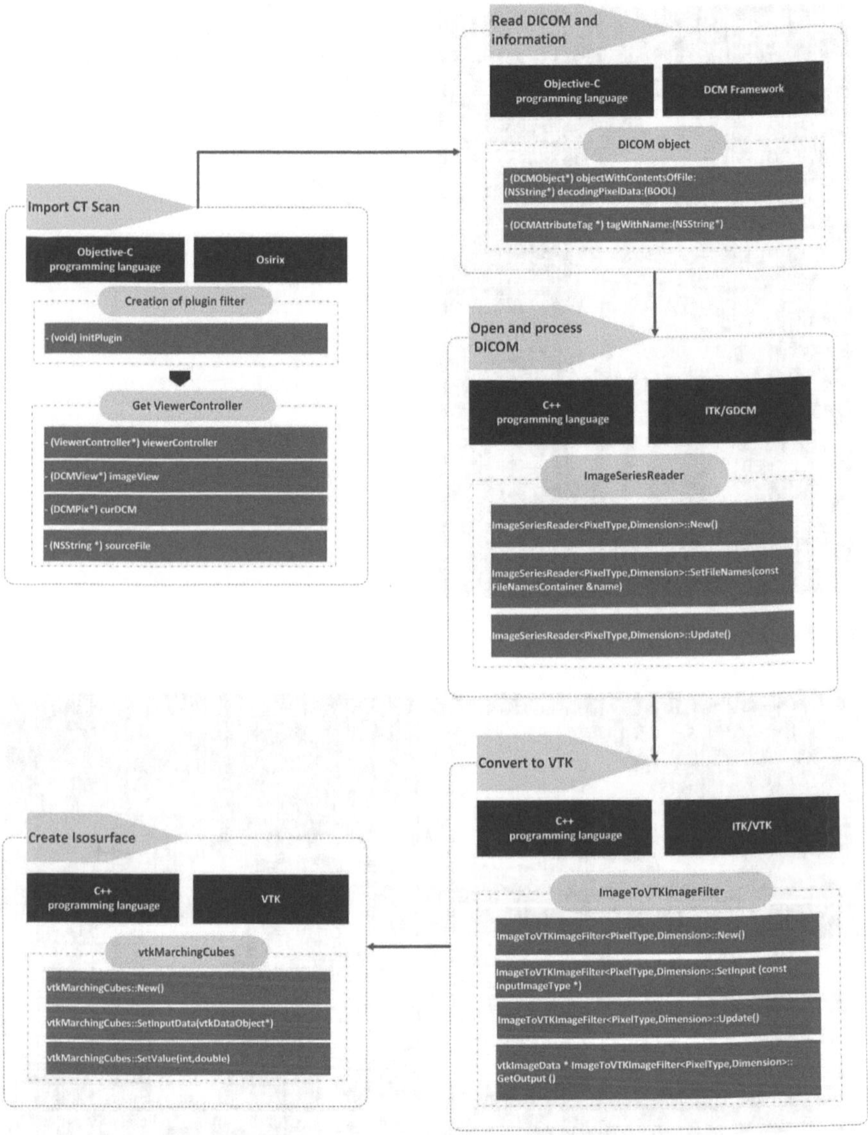

Fig. 4 `OrthoMED`'s internal workflow to create an isosurface from a CT scan

to read the DICOM files and their metadata, ITK and GDCM, to parse and process each DICOM file and VTK, to implement the MC algorithm and 3D visualization [6, 7, 11]. OsiriX was chosen since it is a widely used viewer for medical purposes, allowing a minimized learning curve associated with the usage of this new tool.

Figure 4 presents the application's internal workflow to create an isosurface from a CT scan. For OsiriX to detect `OrthoMED` as a plugin it is necessary to create

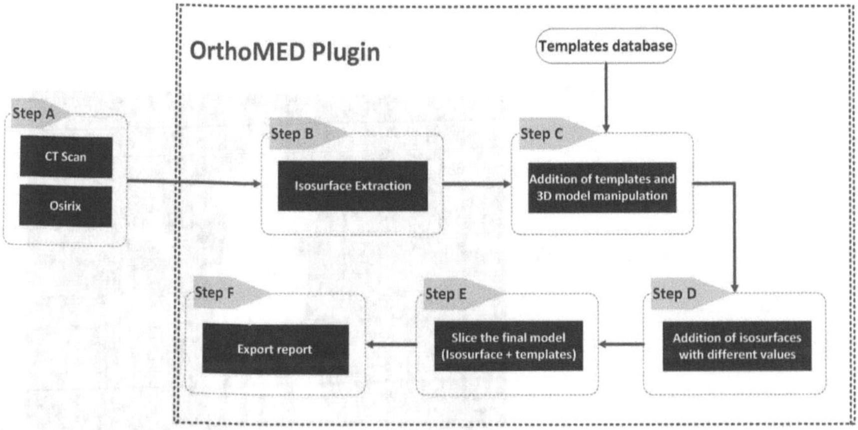

Fig. 5 `OrthoMED`'s workflow

a sub-class of `PluginFilter`. That way it is possible to open the plugin from the OsiriX's main menu and import the CT scan from its `ViewerController`. Then, to read and extract meta-information from de CT scan (e.g., Patient's name, Patient's age) the OsiriX DCM Framework was used. By creating an instance from `DCMObject` all the meta-information associated to the CT study can be retrieved. With ITK and the GDCM libraries, the CT scan can be read and converted to a VTK object to be displayed on screen.

VTK has an implementation of the MC algorithm that when executed results in an isosurface of chosen HU where the templates can later be added.

Figure 5 presents the application's workflow, beginning with the CT scan's upload and ending with the report export. Since the isosurfaces and the templates are now structurally compatible, with VTK they can be resized and its position changed in the same geometric plane.

The proposed solution workflow can be divided in six steps:

Step A Select the imaging study (i.e. CT scan) and run the `OrthoMED` plugin. This step is done within the OsiriX environment;

Step B The current imaging study is transferred to the plugin that as a first interaction asks for the initial HU value for the isosurface to be created. Once this value is entered, the isosurface is generated and displayed. This isosurface is extracted using the MC algorithm;

Step C Add surgical templates and handle them, changing their positions in a 3D space. These templates model the implants that will be used in the surgery;

Step D Add different isosurfaces, enabling the analysis of existing intersections in the surrounding tissues;

Step E Slice the generated model that includes all the surgical templates. These slices are made in a chosen plane and in the initial isosurface;

Step F Export the report with the patient's info, a list of the physical implants used, selected images and notes that the surgeon included.

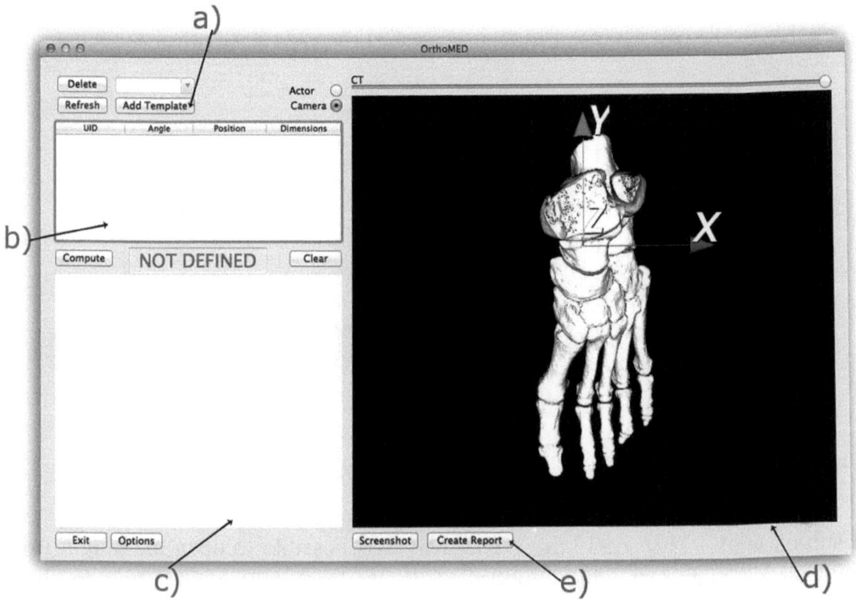

Fig. 6 `OrthoMED`'s main window

During **Step C** the surgeon is able to visualize the patient's CT scan with MPR, allowing its analysis in three different planes. By moving the related plane, the surgeon is now able to visualize each slice from the chosen plane. This is very helpful because it allows the precise location of the fracture.

Figure 6 presents a screenshot of `OrthoMED`'s main window with its five sections:

a) Opens the window with the surgical templates database, where the surgeon can choose which template he wants to add. These templates are the 3D digital representation of a real template. They have the same shape and size;
b) Table with the surgical templates added, with their corresponding positions and angles;
c) Section where the final 3D model slices are displayed. Scrolling up and down shows the whole array;
d) Main section, where the surgeon handles the 3D isosurface as well as the templates, always in a 3D space;
e) Exporting section of the report with the surgery plan.

The upper slider can be used to change the isosurface's opacity, helping the visualization of the internal interceptions (Fig. 7).

The two radio buttons on the side are used to select which structure the user wants to move. If 'Actor' is selected, then the surgeon can select, move or rotate any independent 3D object (i.e., any template added). If 'Camera' is selected, then the point of view from all scene is moved or rotated. Fig. 8 presents the window with all available templates. Here the user can select a template and check its data on the

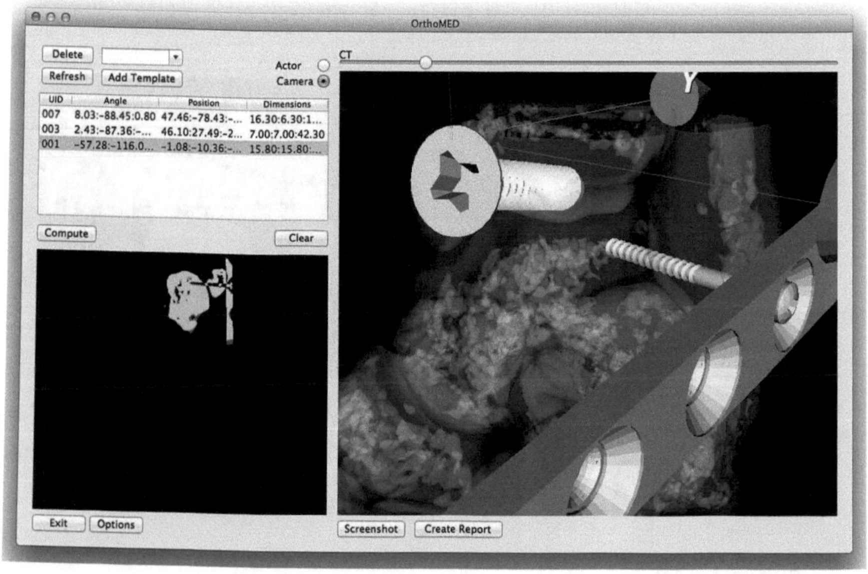

Fig. 7 `OrthoMED`'s main window with the 3D view zoomed

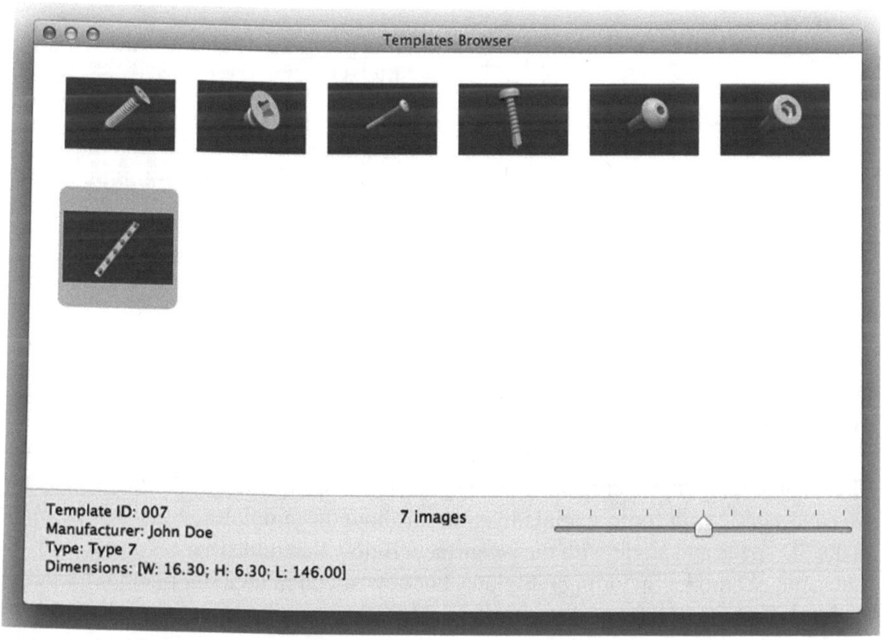

Fig. 8 `OrthoMED`'s templates database window

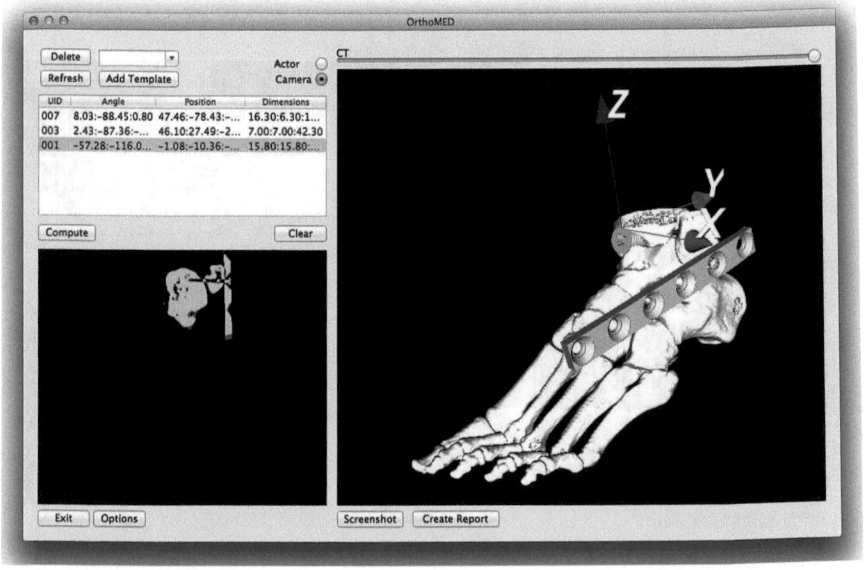

Fig. 9 `OrthoMED`'s main window with some templates on the generated isosurface

Fig. 10 Options window

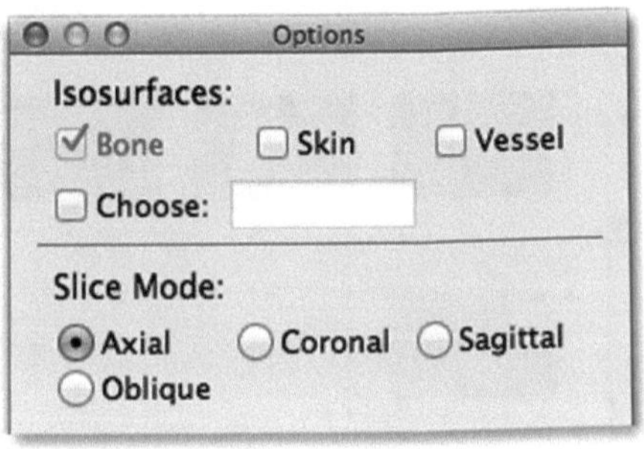

bottom. Double-clicking the chosen template, it will automatically be added to the main section, in the (0,0,0) position.

In the main section in Fig. 6, one can see an isosurface of value 300 in HU scale. Then, some templates were added and positioned as wanted (Fig. 9). On the left side we have a table with some spatial information about the templates, e.g., their position in the 3D space and angle with the isosurface. Below that table there is a section with that same 3D model including templates but now sliced in an axial plane for a better analysis of the templates real positioning. This plane can be selected on the options window (Fig. 10).

Figure 11 presents some elements of the array with the slices of the final 3D model. Zooming and decreasing the opacity of the isosurface, the surgeon is able to analyze the exact spot where the template is positioned (Fig. 7). Figure 12 shows a

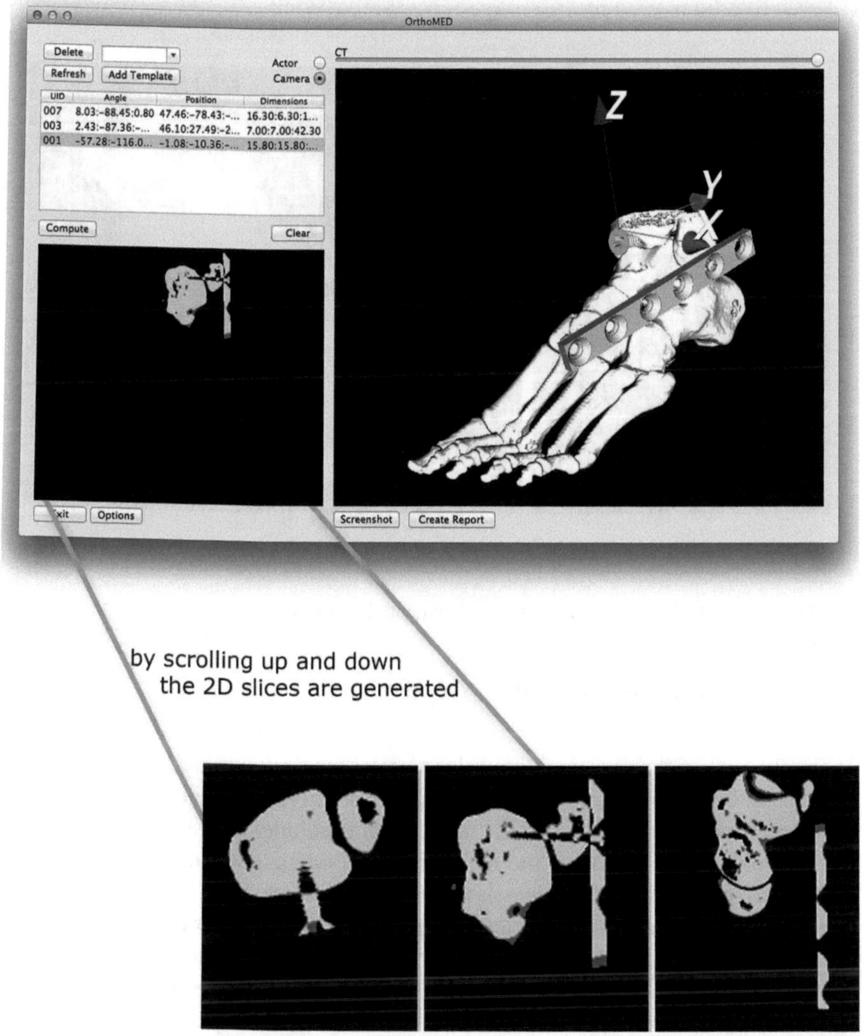

Fig. 11 2D slices generated from the planned 3D model

new isosurface added. In that way, the surgeon is now able to evaluate his plan and how it will affect the surrounding tissues. This is quite useful for his analysis. This isosurface and its value could be entered in the options window (Fig. 10).

After the planning process, the surgeon is able to export a report with all the information needed, e.g., a table with the templates information and their position in the 3D space, some screenshots taken from the final 3D model as well as the patient's specific information (Fig. 13).

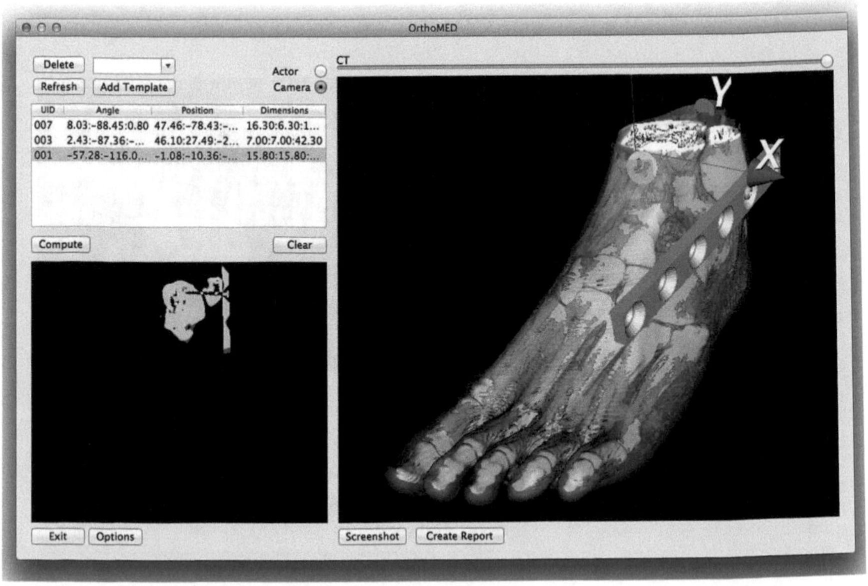

Fig. 12 `OrthoMED`'s main window with the generated isosurface

4 Conclusion/Discussion

The main goal of the presented work is to create a solution which allows the interoperability between images in two different format types. The currently available solutions have limitations, some of them do not include 3D modeling or when is that available, the creation of the model is based on standard models or the intervention of specialized technicians is required. The `OrthoMED` plugin enables the interoperability between a CT scan 3D model and surgical templates representing orthopedic physical implants. Since we are dealing with different types of image (i.e. the CT study is a matrix of voxels and the surgical templates are vector graphics) it was necessary to develop a method to join them in the same planes. These surgical templates are STL files, created from CAD models of physical implants provided by medical implants suppliers. The advantage in using this kind of files is due to its wide use by the implants industry. Comparing the proposed solution with the described commercial ones, `OrthoMED` presents an alternative approach, delegating the task entirely to the surgeon. With this plugin, the surgeon is able to add templates and handle their position always in a 3D space, which allows a constant evaluation of the best positioning. He can also slice the final 3D model with templates on it. After choosing the slicing plane (e.g. Axial, Sagittal, Coronal, Oblique), the surgeon can evaluate his surgical solution in a 2D view that gives him more detailed information. Finally he can export the surgery report plan. The developed solution becomes advantageous for the surgeons. Thus, they can manipulate the generated 3D model, composed by one or more isosurfaces, and they can add the implants templates from

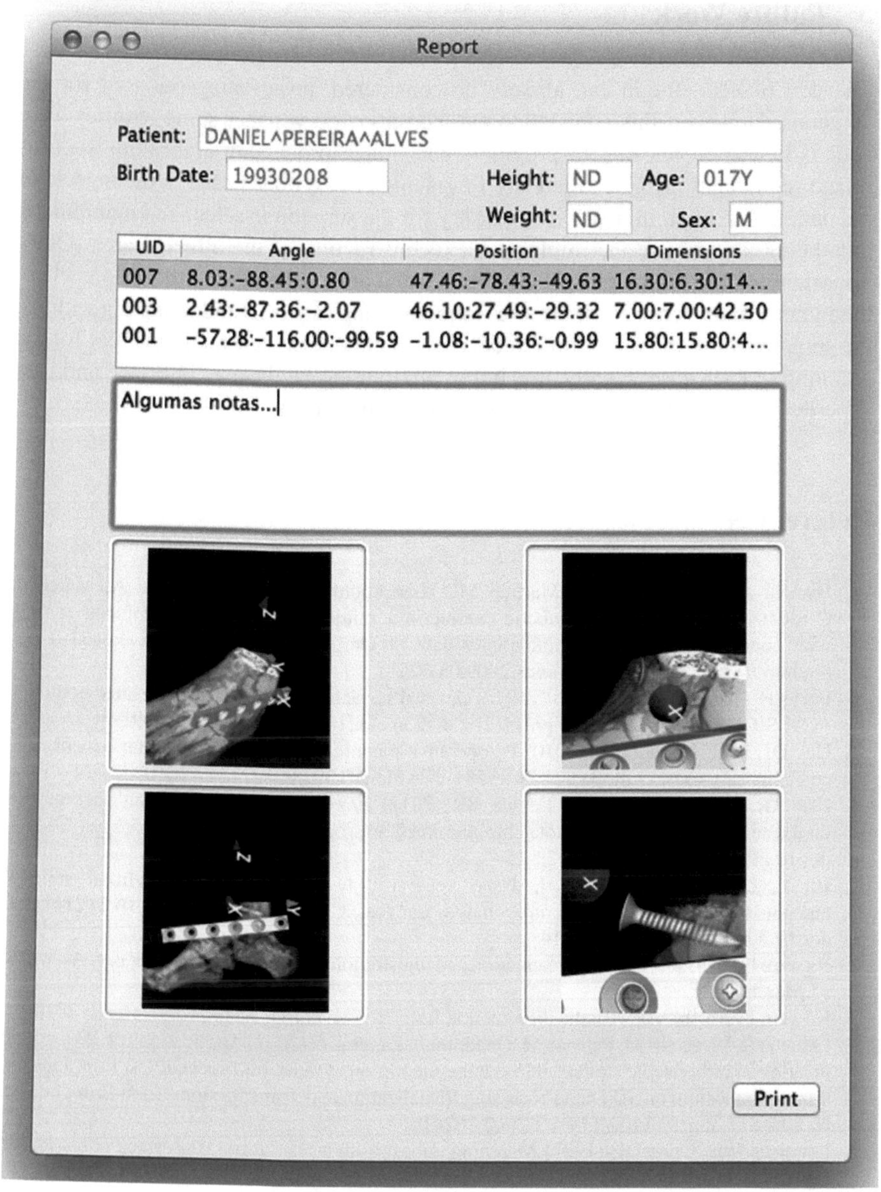

Fig. 13 Surgery planning report export window

the database. Comparing this solution with others, `OrthoMED` brings a different, enhanced and complementary solution to orthopedic surgical planning.

5 Future Work

The `OrthoMED` plugin can already be considered an advantageous tool for the surgeons. However, this application can be improved whether some features were added. It will be relevant to provide some image processing algorithms such as image segmentation. When there are fragments of free bone tissue in the muscle of the patient due to an injury, it is necessary for the surgeon to select and manipulate, thus being able to use the implants for reconstruction of the affected area. Other important feature is to highlight the intersection area, determining the points where the intersections occur. Furthermore, implementing more 3D modeling algorithms, the surgeons have the possibility to decide and choose the most suitable tool for the planning of each case. Finally, it is important to improve the user interface and user experience of the application, making it more intuitive and simpler to operate.

References

1. Bianchi A, Muyldermans L, Martino MD, Lancellotti L, Amadori S, Sarti A, Marchetti C (2010) Facial soft tissue esthetic predictions: validation in craniomaxillofacial surgery with cone beam computed tomography data. J Oral Maxillofac Surg 68(7):1471–1479. doi:http://dx.doi.org/10.1016/j.joms.2009.08.006
2. Fuchs H, Kedem ZM, Uselton SP (1977) Optimal surface reconstruction from planar contours. ACM SIGGRAPH Comput Graph 11(2):236–236. doi:10.1145/965141.563899
3. Hak DJ, Rose J, Stahel PF (2010) Preoperative planning in orthopedic trauma: benefits and contemporary uses. Orthopedics 33(8):581–584. doi:10.3928/01477447-20100625-21
4. Hsu AR, Kim JD, Bhatia S, Levine BR (2012) Effect of training level on accuracy of digital templating in primary total hip and knee arthroplasty. Orthopedics 35(2):e179–183. doi:10.3928/01477447-20120123-15
5. Hu Y, Li H, Qiao G, Liu H, Ji A, Ye F (2011) Computer-assisted virtual surgical procedure for acetabular fractures based on real CT data. Injury 42(10):1121–1124. doi:10.1016/j.injury.2011.01.014
6. Kitware I (2014) Itk-insight segmentation and registration toolkit. http://www.itk.org. Accessed 31 March 2014
7. Kitware I (2014b) Vtk-visualization toolkit. http://www.vtk.org. Accessed 31 March 2014
8. Lattanzi R, Viceconti M, Petrone M, Quadrani P, Zannoni C (2002) Applications of 3D medical imaging in orthopaedic surgery:introducing the hip-op system. In: Proceedings. First International Symposium on 3D Data Processing Visualization and Transmission, IEEE Comput Soc, pp 808–811. doi:10.1109/TDPVT.2002.1024165
9. Lorensen WE, Cline HE (1987) Marching cubes: a high resolution 3D surface construction algorithm. ACM SIGGRAPH Comput Graph 21(4):163–169
10. Mabrey JD, Reinig KD, Cannon WD (2010) Virtual reality in orthopaedics: is it a reality? Clin Orthop Relat Res 468(10):2586–2591. doi:10.1007/s11999-010-1426-1
11. Malaterre M et al JPR (2014) Gdcm-grassroots DICOM library. http://gdcm.sourceforge. net/. Accessed 31 March 2014
12. Rosset A (2014) Osirix imaging software - advanced open-source PACS workstation DICOM viewer. http://www.osirix-viewer.com. Accessed 31 March 2014
13. Rosset A, Spadola L, Ratib O (2004) OsiriX: an open-source software for navigating in multidimensional DICOM images. J Digit Imaging J Soc Comput Appl Radiol 17(3):205–216. doi:10.1007/s10278-004-1014-6

14. Roth SD (1982) Ray casting for modeling solids. Comput Gr Image Process 18(2):109–144. http://dx.doi.org/10.1016/0146-664X(82)90169-1
15. Shiha A, Krettek C, Hankemeier S, Liodakis E, Kenawey M (2010) The use of a professional graphics editing program for the preoperative planning in deformity correction surgery: a technical note. Injury 41(6):660–664. doi:10.1016/j.injury.2009.10.051
16. Sikorski JM, Chauhan S (2003) Aspects of current management. J Bone Joint Surg 85(3):319–323
17. Steen A, Widegren M (2013) 3D Visualization of Pre-operative Planning for Orthopedic Surgery. In: Ropinski T, Unger J (eds) Proceedings of SIGRAD 2013, visual computing, June 13–14. Linköping University Electronic Press, Sweden, pp 1–8
18. Steinberg EL, Shasha N, Menahem A, Dekel S (2010) Preoperative planning of total hip replacement using the TraumaCad system. Arch Orthop Trauma Surg 130(12):1429–1432. doi:10.1007/s00402-010-1046-y
19. Suero EM, Hüfner T, Stübig T, Krettek C, Citak M (2010) Use of a virtual 3D software for planning of tibial plateau fracture reconstruction. Injury 41(6):589–591. doi:10.1016/j.injury.2009.10.053
20. The B, Verdonschot N, van Horn JR, van Ooijen PMA, Diercks RL (2007) Digital versus analogue preoperative planning of total hip arthroplasties: a randomized clinical trial of 210 total hip arthroplasties. J Arthroplast 22(6):866–870. doi: http://dx.doi.org/10.1016/j.arth.2006.07.013
21. Wade RH, Kevu J, Doyle J (1998) Pre-operative planning in orthopaedics: a study of surgeons' opinions. Injury 29(10):785–786
22. Wang H (2009) Three-dimensional medical CT image reconstruction. In: 2009 international conference on measuring technology and mechatronics automation, IEEE, pp 548–551. doi:10.1109/ICMTMA.2009.10

Preoperative Planning of Surgical Treatment with the Use of 3D Visualization and Finite Element Method

Wojciech Wolański, Bożena Gzik-Zroska, Edyta Kawlewska, Marek Gzik, Dawid Larysz, Józef Dzielicki and Adam Rudnik

Abstract This chapter describes a method of engineering support of preoperative planning of surgical procedures with the use of engineering tools, such as state-of-the-art software for medical image processing, or a finite element method. The procedure of pre-operative planning consists in matching individual cases of incision sites and directions, visualization and selection of areas for resection as well as planning the technique of implant positioning and fixation. Also, the final visualization of the result of the planned medical procedure can be performed. This paper presents procedural propositions in surgery planning in the cases of corrections of the head shape in patients with craniosynostosis, corrections of the chest deformity such as pigeon chest and stabilization of the lumbar spine. 3D models created on the basis of computer tomography (CT) or magnetic resonance imaging (MRI) enabled it to conduct a biomechanical analysis as well as an objective quantitative and qualitative virtual evaluation of the surgical procedure. Preoperative planning support gives the physician an opportunity to prepare for the operation in a better way, which results in the selection of the best possible variant of an operative technique, reduction of time of the surgical procedure and minimization of the risk of intraoperative complications.

W. Wolański (✉) · E. Kawlewska · M. Gzik
Biomechatronics Department, Faculty of Biomedical Engineering,
Silesian University of Technology, Zabrze, Poland
e-mail: wwolanski@polsl.pl

B. Gzik-Zroska
Department of Biomaterials and Medical Devices Engineering, Faculty of Biomedical Engineering, Silesian University of Technology, Zabrze, Poland

J. Dzielicki
Medical University of Silesia, School of Medicine in Katowice, Katowice, Poland

D. Larysz
Department of Radiotherapy, Maria Sklodowska-Curie Memorial Cancer Center and Institute of Oncology, Gliwice, Poland

A. Rudnik
Department of Neurosurgery, Medical University of Silesia, Katowice, Poland

J. M. R. S. Tavares, R. Natal Jorge (eds.), *Developments in Medical Image Processing and Computational Vision,* Lecture Notes in Computational Vision and Biomechanics 19,
DOI 10.1007/978-3-319-13407-9_9

1 Introduction

Engineering support in medicine can be observed on a daily basis in a form of measuring apparatuses, hospital equipment or new materials used for the manufacturing of surgical tools, implants or prosthetic appliances. However, apart from technical facilities a new methodology has been being developed aiming at the support of surgical procedures with the use of engineering software. Such procedures are used in some medical centres, mainly in the field of neurosurgery, orthopaedic surgery and cardiosurgery. At the planning stage an engineer may indicate elements which should be taken into consideration during an operation in order to achieve the desired treatment effects. It is nevertheless the doctor who makes the final decision on the operative technique and methods of surgical procedure. The possibility of a 3D visualization of the surgical procedure and prediction of the course of the operation as well as evaluation of the results undoubtedly provides a perfect assistance to the physician. Virtual training before a real-life procedure in the operating theatre enables the doctor to prepare for the operation in a precise way. It is essential in the case of young surgeons who are only beginning to develop their skills and technique. It is also vital that surgical procedures be planned individually for each patient. While performing the simulation it is possible to take into account certain ontogenetic features which could not be fully determined in a standard way, such as thickness of the bones in the sites of planned incisions or drilling.

Medical imaging technology enables it to export images of diagnostic examinations, e.g. CT or MRI, to the computer. Thanks to that a 3D model can be generated and subsequently modified. Nowadays, new systems are being created which support the doctors in the scope of the selection of a surgical technique or a proper implant. The system VIRTOPS (Virtual Operation Planning in Orthopaedic Surgery) may be one of the examples of the above-described software. It is used to plan operations of bone tumours with endoprosthetic reconstruction of the hip based on multimodal image information [17]. The chief objective of the programme is to match a proper endoprosthesis to an individual case as well as to provide a very thorough visualization of the tumour located in the bone. 3D images or films developed during the planning stage of the operation may serve as medical documentation as well as be used for the patient's preoperative information. CT and MRI images are imported to VIRTOPS system. On the basis of the generated models virtual operation planning is carried out (Fig. 1).

Another programme which is used for preoperative planning of surgical procedures is SQ PELVIS. It enables virtual planning of operations of pelvis injuries on the models created on the basis of DICOM images [5]. The segmentation of tissues on the grounds of the Hounsfield scale plays an essential role in the planning process. Having generated a satisfactory model one may position implants and match them to the individual needs of the examined patient (Fig. 2).

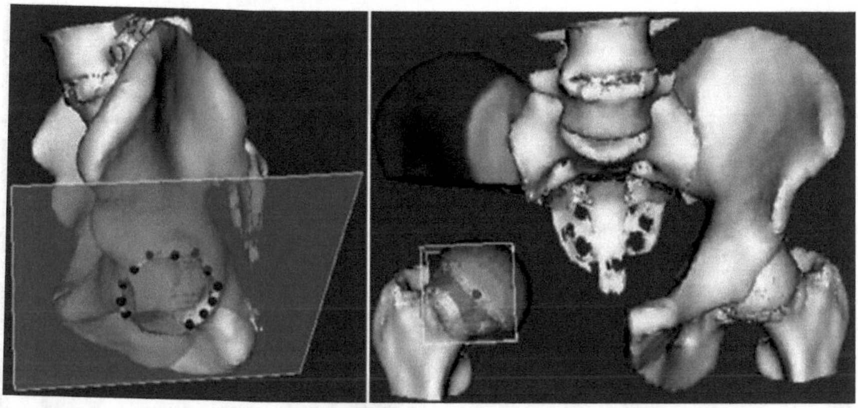

Fig. 1 *Left*: The marked points on the hip joint border and the approximated plane are shown. *Right*: Resulting position of the artificial hip joint in correspondence to the mirrored, healthy hip part [16]

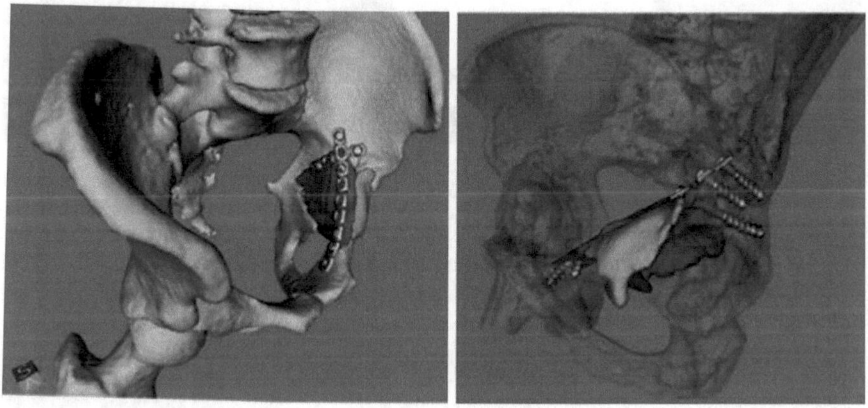

Fig. 2 Virtual planning of pelvis stabilization with the use of SQ PELVIS system. *Left*: Virtual reduction and fixation of the fractured bone. *Right*: The direction and length of the screws [5]

Another approach aims to support the surgeon by providing them with templates which facilitate technical aspects of carrying out the operation, for instance, a navigation system (Fig. 3) which was used in the work of Gras et al. [13] to plan the position of the stabilizing screws in pelvic ring injuries.

Another example can be provided by operative planning in orthognathic surgery [10]. The standard planning is done on the basis of CT scanning (Fig. 4). However, there are also special programmes, such as Mimics and 3-matic software (Materialise) [23] for planning the corrections of the facial skeleton. Similar procedures supporting treatment in orthognathic surgery were developed, among others, by: Cutting [8, 9], Yasuda [30] and Altobelli [1].

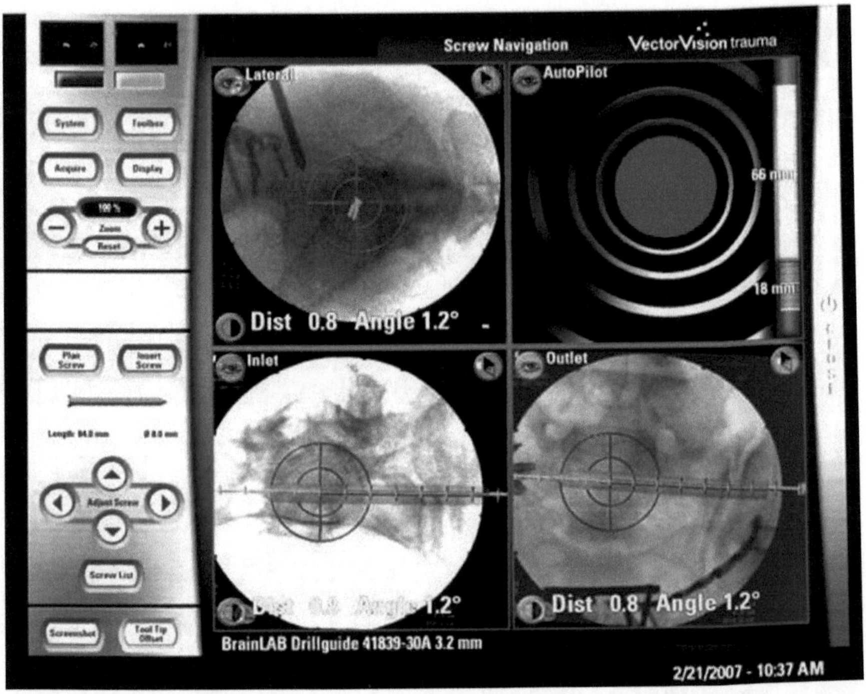

Fig. 3 Sterile touch screen of the navigation system (*Vector Vision, Brainlab*) displaying standard images (*lateral view, inlet, outlet*) and an auto-pilot view. *Red bar*: virtually planned SI-screw; *yellow line*: prospective path of the navigated guide wire (*trajectory*), *green bull's-eye*: reflecting the exact positioning of navigated instruments to achieve the planned screw position [13]

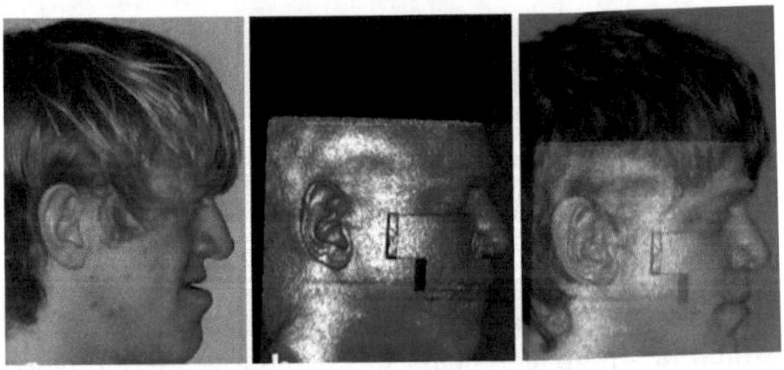

Fig. 4 Example of computer-aided surgery (*CAS*) of a patient with Crouzon syndrome. Simulation and result of Le Fort II distraction before surgery and after CT planning [10]

In more advanced research new devices are being developed with the purpose of supporting the doctor during the surgical procedure, for example: a neck jig device presented in the work of Raaijmaakers et al.[25]. The Surface Replacement Arthroplasty jig was designed as a slightly more-than-hemispherical cage to fit the anterior part of the femoral head. The cage is connected to an anterior neck support. Four knifes are attached on the central arch of the cage. A drill guide cylinder is attached to the cage, thus allowing guide wire positioning as pre-operatively planned (Fig. 5).

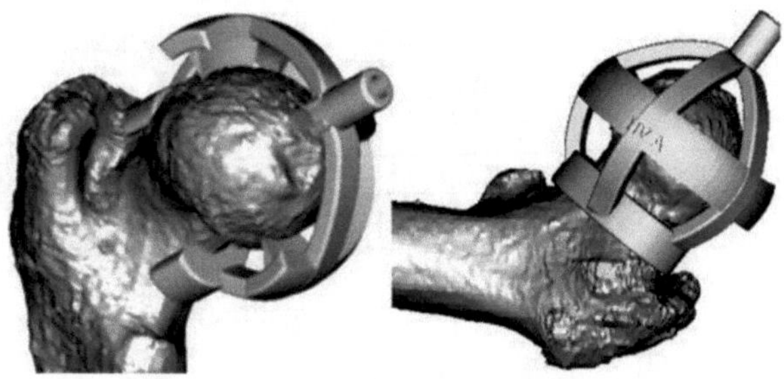

Fig. 5 Neck jig designed to drill a guide wire in a pre-determined position and direction, seen from medioposterior (*left*) and anterolateral (*right*) [25]

Apart from planning a procedure for an individual patient, new methods of engineering support make it possible to choose optimal parameters for the operation. An example can be provided by the application of a method of finite elements in the biomechanical analysis of the system after simulated virtual treatment. In the research of Jiang et al. [19] planning of corrective incisions (scaphocephaly) was done as well as biomechanical analysis of the obtained models was performed (Fig. 6). Thanks to that, it is possible to choose the most favourable variant of the operation. In addition to that, the research of Szarek et al. [27] analysed the level of stress in the hip joint endoprosthesis resulting from variable loads during human motor activity.

Analysing the influence of preoperative planning and 3D virtual visualization of the examined cases on the quality of treatment, it can be stated that the engineering support provides assistance for the vast majority of doctors in the scope of complex assessment of the phenomenon and preparation for a real-life procedure. The conducted research has proven that [18] both the planning time and labour intensity are reduced by around 30 % if 3D models are available. In addition to that, the precision (accuracy) of predicting the size of the resection area (e.g. in the case of tumours) increases by about 20 % (Fig. 7). Moreover, according to subjective feelings of the examined doctors their confidence in the established diagnosis has risen by around 20 % in the case of 3D planning.

2 Engineering Support Procedure for Preoperative Planning

Surgical treatment within the skeletal system is always the last resort in the case when other preventive methods have failed. For instance, when the application of orthopaedic equipment has not brought the desirable effects. On the basis of several-year tests carried out in co-operation with surgeons a general scheme of engineering support procedure has been developed for pre-operative planning of surgical operations (Fig. 8).

In the first phase the attending physician gives a diagnosis of the disease. Usually, within the framework of a regular diagnosis a CT or MRI examination is done, thanks to which 2D images of individual cross sections are obtained. On the grounds of the Hounsfield scale, in the programme Mimics® Materialise [31] it is possible to segment the tissues of interest (e.g. bones, cartilages) and then generate a 3D model.

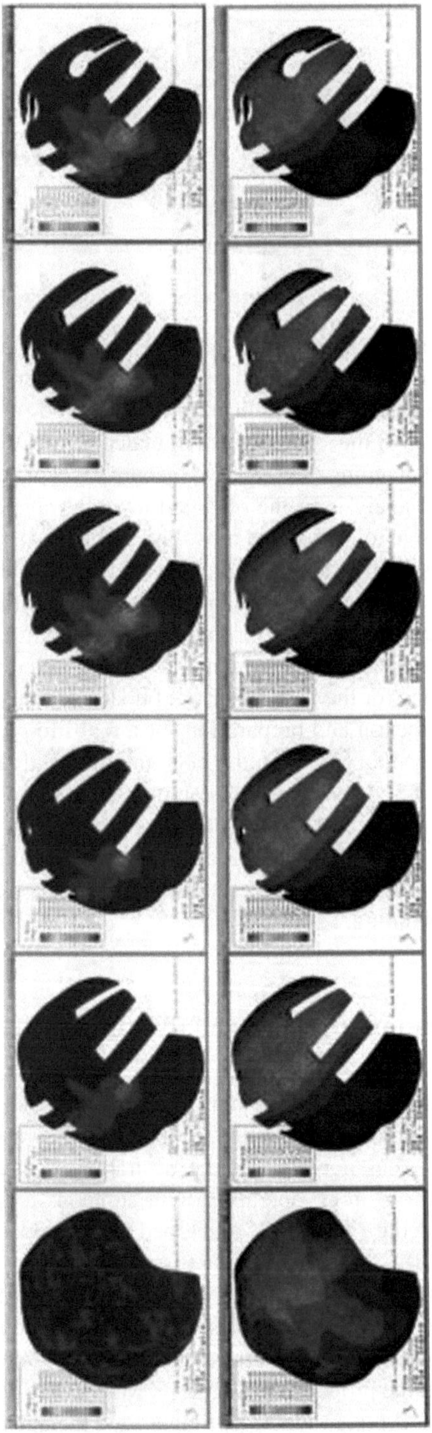

Fig. 6 Distribution of stress (*top*) and displacements (*bottom*) in the skull vault before the surgery and in five variants of corrective incisions [19]

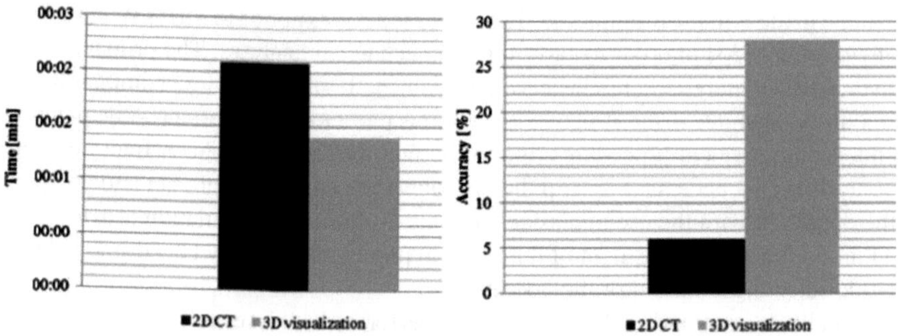

Fig. 7 Comparison between viewing 2D CT images and 3D displays of thoracic cavities in determining the resectability of lung cancer. *Left*: Planning time. *Right*: Accuracy of predicted resectability [18]

Fig. 8 Developed procedure of engineering support procedure for preoperative planning

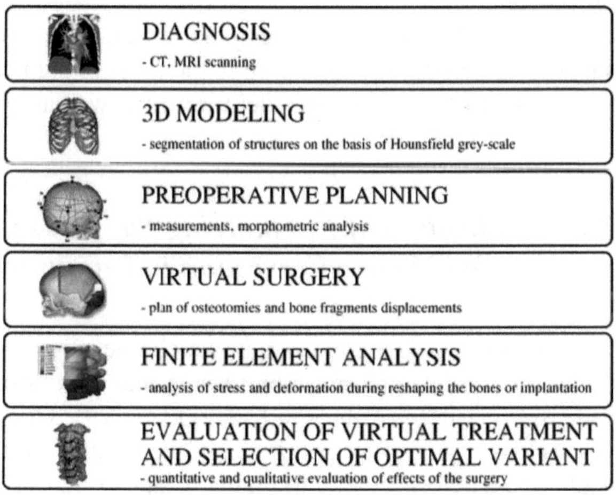

In the next stage, on the basis of the constructed geometrical model it is possible to carry out detailed morphological measurements in order to determine the type of the defect and degree of the disease progression.

On these grounds the patient is qualified for the surgical procedure by the doctor. Additionally, the programme 3-matic® Materialise [32] makes it possible to do the analysis of bone thickness, which is very helpful in the selection of surgical tools for the operation. Mimics programme enables all sorts of modifications of the obtained model as well as simulations of the planned operation. In consultation with the doctor, bone incisions and displacements are simulated with the purpose of obtaining the desirable treatment effects. After the correction has been planned, it is advisable to conduct the morphometric analysis once again in order to check the values of indexes which were used in the preoperative evaluation.

Next, the model is prepared to be introduced into computing environment. Discretization of the model, i.e. the creation of the volumetric mesh and its optimization is done in the 3-matic programme. Then, the model is exported to Ansys Workbench® environment [33] in order to carry out biomechanical analyses. The primary objective of FEM analysis is to check whether during bone modelling or implanting no fracture or damage to the structure occurs. It is particularly important while planning endoscopic surgical procedures due to the fact that any unforeseen fracture of the bones makes it necessary to stop the microinvasive surgical treatment and complete the operation with the use of classic methods. A numerical simulation provides thus an individual risk assessment of the surgical procedure and may be a decisive factor while selecting a variant of the operation.

Finally, by comparing the results of the performed analyses it is possible to make the most advantageous and the safest choice of the operative variant. It must be emphasized that preoperative planning is an absorbing and time-consuming process, and therefore, not suitable for all kinds of operations. Its application is justified and brings many notable benefits in the case of particularly complicated surgical procedures.

In the further part this paper presents examples of procedures of engineering support for preoperative planning in the cases of surgical corrections of head shape in infants, corrections of chest deformities as well as spine stabilization.

2.1 Application of Engineering Support in Preoperative Planning of Head Shape Correction in Infants with Craniosynostosis

Craniosynostosis is a condition in which one or more of the fibrous sutures in an infant skull prematurely fuse by turning into bone (ossification), thereby changing the growth pattern of the skull [2, 20, 21, 29]. One of the most common cases of craniosynostosis is trigonocephaly, i.e. premature fusion of the metopic suture leading to a deformity of a triangular shaped forehead. Planning of the endoscopic correction of trigonocephaly in a two-month boy was done. CT images of the head were imported to *Mimics* environment in order to generate a 3D model of the skull. The primary task was to decide on the basis of a morphological analysis whether to qualify the patient for the classic surgical procedure or microinvasive one. The bone incisions and displacements were planned as well as possible variants of correction were developed.

In the first place, the analysis of bone thickness was performed in order to initially determine a type of the operation [22]. Maximum and minimum thickness was measured in the sites of fusion of the metopic suture subject to resection. Thickness in those points was respectively: max 7.01 mm, 4.46 mm and min 2.02 mm (Fig. 9). Thickness points of the whole skull were also determined. Average thickness of bones equalled 2.0 mm with a standard deviation of 1.2 mm.

Subsequently, points necessary for setting indexes determining an incorrect shape of the head were marked on the model [28]. These are the following points: *euryon, metopion, sphenion c, lateralis orbitae, medialis orbitae, nasion* (Fig. 10).

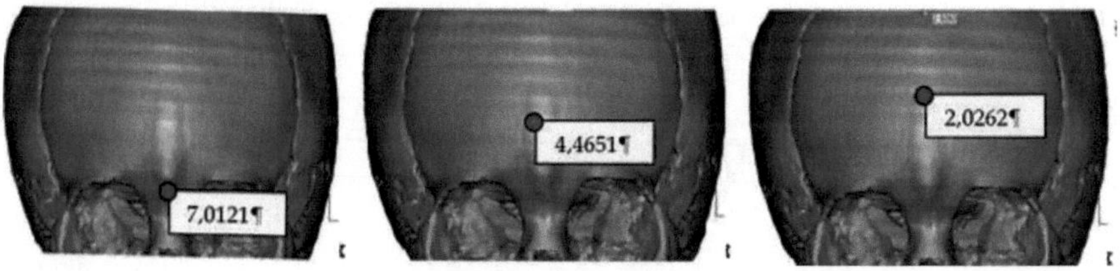

Fig. 9 Bone-thickness analysis performed in 3-matic software

Fig. 10 Three-dimensional model of skull with trigonocephaly with marked anatomic points

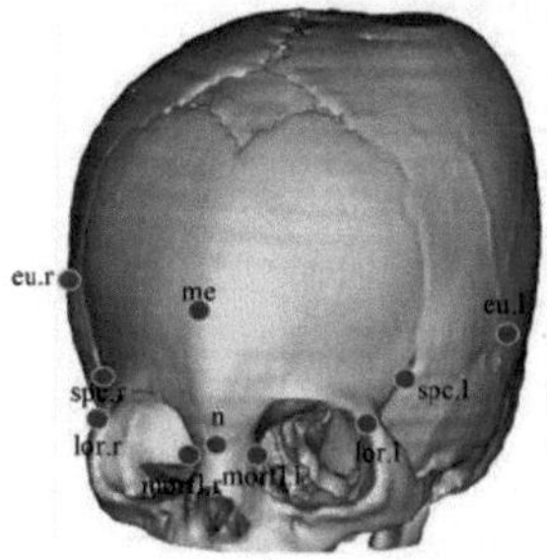

Legend:

eu	*euryon*
me	*metopion*
spc	*sphenion c*
lor	*lateralis orbitae*
morfl	*medialis orbitae*
n	*nasion*

One set the values of indexes determining an incorrect shape of the skull in trigonocephaly. Those values were next compared to the standard values of children with a regular skull shape at the age of 0–2 months old in order to determine the way the correction should be performed. The results have been presented in Table 1. The measurements showed that the frontal angle was too acute but other indexes were within regular limits. No hypertelorism was detected, therefore the correction was going to be made only on the frontal bone without any interference in the orbital cavities. In this way it was determined that it was possible to carry out a microinvasive procedure. The main decisive factors at that stage of planning were as follows: the patient's age, bone thickness (within 5 mm in the sites of potential incisions) as well as a correct distance between orbital cavities and a lack of deformities within facial skeleton. The doctor made a decision that the correction of the skull shape was going to consist in the cutting of the fused metopic suture and parting of the bones in order to obtain an optimum shape of the head.

The virtual correction was performed in two stages. In the first one the frontal bone was separated from the rest of the skull alongside frontoparietal sutures. The lower limit was provided by the nasal bone and frontozygomatic sutures. The incisions of the frontal bone were planned in *Mimics* environment in the way guaranteeing an optimum forehead shape (Fig. 11). Dislocations, in fact rotations, of the fragments of the bones were done manually taking into consideration the doctor's suggestions and actual conditions of the operation. Point *nasion (n)* on the nasal bone was defined to be a fixed point according to which the bones were parted to make the head shape round.

Table 1 Craniometric measurements results in patient with trigonocephaly

Index	Figure	Measured value	Normative value	Guidelines for surgery
Frontal bone angle	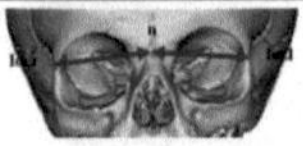	121,8°	133,1° ± 5,6	increase
Naso-orbital angle	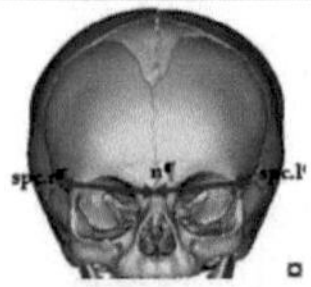	103,5°	104,9° ± 5,9	regular
Index of the width of the inner orbits and the width of the skull	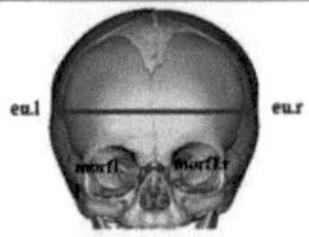	0,14	0,16 ± 0,02	regular
Index of the width of the outer orbits and the width of the skull	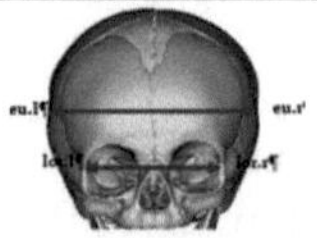	0,62	0,65 ± 0,03	regular

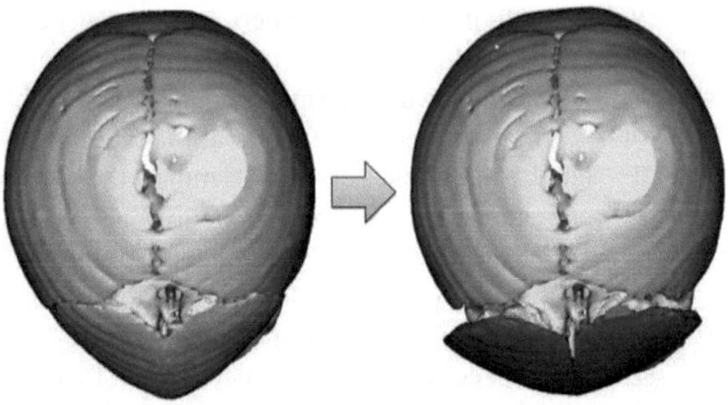

Fig. 11 Virtual correction of forehead performed in Mimics

Having obtained an optimal visual effect of the correction, one measured displacement of several bone points which in the further planning phase were introduced into *Ansys* environment as boundary conditions. In the end, the average displacement of the bones from their initial position equalled 11 mm. The value of the frontal bone angle was checked once again in order to evaluate if it was now close to standard. After the procedure the angle was increased up to 132.7°, which produced a satisfactory effect of the correction (Fig. 12).

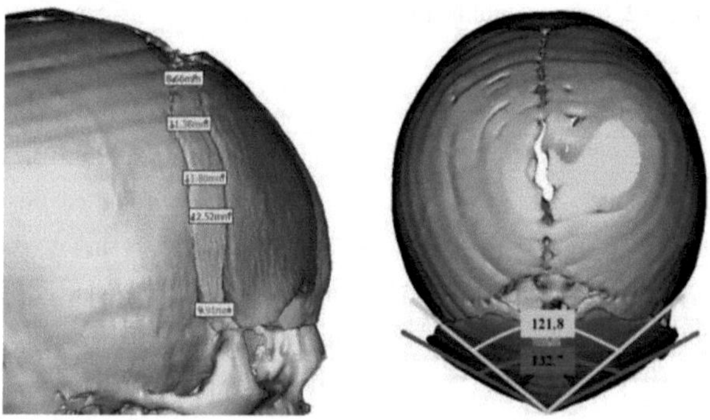

Fig. 12 Measurements of skull after virtual correction. *Left*: Displacement necessary to correct the forehead shape. *Right*: Forehead angle before (*121,8°*) and after (*132,7°*) the surgery

Numerical simulations were carried out in *Ansys* environment. However, before that discreet models of individual bones had been prepared in *3-matic* programme compatible with *Mimics* software.

For the examined models simplifications were adopted in three basic categories: geometry, material and boundary conditions. Skull geometry, which was generated on the basis of CT images, was imported from *Mimics* programme without skin, blood vessels and other structures. Also, one did not take into consideration joints between the anatomical elements of the skull, such as cartilages, sutures, etc. Preparatory proceedings were similar for all of the below-mentioned cases. The generated bone models with adequate incisions were digitalized. In order to optimize the model, Laplace's method of approximating integrals was used several times (an inbuilt function of the software) with a coefficient equal to $0.4 \div 0.7$. Next, they were divided into tetrahedral finite elements of Solid 72 type, whose maximum length of edges did not exceed 3 mm. Then, a volumetric mesh was generated in order to finally export the model to **.cdb* format. Such actions caused the loss of geometrical details which were deemed irrelevant.

Material properties of the skull were adopted as isotropic in the process of modelling. It is evident that in the modelling of long bones or adult bones the bone should be treated as anisotropic material. However, both in this work and other research works [3, 6, 7] such simplification was accepted. The value of Young's modulus was adopted at the level of 380 MPa and Poisson's ratio equal to 0.22, which had been determined in earlier research [14]. These values are close to the results obtained by other researchers.

The last category of the simplification premises includes the boundary conditions of the model. After the introduction of the model into *Ansys* environment, the skull bones were fixed in the sites where there are natural joints: fusion of bones and cartilages. It should be pointed out that these joints are elastic joints (sutures), while in the static analysis a rigid fixation is necessary, which can on the other hand cause the occurrence of local concentration of stress. Further displacements were subsequently set. They had been measured during the correction planning done in cooperation with the doctor. The values of displacements were also averaged with a view to avoiding additional calculation errors.

Table 2 List of simplification assumptions

Category	Description
Model geometry	Models were digitalized by means of tetrahedral elements Solid 72
	Skin and other adjacent soft tissues were omitted
	Anatomic joints were omitted: fusions of bones and cartilages
	Geometrical model was smoothed by means of Laplace function
Material characteristics	Skull bone material was adopted as isotropic [12, 14]
	Young modulus E = 380 MPa
	Poisson's ratio $\mu = 0{,}22$
Boundary conditions	Models were fixed in the sites of sutures
	Averaged values of displacements were introduced, which had been determined in Mimics software during the correction planning
	Impact of adjacent structures was omitted
Solution	Total deformation
	Reduced strain (von Mises Hypothesis)
	Reduced stresses (von Mises Hypothesis)

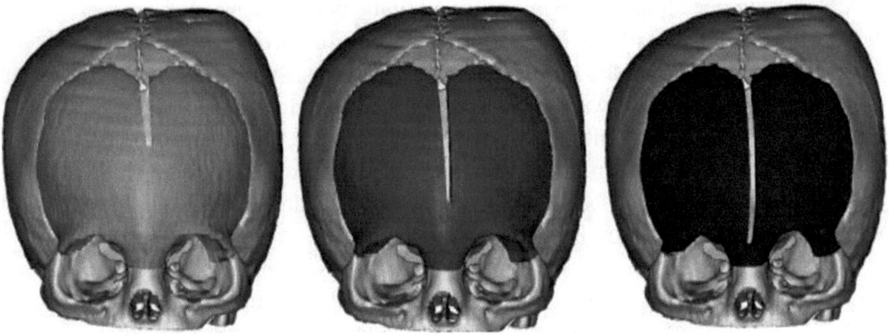

Fig. 13 Applied variants of frontal bone incisions being 30, 50 and 70 mm long

The analysis determined the total deformation, reduced strain and stresses with the use of von Mises hypothesis. An abridged list of simplification assumptions has been presented in Table 2.

Three variants of incisions were prepared for the analysis (Fig. 13) being 30, 50 and 70 mm long respectively. Simulation was performed in order to ensure that no damage to the bones occurs during the medical procedure due to the deformation done by a certain value.

After the model geometry had been introduced, a rigid fixation was placed in the site of the frontal bone (in the vicinity of *nasion* point)—(Fig. 14). Moreover, the displacements in axes x and z were completely restricted in the sites of the

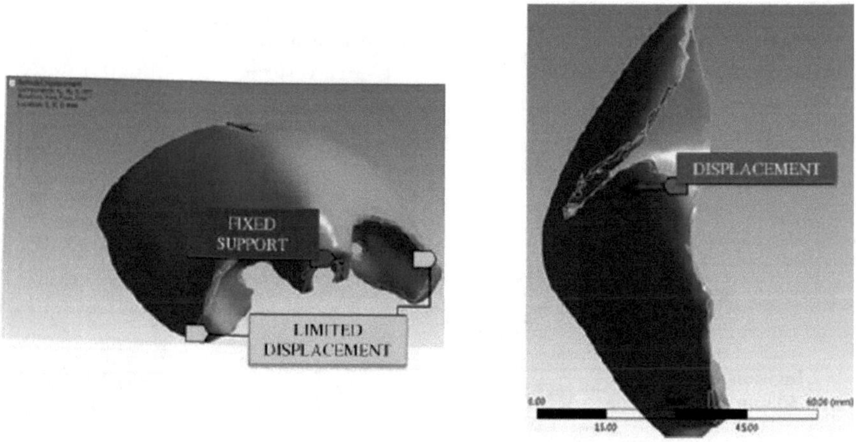

Fig. 14 Boundary conditions of trigonocephaly correction. *Left*: Fixation of model. *Right*: Points of application of displacement equal to 11 mm in y axis

frontoparietal suture. Also, the dislocation of these sites in *y* axis was partially limited (a maximum value of 6 mm was determined on the basis of the simulation results in Mimics software). It was calculated that displacement of upper parts of the incised halves of the frontal bone necessary to obtain an optimum shape of the skull equals 11 mm in the direction of *y* axis.

The results of numerical analysis have been presented in Table 3. The distribution of displacements has been taken into consideration as well as the maps of stresses occurring in the frontal bone in different incision variants. The case subject to examination is an example of one of the simplest methods of treatment in the context of incision technique. It results mainly from the fact that this is a microinvasive procedure, therefore the possibilities to use different incisions are small due to the limitations connected with the operative field and the applied surgical tools. Further part of this work presents an example of a classic surgical procedure of trigonocephaly correction.

Analysing the results of the simulation it was stated that the distribution of bones displacement is very similar in all three variants. Considerable differences may be noticed in maximum values of stresses occurring at the time of bone modelling. In the first variant they are the smallest and equal max 43 MPa, in the second variant 54 MPa. In both cases the stresses do not exceed permissible values, therefore it can be assumed that no bone damage will occur during the surgical procedure. In the third variant, maximum stresses equal 62.5 MPa. This variant was rejected due to the fact that too deep incision is always more risky as to the fracture of the bone in the vicinity of *nasion* point. At the same time, the visual effect does not differ much from the result obtained in variant 2. Variant 1 was also rejected as in this case the incision could prove too small to enable further correct growth of the skull. Finally, on the grounds of the quantitative and qualitative assessment variant 2 of the correction was adopted as optimal.

Table 3 Results of numerical simulations for skull with trigonocephaly

Variant	Model	Total deformation	Reduced stress
„1" **Incision:** **30 mm**	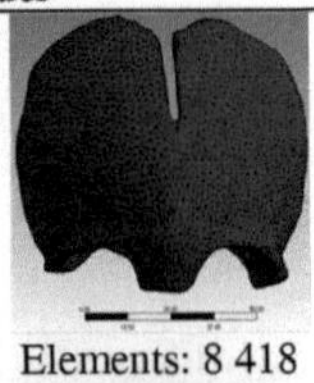 Elements: 8 418 Nodes: 46 779	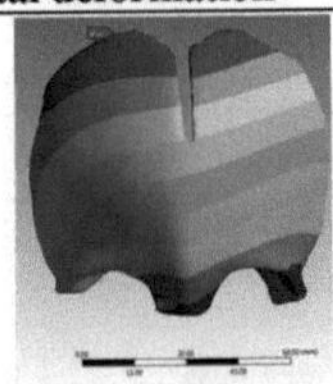 Max: 11,56 mm	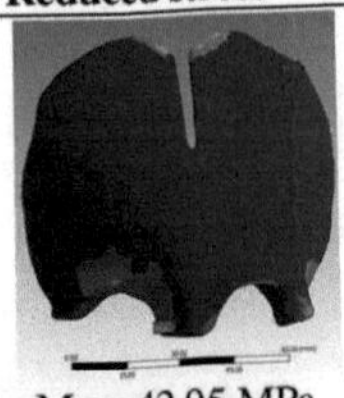 Max: 42,95 MPa
„2" **Incision** **50 mm**	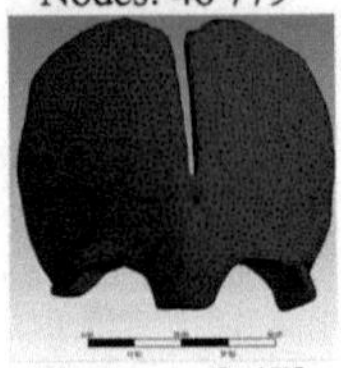 Elements: 8 478 Nodes: 47 108	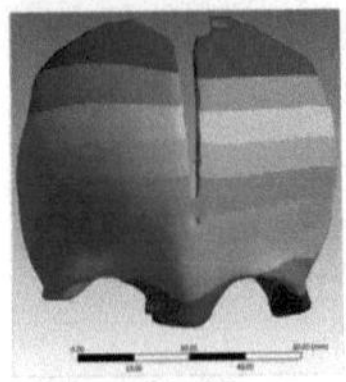 Max: 11,43 mm	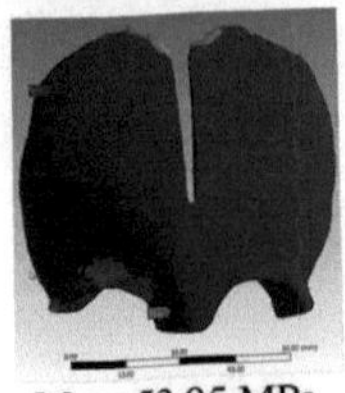 Max: 53,95 MPa
„3" **Incision:** **70 mm**	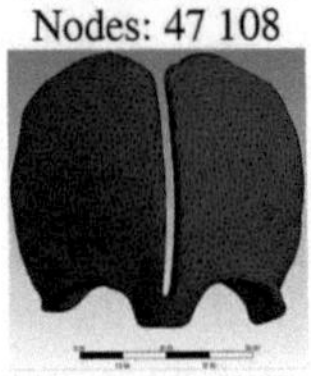 Elements: 8 369 Nodes: 46 369	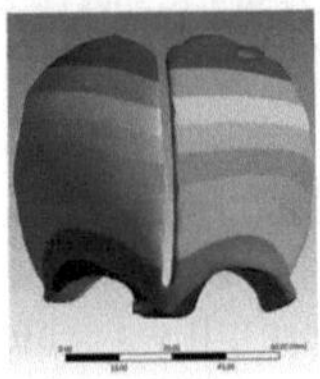 Max: 11,53 mm	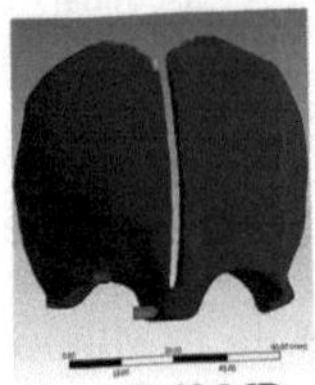 Max:62,48 MPa

2.2 *Application of Engineering Support in Preoperative Planning of Pigeon Chest Correction*

The most common chest deformities (considered developmental anomalies) in children include funnel chest (pectus excavatum) and pigeon chest (pectus carinatum). Funnel chest usually requires surgical treatment in order to restore correct breathing parameters [15]. Whereas, in the case of pigeon chest an early discovery of the defect makes it possible to undertake a non-invasive treatment, for instance by means of orthoses. Pigeon chest is a deformity of the anterior wall of the chest characterized by a strong deformation of the sternum and parasternal fragments of the ribs. The authors of this work present in cooperation with thoracic surgeons preoperative planning of the correction procedure of pigeon chest in a 13-year-old boy.

In the first place, the evaluation of the malformation degree was carried out with the use of the Haller index (Fig. 15) defined as a relationship of the chest width in the transverse plane to the distance between the sternum and spine. That was done in order to decide if a surgical procedure was necessary. The Haller index equals 2.5 for a normally formed chest, whereas in the examined patient it amounted to 1.71, which confirmed the increased anterior and posterior dimension.

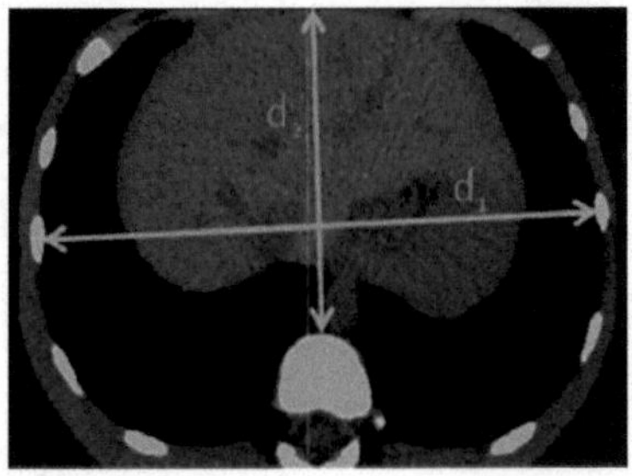

Fig. 15 Determining haller index

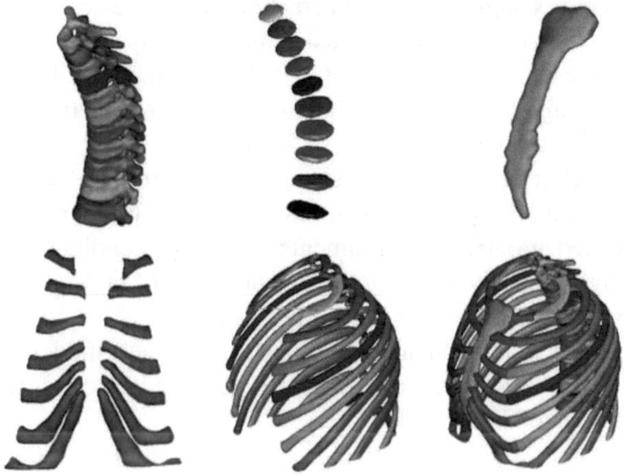

Fig. 16 Three-dimensional geometrical models of human pigeon chest elements

In the next stage, a geometrical model of the chest was started to be developed. On the basis of the patient's CT images using *Mimics* software a three-dimensional model of individual structures of the chest was developed. The process of building a geometrical model consisted in generating and editing masks of individual elements. The creation of a mask in *Mimics* environment consists in segmentation by means of partition of homogeneous areas as to grey shades in a previously defined search area. In the process of segmentation of the pigeon chest model the following items were distinguished (Fig. 16):

- 22 Bone ribs,
- 11 Thoracic vertebrae,
- 10 Intervertebral discs,
- 14 Cartilage ribs
- Sternum.

The algorithm of creating the above-mentioned elements was very similar in each case except for intervertebral discs and cartilage ribs which required more correction with the use of masks editing tools due to a heterogeneous grey shade.

Next, one began planning of the correction treatment of the defect by means of Ravitch's method. It consisted in resection of the elements of the cartilage ribs

Fig. 17 Comparison of chest shape before and after the virtual correction

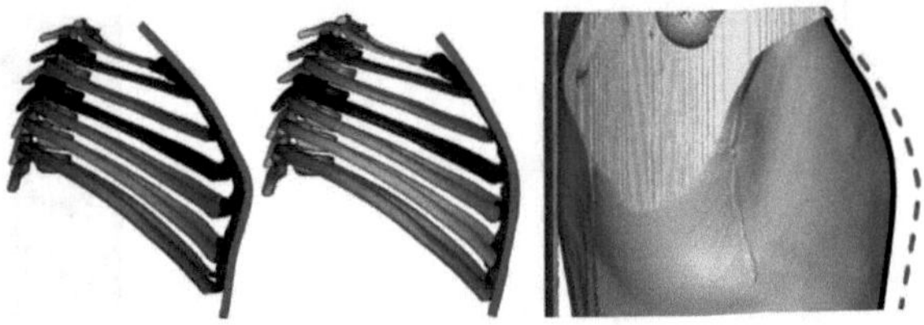

and sternum as well as their adequate rotation and repositioning. Displacement and rotation of the fragments of the bones were set manually taking into consideration the doctor's suggestions and actual circumstances of the surgical procedure. A correct position of the sternum was obtained by repositioning it in the direction towards the spine by about 30 mm (Fig. 17). At the same time, by removing the fragments of the cartilage ribs and by moving them one decreased the inclination angle of the sternum to the median plane from 24.26° to 13.05.

After obtaining an optimum visual effect of the correction, the dislocations of several bone points were measured. In the further phase of planning they were introduced into *Ansys* environment as boundary conditions. All elements of the chest were digitalized by tetrahedral elements Solid72 in 3-matic programme. The volumetric mesh was created and optimized (Fig. 18).

The numerical analysis of the pigeon chest model was performed with the use of *Ansys Workbench* environment. The boundary conditions of the analysis have been presented in Table 4.

With a view to carrying out simplification of the numerical model one omitted the impact of internal organs as well as pressure inside the thorax. The total number of finite elements amounted to 299 974, which were connected in 550 482 nodes. Contacts between individual elements were done automatically in the first stage, then their surfaces were corrected manually. The surfaces were linked by means of a 'Bonded' type connection, which does not allow the elements to dislocate in relation to each other. The total number of all connections amounted to 70. The model was fixed by means of taking away the degree of freedom in the nodes on the upper surface of the first thoracic vertebra and the lower surface of 11-th vertebra.

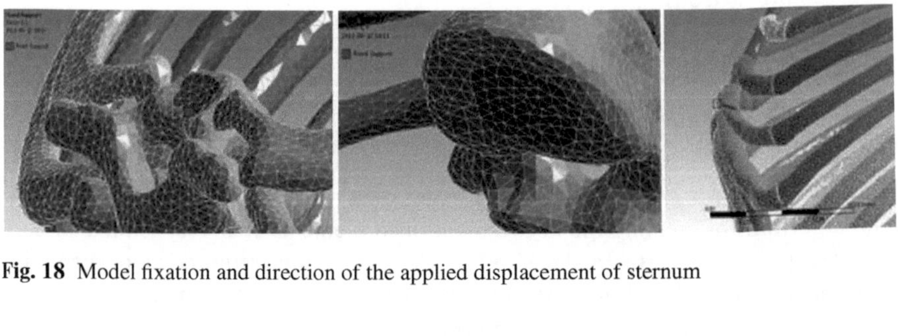

Fig. 18 Model fixation and direction of the applied displacement of sternum

Table 4 List of boundary conditions for numerical analysis of pigeon chest

Category	Description		
Model geometry	Models were divided into tetrahedral elements Solid 72		
	It was omitted impact of internal organs and pressure inside the thorax		
	Surfaces were joined by bonds of a 'bonded' type		
	Finite element mesh was smoothed by Laplace's function		
Material characteristics	bone material was adopted as isotropic [4, 11]		
		Young modulus [MPa]	*Poisson's ratio*
	Bony rib	5000.0	0.3
	Cartilage rib	24.5	0.3
	Sternuin, vertebrae	11500.0	0,.3
	Intervertebral disc	110.04	0.4
Boundary conditions	Models were fixed in 1 and 11 thoracic vertebrae		
	Displacement of the sternum by 30 mm, which was determined in *Mimics* software during the correction planning, was introduced		

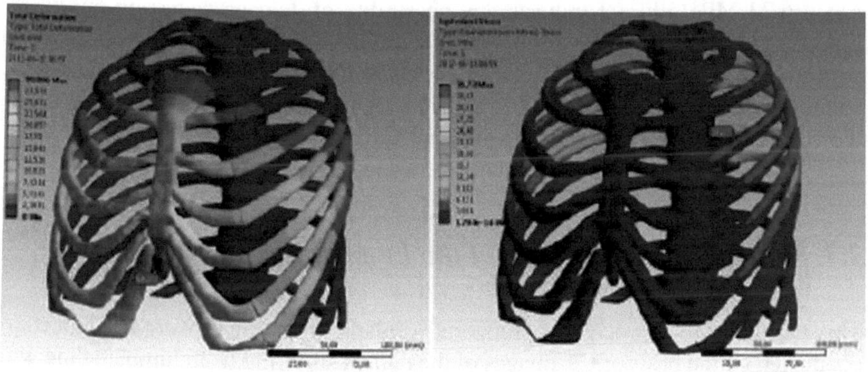

Fig. 19 Results of numerical simulation of correction. *Left*: Map of deformation. *Right*: Map of equivalent stresses

During the numerical analysis, reduced strain and stresses were determined with the use of von Mises hypothesis. The results of the numerical analysis have been shown in Fig. 19.

On the basis of the performed numerical calculations the index of the model stiffness was determined. It was defined according to the below formula (1) which equalled 2.86 for the analyzed case.

$$k = \frac{F}{d} \left[\frac{N}{mm} \right] \tag{1}$$

where F is the measured force and d is the measured displacement

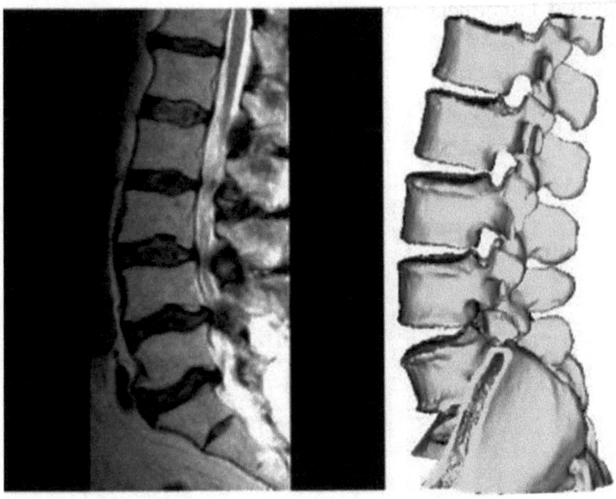

Fig. 20 Lumbar spine with degeneration process and spondylolisthesis. *Left*: CT examination. *Right*: 3D model

While analyzing the findings of the simulation it was stated that the distribution of maximum stresses in the sternum (6.92 MPa), cartilage ribs (8.39 MPa) and bone ribs (36.73 MPa) did not indicate any possibility of damage occurring during the procedure of the pigeon chest correction by Ravitch's method as they were all lower than 87.0 MPa, which was adopted as a permissible value. The obtained maximum values of main deformations 0.0012 in bone elements of the chest were also below the values suggesting the bone destruction [24].

2.3 Preoperative Planning of the Lumbar Spine Stabilization

This part presents a process of preoperative planning of a neurosurgical procedure conducted on the basis of CT images of the patient suffering from lumbar spine with degeneration process and spondylolisthesis.

In the presented case preoperative planning concerned the lumbar spine degeneration and mild form of bulging of L4/L5 intervertebral disc.

CT images processing was done with the use of *Mimics* software. The spine structures, which were important due to mechanical aspects, were segmented on the basis of masks assigned to them. The development of the masks consisted in matching the upper and lower threshold of the grey shade level corresponding to individual structures. The vertebrae segmentation was performed using masks covering the areas in which given vertebrae were located. The effect of the performed operations has been presented in Fig. 20.

The created geometrical models of the anatomical structures of the spine constitute the basis for further procedures aiming to check the degree of the implant matching by means of the simulation of a surgical procedure. At this stage a 3D model of stabilization executed in CAD software can be transferred to *Mimics* programme (in STL format). Next step is to adjust the implant in the site of the predicted stabilization.

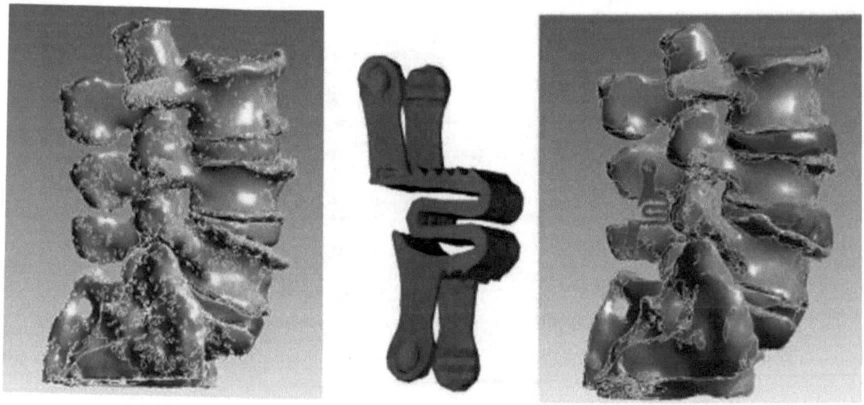

Fig. 21 Model of spine segment before and after stabilization with the Coflex implant

Precise positioning of the implant in the spine as well as the fact that the surgical procedure is microinvasive play an essential role during the implant insertion. The performed simulation makes it possible to verify the construction by checking compatibility of main stabilization measurements with individual anatomical features of the patient. In this case it was used an implant by Coflex company which is used in clinical practice for lumbar spine stabilization with posterior intervertebral systems (Fig. 21).

In the case of application of ready-made implants available on the market, the preoperative planning enables it to choose from the catalogued series of types the best kind and type of stabilization matching an individual patient. Geometrical models of L4 and L5 vertebrae were modified in the site of the implant positioning, exactly like during a surgical procedure. Material properties were attributed to stabilization. They were determined as follows: titanium alloy Ti-6Al-4 V, i.e. Young modulus equal to 115 GPa and Poisson's ratio equal to 0.3 [23].

For the sake of subsequent strength analysis the model was digitalized with the use of a finite element method MES. Each element of the performed model had a mesh created by means of tetragonal elements of an average edge distance of 3 mm. Then, material properties were determined for individual elements. The programme *Mimics* by the firm *Materialise*, which was used in this research, makes it possible to define proportions and distribution of the material within the object. The programme enables it to attribute to each spatial element as many properties as defined by the designer. Cortical bone tissue is different from compact bone not only in its structure but also in mechanical properties. That is why cortical bone and spongy bone were distinguished within each vertebra. In order to segment the spongy bone tissue the functions available in *Mimics* software were applied. To achieve that it was necessary to make the mask areas of spongy bone on the vertebra contours in all cross sections

The masks served the purpose of providing the areas covered by defined masks with spongy bone material properties. This tool of the programme was used while defining material properties of other anatomical structures on the basis of the already

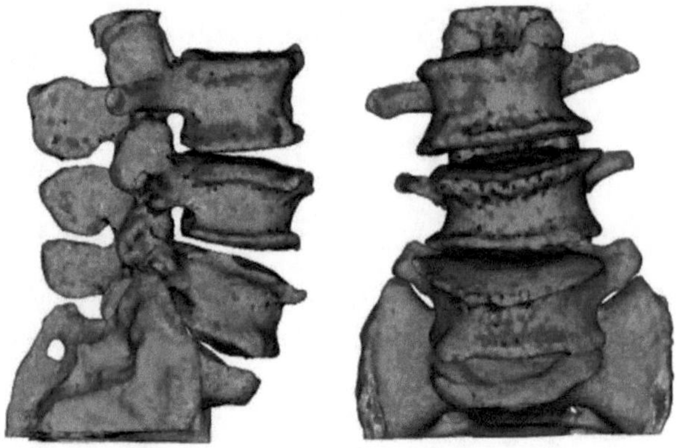

Fig. 22 Spine model revealing differentiation of bone tissue

Table 5 Material properties of spinal structures used in numerical simulations

Structure	Young modulus [MPa]	Poisson's ratio
Compact bone (vertebrae)	10000,0	0,3
Spongy bone (vertebrae)	100,0	0,3
Intervertebral disc	200,0	0,49
Nerves	10,0	0,3

created masks. The values of the determined properties have been placed in Table 5, whereas the graphic distribution of tissues has been presented in Fig. 22.

A key factor taken into consideration in the selection of a stabilization type for the lumbar spine is the impact it will exert on the stabilized section. Numerical simulations of the models of the physiological section of the human lumbar spine as well as numerical simulations of the posterior interspinal stabilization make it possible to analyse the degree of load on the spine and the influence of implantation on spinal properties. The analysis of the spinal load and of the impact of the conducted implantation on the lumbar spine properties was made in *ANSYS* programme. In order to achieve that, the executed models, both physiological one and stabilized one, were imported to that programme. Calculations were carried out with the set boundary conditions equal to loads occurring in a natural standing position. The load amounting to 1000 N was set on the upper surface of vertebra L3 while fixation was set on the lower surface of vertebra L5/S1 (Fig. 23).

While analyzing the obtained results of compression it was noticed that resultant values of displacements are higher for the physiological spine model than in the case of the implant model. Their maximum values equal respectively 0.45 mm for the model without implant, and 0.22 mm for the model with implant. The biggest reduction of stresses determined according to Huber-Mises hypothesis occurred in the bone tissue, at the vertebral pedicle. The values did not exceed 36 MPa for the physiological model. However, for the spine-and-implant system the highest

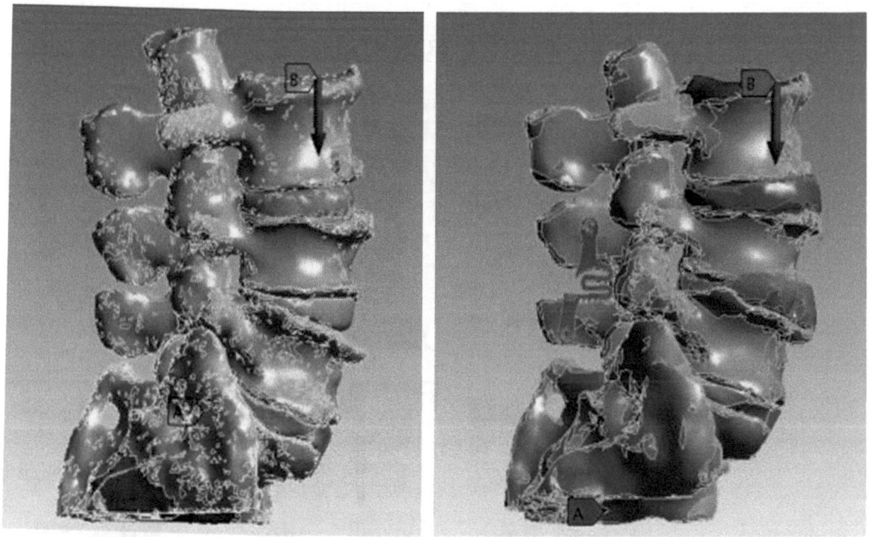

Fig. 23 Boundary conditions (*A-support, B-load*) before and after stabilization

intensity of stresses occurred in the very implant amounting to 37 MPa. In the spine-and-implant system one observed lower values of strain than in the physiological model. Maximum values of strain equalled respectively 0.016 and 0.008 (Table 6).

The conducted analyses make it possible to state that the implanted stabilization has improved the spine stability. After the implant positioning the values of resultant displacements decreased during strength simulations. It resulted from the fact that the degenerated movable segment was stabilized with the use of the implant as well as due to the material properties forming the implant. Also it is significant that after stabilization the cross-section areas of spinal nerves increase (Fig. 24), therefore it can be concluded that the patient's pain will decrease.

The performed research shows how medical and biomechanical interpretation of numerical simulations can be used to plan neurosurgical procedure of spine stabilization. Biomechanical analyses of strength and forces can ascertain the durability and stability of the implant connection with the stabilized section of spine and also determine places that require reconstruction of bone. With finite element method, surgical prediction can be made to guide surgeons to make the decision of improving surgical treatment. Virtual planning of the treatment is helpful for the neurosurgeons, because it increases the quality of treatment and safety during the operation.

3 Conclusions

Preoperative planning of medical procedures with engineering support definitely facilitates the achievement of desirable effects of treatment. Contemporary technical and technological advances, particularly in bone surgery, encourage the implemen-

Table 6 Results of numerical simulations

	Total deformation	Reduced strain	Reduced stress
Before stabilization	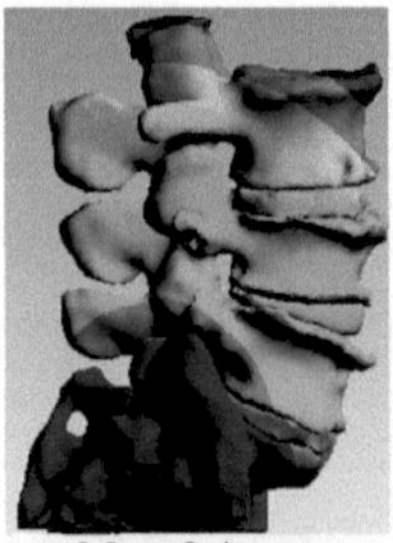 Max: 0,4 mm	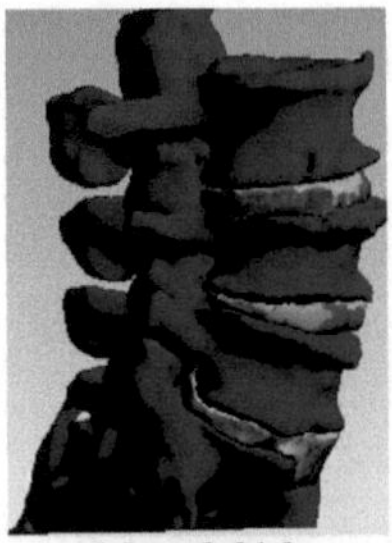 Max: 0,016	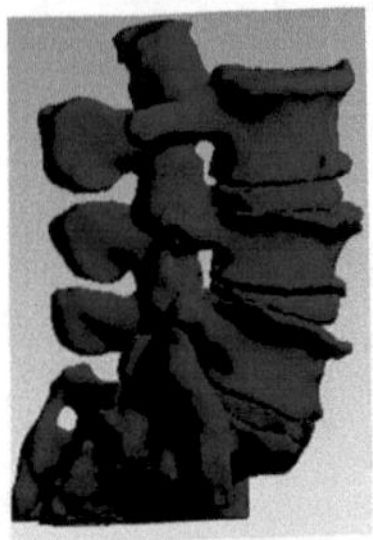 Max: 36 MPa
After stabilization	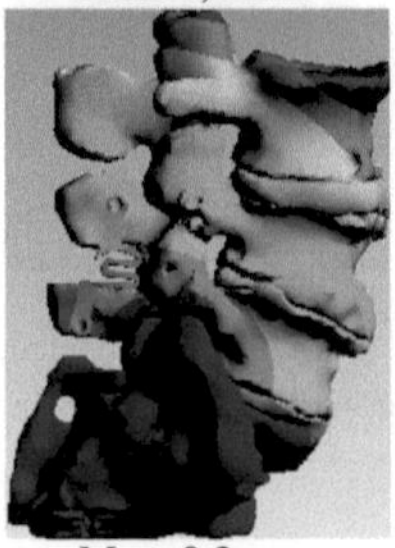 Max: 0,2 mm	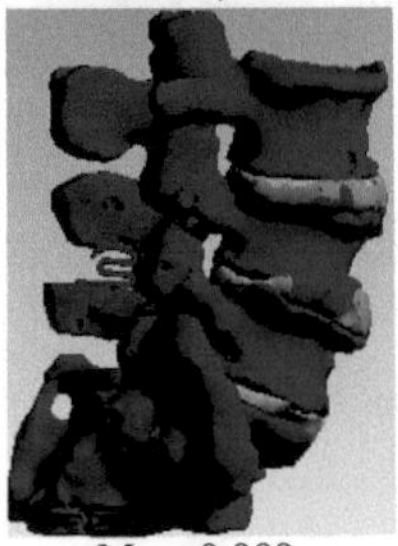 Max: 0,009	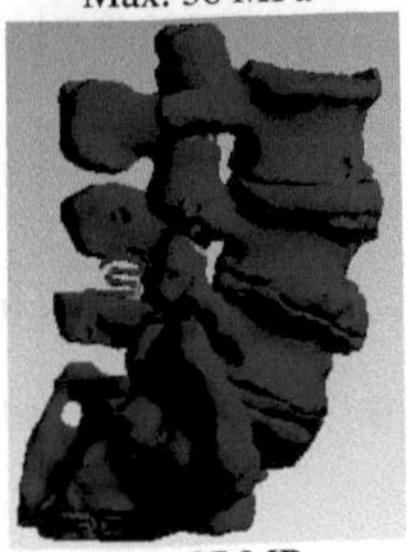 Max: 37 MPa

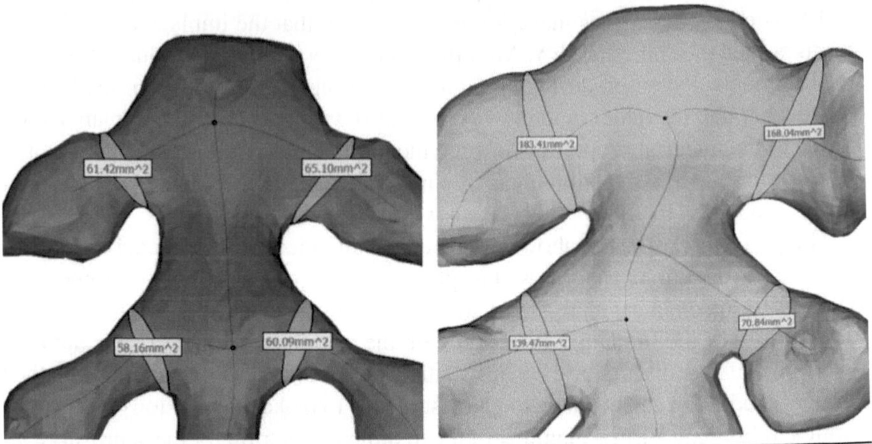

Spinal level	Right		Left	
	Before	After	Before	After
L3-L4	61 mm^2	183 mm^2	65 mm^2	168 mm^2
L4-L5	58 mm^2	139 mm^2	60 mm^2	71 mm^2

Fig. 24 Cross-section areas of the spinal nerves before and after stabilization

tation of new innovative ideas and cutting edge technology into operative technique aiming at the application of microinvasive procedures. There are several CAD programmes which could become a perfect biomechanical tool complementing medical knowledge. Such software makes it possible to do, among other things, mechanical analyses as well as to plan surgical procedures. Preoperative planning may be supplemented by an additional procedure of reconstructing anatomical structures and performing a virtual medical operation (simulation) in the computer system. The models obtained in such a way may also serve the purpose of engineering analysis which aims at characterizing the interaction of tissues in time as well as assessing the risk of bone damage or fracture during a surgical procedure. The developed method of engineering support makes it easier for the doctors to make right decisions at each stage of treatment. This kind of support may have a significant importance for young inexperienced surgeons or medical students. However, even experienced doctors may practise each phase of the surgical procedure virtually, which considerably shortens the duration of the operation. The application of a complex planning procedure is simply indispensable in the case of complicated, multi-phase surgical procedures. Its major advantage is an individual approach to each patient. The examples of planning surgical procedures show that engineering support increases patients' safety during the operation and improves the quality of treatment. Interdisciplinary collaboration between doctors and engineers brings desirable benefits and results in well-performed operations.

References

1. Altobelli DE, Kikinis R, Mulliken JB, Cline H, Lorensen W, Jolesz F (1993) Computed-assisted three-dimensional planning in craniofacial surgery. Plast Reconstr Surg 92:576–585
2. Barone CM, Jimenez DF (2004) Endoscopic approach to coronal craniosynostosis. Clin Plast Surg 31:415–422
3. Baumer TG, Powell BJ, Fenton TW, Haut RC (2009) Age dependent mechanical properties of the infant porcine parietal bone and a correlation to the human. J Biomech Eng 131(11):111–116
4. Bruchin R, Stock UA, Drucker JP, Zhari T, Wippermann J, Albes JM, Himtze D, Eckardt S, Konke C, Wahlers T (2005) Numerical simulation techniques to study the structural response of the human chest following median sternotomy. Ann Thorac Surg 80:623–630
5. Cimerman M, Kristan A (2007) Preoperative planning in pelvic and acetabular surgery: the value of advanced computerized planning modules. Injury 38(4):442–449
6. Coats B, Margulies SS (2006) Material properties of human infant skull and suture at highrates. J Neurotrauma 23:1222–1232
7. Couper ZS, Albermani FG (2005) Biomechanics of shaken baby syndrome: physical testing and numerical modeling. In: Deeks Hao (eds) Developments in mechanics of structures and materials. Taylor Francis Group, London, pp 213–218
8. Cutting C, Bookstein Fl, Grayson B, Fellingham L, Mccarthy JG (1986) Three dimensional computer-assisted design of craniofacial surgical procedures: optimization and interaction with cephalometric and CT-basedmodels. Plast Reconstr Surg 77:877–885
9. Cutting C, Grayson B, Bookstein F, Fellingham L, Mccarthy JG (1986) Computer-aided planning and evaluation of facial and orthognathic surgery. Clin Plast Surg 13:449–462
10. Ehmer U, Joos U, Flieger S, Wiechmann D (2012) The University Münster model surgery system for Orthognathic surgery. Part I—the idea behind. Head Face Med 8:14

11. Furusu K, Watanabe I, Kato Ch, Miki K, Hasegawa J (2001) Fundamental study of side impast analysis using the finite element model of the human thorax. JSAE 22:195–199
12. Gzik M, Wolański W, Kawlewska E, Larysz D, Kawlewski K (2011) Modeling and simulation of trigonocephaly correction with use of finite elements method. Proceedings of the III ECCOMAS thematic conference on computational vision and medical image processing: VipIMAGE, Portugal, pp 47–50
13. Gras F, Marintschev I, Wilharm A, Klos K, Mückley T, Hofmann G (2010) O: 2D-fluoroscopic navigated percutaneous screw fixation of pelvic ring injuries—a case series. BMC Musculoskelet Disord 11:153
14. Gzik M, Wolański W, Tejszerska D, Gzik-Zroska B, Koźlak M, Larysz D (2009) Interdisciplinary researches supporting neurosurgical correction of children head deformation. Model Optim Phys Syst 8:49–54
15. Gzik-Zroska B, Wolański W, Gzik M (2013) Engineering-aided treatment of chest deformities to improve the process of breathing. Int J Numer Method Biomed Eng 29:926–937
16. Handels H, Ehrhardt J, Plötz W, Pöppl SJ (2001) Three-dimensional planning and simulation of hip operations and computer-assisted construction of endoprostheses in bone tumor surgery. Comput Aided Surg 6(2):65–76 (Wiley Online Library)
17. Handels H, Ehrhardt J, Plötz W, Pöppl SJ (2000) Virtual planning of hip operations and individual adaption of endoprostheses in orthopaedic surgery. Int J Med Inform 58–59:21–28
18. Hu Y, Malthaner RA (2007) The feasibility of three-dimensional displays of the thorax for preoperative planning in the surgical treatment of lung cancer. Eur J Cardiothorac Surg 31:506–511
19. Jiang X, You J, Wang N, Shen Z, Li J (2010) Skull mechanics study of PI procedure plan for craniosynostosis correction based on finite element method, Proceedings of 4th International Conference on Bioinformatics and Biomedical Engineering (iCBBE)
20. Jimenez DF, Barone CM, Cartwright CC et al (2002) Early management of craniosynostosis using endoscopic-assisted strip craniectomies and cranial orthotic molding therapy. Pediatrics 110:97–104
21. Larysz D, Wolański W, Gzik M, Kawlewska E (2011) Virtual planning of the surgical treatment of baby skull shape correction. Model Optim Phys Syst 10:49–52
22. Larysz D, Wolański W, Kawlewska E, Mandera M, Gzik M (2012) Biomechanical aspects of preoperative planning of skull correction in children with craniosynostosis. Acta Bioeng Biomech 14:19–26
23. Marchetti C, Bianchi A, Muyldermans L, Di Martino M, Lancellotti L, Sarti A (2011) Validation of new soft tissue software in orthognathic surgery planning. Int J Oral Maxillofac Surg 40:26–32
24. Nackenhorst U (1997) Numerical simulation of stress stimulated bone remodeling. Technische Mech 17(1):31–40
25. Raaijmaakers M, Gelaude F, de Smedt K, Clijmans T, Dille J, Mulier M (2010) A custom-made guide-wire positioning device for hip surface replacement arthroplasty: description and first results. BMC Musculoskelet Disord 11:161
26. Sacha E, Tejszerska D, Larysz D, Gzik M, Wolański W (2010) Computer method in craniosynostosis. Proceedings of 12th International Scientific Conference "Applied Mechanics", Technical University of Liberec, pp 111–115
27. Szarek A, Stradomski G, Włodarski J (2012) The analysis of hip joint prosthesis head microstructure changes during variable stress state as a result of human motor activity. Mater Sci Forum 706–709:600–605
28. Tejszerska D, Wolański W, Larysz D, Gzik M, Sacha E (2011) Morphological analysis of the skull shape in craniosynostosis. Acta Bioeng Biomech 13(1):35–40
29. Wolański W, Larysz D, Gzik M, Kawlewska E (2013) Modeling and biomechanical analysis of craniosynostosis correction with the use of finite element method. Int J Numer Method Biomed Eng 29:916–925
30. Yasuda T, Hashimoto Y, Yokoi S, Toriwaki JI (1990) Computer system for craniofacial surgical planning based on CT images. IEEE Trans MedImaging 9:270–280

31. Materialise software & services for biomedical engineering: mimics software. http://biomedical.materialise.com/mimics. Accessed 13 March 2014
32. Materialise software & services for biomedical engineering: 3-matic software. http://biomedical.materialise.com/3-metic. Accessed 13 March 2014
33. ANSYS software. http://www.ansys.com/. Accessed 13 March 2014

Pretreatment and Reconstruction of Three-dimensional Images Applied in a Locking Reconstruction Plate for a Structural Analysis with FEA

João Paulo O. Freitas, Edson A. Capello de Sousa, Cesar R. Foschini, Rogerio R. Santos and Sheila C. Rahal

Abstract The concept about fracture stabilization by compression and the use of locking plates have been the interest of many studies. An understanding of the bone-plate construct stability is important for clinical use. Differences in plate geometries and materials have influenced in the results obtained. Thus, the present study evaluated the acquisition of images and geometric reconstruction seeking a more detailed study of its structure through the application of numerical methods such as finite elements. A seven-hole locking reconstruction plate manufactured with stainless steel was used as material model. Acquisition of geometric information was obtained from the profile projection method for simplified shapes such as curves and external rays. The micro CT (computed tomography) worked as additional information on details of the structure as volume and validation of data obtained from the projection profile.

1 Introduction

1.1 Bone Plate and Biological Considerations

There are many different sizes and shapes of bone plates available for fracture immobilization [15]. The dynamic compression plate (DCP) has oval holes to allow axial compression of the fracture site during screw tightening [6] and the construct stability requires plate-to-bone compression [15, 3]. Despite being widely used, the DCP may present disadvantages such as cortical loss under the plate, delayed union, and refracture after plate removal [15, 3, 6].

J. P. O. Freitas (✉) · E. A. C. de Sousa · C. R. Foschini
Faculdade de Engenharia de Bauru, Universidade Estadual Paulista—Unesp, Bauru, São Paulo, Brazil
e-mail: joaopaulo.web@gmail.com

R. R. Santos · S. C. Rahal
School of Veterinary Medicine and Animal Science, Universidade Estadual Paulista—Unesp, Botucatu, São Paulo, Brazil

J. M. R. S. Tavares, R. Natal Jorge (eds.), *Developments in Medical Image Processing and Computational Vision*, Lecture Notes in Computational Vision and Biomechanics 19,
DOI 10.1007/978-3-319-13407-9_10

The biological concept of the internal fixation of the fracture stimulated the development of a new approach to the plate fixation [9, 15]. Different from the conventional plate, in a locked plate the screw is locked into the plate and the forces are transferred from the bone to the plate through the threaded connection [15, 7, 6]. In addition, the plate compression on the bone is not required with this system and bone blood supply is preserved, but the stiffness of the construct determines the fracture stability [15].

The locked plate was initially developed to stabilize fractures with poor bone quality, such as osteoporosis, osteomalacia or comminution [11], but its use has been widespread [7]. Several modifications have been performed in locked plate designs [7, 3]. However, concerns about the adequate use of these plates have been raised [11]. Pre-operative planning and care with biomechanical principles are important to locked compression plate be successful [12]. Factors such as number, orientation angle, and monocortical or bicortical placement of the locked screws may influence fixation strength [13, 10, 4, 3, 8]. Furthermore, the use inadequate of locked screws can produce a more stiff construct that may compromise fracture healing [11].

Thus, an understanding of the bone-plate construct stability is important for clinical use. Biomechanical studies performed by static and dynamical tests are necessary to determine the construct stiffness, strength and failure mode of the plating configurations [13, 10, 4, 2, 8]. Mechanical properties may also be evaluated by using numerical models such as Finite Element Analysis [13, 14]. A first step in a study is to analyze the geometry of plates already manufactured.

1.2 Geometry

Biomechanical geometries are a constant study focus, because it is common to have problems in their reconstruction. Many studies suggest the process using computed tomography (CT), manual measurements, 3D scan, and others. When the object has a complex geometry the method with 3D scan and CT are more required. If only the surface is the center of study, scan 3D can be used if the surfaces are not polished. However, if the internal layers are important, CT is used. In this case is necessary more knowledge in medical softwares.

Simple geometries do not require so much. Measurementments can be made both by simple instruments such as a caliper rule or a profile projector and by sophisticated equipment such as a scanner and computed tomography.

These methods are appropriate when the product is simple and do not want to spend much time.

However, in order to obtain the quality in the measurements and in the same time the geometry with simple surfaces, both methods can be merged. Manual and visual measurements show the large sizes and the global shape, and micro CT gives details about small sizes and local shapes, like radius of curvatures.

For the analysis of the structure, it is necessary to have a geometry with volumetric information, i.e. through a solid model.

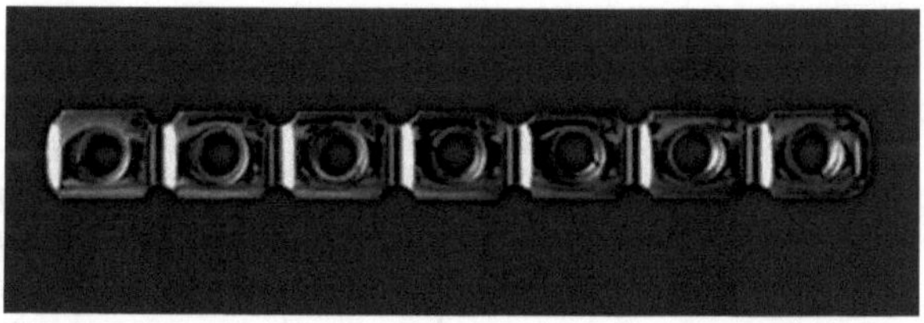

Fig. 1 Seven-hole locking reconstruction plate

Computer Aidded Design (CAD) is the ideal type of software for this. With CAD software is possible to model the geometry from measurement data already obtained and the final geometry is the base for Finite Element Analysis.

1.3 Finite Element Analysis (FEA)

When designing a structure, know all details about the actual problem is really important. A first analysis is made to create a model able to represent the current structure. This model provides all balance equations from mathematical relationships known by mechanical studies. These equations translate the physics behavior of the structure. The mathematical manipulation provides enough data to study internal strength, showing all displacements, deformations and stresses. These data need analyses, comparing the results with what was expected in the proposed model.

This procedure is valid for any beginning of the project, as well as its development, but when geometries are more complex (when compared with simple problems from mechanical classic) the solution is not accurate and it is in this context that the finite element method provides an approximate solution from the discretization of a continuous system.

The parameters that describe the behavior of the system are the nodal displacements [1]. From them it is possible to analyze the internal forces, stresses, and evaluate the strength of the analyzed structure.

Finite Element Method (FEM) calculation had been showed as a valid method applied in biomechanics systems when the results can be used for fixing problems in prostheses [5].

Applying FEM with computer support, the solver (part of FEA responsible for the calculation) can calculate many equations in a short time. Impossible problems to be answered with manual calculation in the past, now have good results for complex problems.

2 Material and Methods

2.1 Plate

A seven-hole locking reconstruction plate manufactured with stainless steel (Free Block—Biomechanical) was used as material model to the study (Fig. 1). The locking

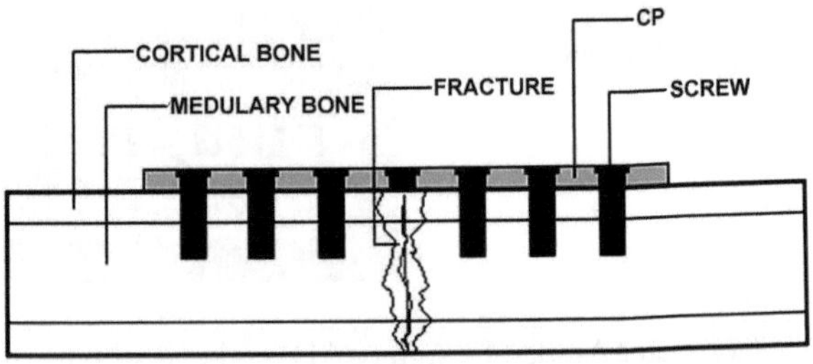

Fig. 2 Schematic illustration of the bone–plate fixation using monocortical locked screws

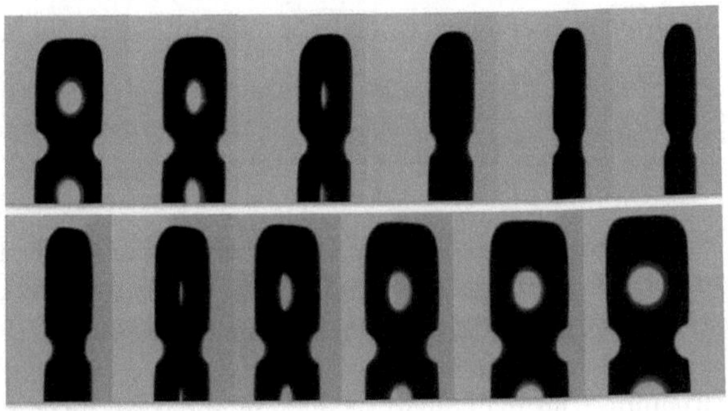

Fig. 3 Some projection images from process of micro CT

reconstruction plate may be used to treat certain types of fractures using bicortical or monocortical locked screws (Fig. 2).

2.2 *Data Acquisition*

The information about the geometry was obtained with two methods. The first method was the profile projection and the second one was the micro CT. The profile projector used was a Mitutoyo PJ311.

With this information, it was possible to evaluate the larger sizes such as length, thickness, diameters, and others. These values were compared with the ones obtained with the digital caliper rule Western DC-60.

The micro CT SkyScan 1176 was used to obtain details about curves and radius. It is important to remember that with the files generated with micro CT, it is possible to reconstruct the 3D file using medical softwares and export the results in Stereolithography (stl) files. However, in the present study the main objective was to develop the geometry using only direct measurements, a type of method more efficient for simple geometries and resulting in fewer problems with surfaces in meshing for FEA.

In order to show an example of SkyScan results in micro CT, the Fig. 3 presents some projected images from the process. These projections need to be transformed into slices for reconstruction.

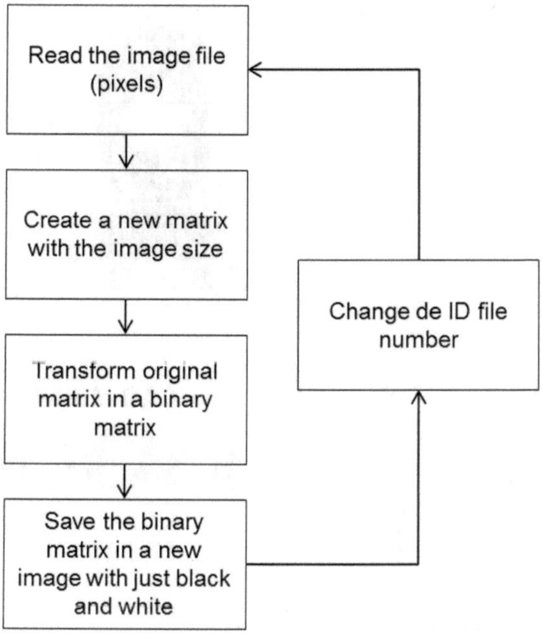

Fig. 4 Matlab routine used to convert the slices of micro CT in binary images for reconstruction

2.3 *Image Treatment*

During the work with images obtained using CT or micro CT, it is common to present noises or contours less defined. If the interest is to reconstruct the three-dimensional image with quality in measurements and details, the image treatment is crucial. For this, there are many ways to convert the files with problems into quality files within the tolerance.

The suggested method for the present study was to use one algorithm written in MATLAB code with a simple algorithm that is able to convert one image file of CT to a binary image which is formed by zero and one that represent the black and white colors.

The control of boundary in the image is made with values obtained from manual and visual measurements already made before. So, if the contour is a resolved problem, the details of geometry can be observed with more precision.

The simple routine used is described in Fig. 4, and an example (one slice image of micro CT) before and after of the treatment with algorithm can be visualized in Fig. 5.

2.4 *CAD Software and Mesh File*

After obtaining all information about the geometry, the next step was to load them in CAD software. There are many types of softwares that can be applicable, but in

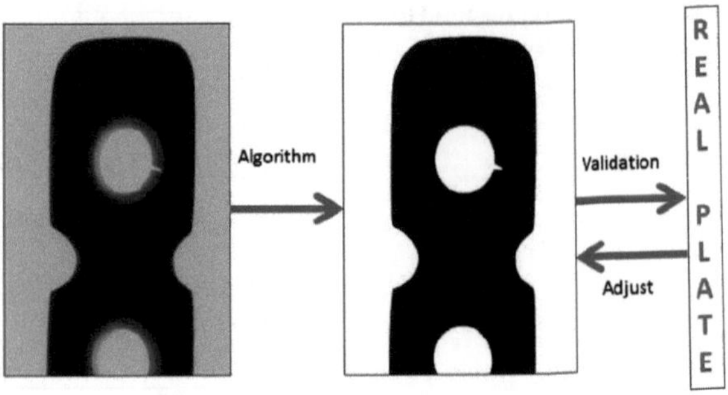

Fig. 5 Image treatment for one slice and validation method

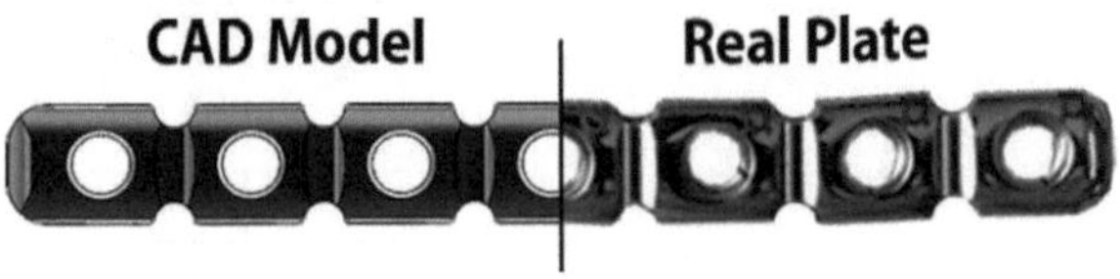

Fig. 6 CAD model and real plate

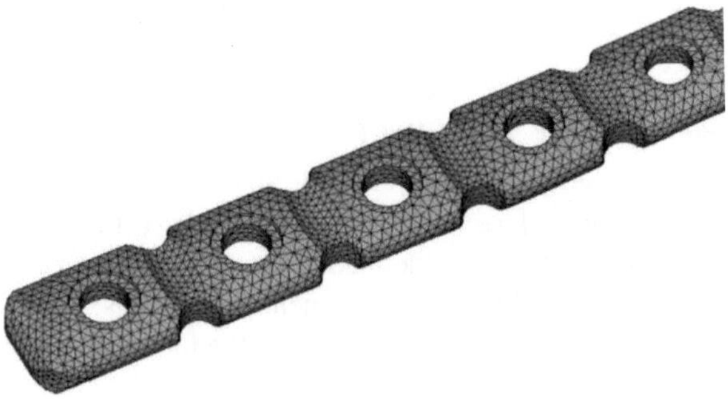

Fig. 7 Partial mesh of plate generated in Ansys

the present study it was chosen Solidworks 2012, because the tools are very simple and the toolbox of surfaces and molds are very useful for reconstructed geometries. In this software is possible to define regions of interest for analysis.

These regions are mapped for the FEM meshing. The mapping is important because it defines the quality of elements, and hence the quality of results.

Figure 6 shows a comparison between the real plate and the model made with Solidworks.

The final geometry is exported in parasolid (*.x_t) extension and imported in the FEM software. In this case was used Ansys APDL 11. The meshing generation was controlled by the finite element size in each line of the geometry. The first mesh created can be visualized in Fig. 7.

3 Results

The image treatment has proved an efficient method to obtain measurements and, in spite of having not been tested, the binary files should be useful for three-dimensional reconstruction with medical softwares support. The Fig. 5 shows the results for one slice.

The model in CAD had good results. Figure 6 shows a qualitative result.

Figure 7 shows how important is the mesh control for a good result in meshing generation. With all models developed like bones and screws, it is possible to apply the boundary conditions in this model and run the solution to provide the behavior of the plate in various conditions.

4 Conclusions

The present study evaluated the acquisition of images and geometric reconstruction seeking a more detailed study of its structure through the application of numerical methods such as finite elements.

A seven-hole locking reconstruction plate manufactured with stainless steel was used as material model. Acquisition of geometric information was obtained from the method of projection profile for simplified shapes such as curves and external rays. The micro CT worked in obtaining additional information on details of the structure as volume and validating the data obtained from the projection profile. Using this method was possible to generate a 3D-model with good quality.

References

1. Alves Filho A (2001) Elementos finitos—A base da tecnologia CAE—Análise dinâmica. ÉRICA, Brazil
2. Cabassu JB, Kowaleski MP, Skorinko JK et al (2011) Single cycle to failure in torsion of three standard and five locking plate constructs. Vet Comp Orthop Traumatol 24:418–425
3. Cronier P, Pietu G, Dujardin C et al (2010) The concept of locking plates. Orthop Traumatol Surg Res 96:17–36
4. Fitzpatrick DC, Doornink J, Madey SM et al (2009) Relative stability of conventional and locked plating fixation in a model of the osteoporotic femoral diaphysis. Clin Biomech 24:203–209
5. Gomes EA, Sousa EAC, Assunção WG (2007) Stress analysis of the prostheses/implant/retention screw set without passive fit using MEF-2D. In: Abstracts of the 19th International congress of mechanical engineering, Brasília, DF, 5–9 November 2007
6. Igna C, Schuszler L (2010) Current concepts of internal plate fixation of fractures. Bulletin UASVM 67:118–123
7. Kubiak EN, Fulkerson E, Strauss E et al (2006) The evolution of locked plates. J Bone Joint Surg Am 88:189–200
8. Merino MKA, Rahal SC, Ribeiro CR, Padovani CR et al (2013) The effect of locked screw angulation on the biomechanical properties of the S.P.S. Free-Block plate. Vet Comp Orthop Traumatol 26:117–122

9. Perren SM (2002) Evolution of the internal fixation of long bone fractures. J Bone Joint Surg Br 84:1093–1110
10. Roberts JW, Grindel SI, Rebholz B et al (2007) Biomechanical evaluation of locking plate radial shaft fixation: unicortical locking fixation versus mixed bicortical and unicortical fixation in a sawbone mode. J Hand Surg Am 32:971–975
11. Scolaro J, Ahn J (2011) Locked plating in practice: indications and current concepts. Univ Pennsylvania Orthop J 21:18–22
12. Sommer C, Babst R, Muller M et al (2004) Locking compression plate loosening and plate breakage: a report of four cases. J Orthop Trauma 18:571–577
13. Stoffel K, Dieter U, Stachowiak G et al (2003) Biomechanical testing of the LCP—how can stability in locked internal fixators be controlled? Injury 34(Suppl. 2):11–19
14. Taheri E, Sepehri B, Ganji R et al (2012) Effect of screws placement on locking compression plate for fixating medial transverse fracture of tibia. Biomed Eng Res 1:13–18
15. Wagner M (2003) General principles for the clinical use of the LCP. Injury 34(Suppl 2):31–42

Tortuosity Influence on the Trabecular Bone Elasticity and Mechanical Competence

Waldir Leite Roque and Angel Alberich-Bayarri

Abstract Osteoporosis is a disease characterized by a remarkable bone mass loss and trabecular bone degradation, which leads to an increase in bone fragility and a higher fracture risk. There are strong evidences that the trabecular microarchitecture degradation impacts the fracture risk. The trabecular bone structure resembles a network composed of tortuous struts and their tortuosity influences the structural stiffness. This work investigates how the trabecular volume fraction, network connectivity, trabecular tortuosity and Young modulus of elasticity can be aggregated in a unique variable to provide information about the trabecular bone fragility. The parameters are estimated for three cohorts, two from *ex vivo* microtomographic (μCT) images and the other one from *in vivo* magnetic resonance imaging (MRI); the μCT image samples are from distal radius and vertebrae, while the MRI samples are also from distal radius. The principal component analysis shows that the principal component, defined as mechanical competence parameter (MCP), can be used to grade the quality of the samples and a visual color spectrum is generated to provide a quality distribution of the samples. The results point out a prevalent direction of the tortuosity along the z direction in all cohorts, which correspond to the most frequent direction of stress and high values of MCP indicating better structured samples. In addition, a remarkable result is the strong correlation between the tortuosity in both x and y horizontal directions and the elasticity in the z vertical direction, evidencing the role that the horizontal trabecular connectivity plays to the mechanical competence of the trabecular bone structure.

W. L. Roque (✉)
Department of Scientific Computation, Federal University of Paraíba, João Pessoa, Brazil
e-mail: roque@ci.ufpb.br

A. Alberich-Bayarri
Biomedical Imaging Research Group, La Fe Health Research Institute, Valencia, Spain
e-mail: angel@quibim.com

J. M. R. S. Tavares, R. Natal Jorge (eds.), *Developments in Medical Image Processing and Computational Vision*, Lecture Notes in Computational Vision and Biomechanics 19,
DOI 10.1007/978-3-319-13407-9_11

1 Introduction

Characterized by bone mass loss and trabecular microarchitecture degradation, osteoporosis is a silent disease which is normally detected by the standard bone mineral density (BMD) in a Dual X-Ray absorptiometry system (DXA). With the increase in longevity, osteoporosis has become a prevalent disease with serious consequences for patients and high cost for health care systems. The BMD essentially estimates the quantity of calcium by unit of bone area—cancellous and trabecular, saying nothing about its internal structure.

It is already known that low value of BMD is an indication of a weaker bone structure and likelihood of fragility fracture; however, it has been noticed that there are cases where different subjects presenting similar BMD, and with the lack of a more precise diagnosis of microarchitecture degradation, have an underestimated risk of fracture [6, 24, 48]. In this sense, the trabecular bone network microarchitecture (solid phase of the cancellous bone) plays an important role to the mechanical behavior and due to that it has become an area of intense investigation.

The trabecular bone analysis used to be carried out through bone biopsies, but with the advent of imaging scanners it has been changing to avoid an invasive procedure preserving the patient physical integrity. Most of these procedures involve imaging techniques like computer tomography (CT), magnetic resonance (MRI), micro computer tomography (μCT), and more recently, high resolution peripheral quantitative computer tomography (HR-pQCT). Unfortunately *in vivo* high resolution imaging is not yet a simple and unexpensive procedure, essentially only MRI and HR-pQCT have been used to scan some trabecular bone sites. μCT is used *in vivo* only for small animals, otherwise just in *ex vivo* studies of human bones due to high radiation exposure. An interesting alternative to such imaging procedures is Quantitative Ultrasound (QUS) [33], which has a lower cost and no radiation problems, but it is currently in its initial clinical steps and has been applied *in vivo* just to the calcaneus.

Boutroy et al. [6] have used HR-pQCT to assess volumetric bone density and some microarchitectural parameters, and in addition to micro Finite Elements (μFE) to investigate bone mechanical properties of the radius. They achieved that bone mechanical properties assessed by μFE may provide information about skeletal fragility and fracture risk not assessed by BMD or architectural measurements alone. Homminga et al. [24] used μCT to relate elastic modulus, anisotropy and volume fraction, basically validating Cowin'law. Tabor [44] determined correlation coefficients among Young modulus and volume fraction, anisotropy and trabecular spacing, thickness and length using μCT and MRI; Saha et al. [18, 42] used CT, μCT and MRI to relate elastic modulus with volume fraction and some parameters established through the samples topological analysis. Roque et al. [37] showed that there is a positive linear correlation among volume fraction, connectivity and Young modulus using CT.

Trabecular bone (TB) histomorphometrical parameters have been largely explored because they are currently well accepted as being among those indicators of bone quality. One of them, the TB volume fraction, BV/TV, plays a fundamental role to

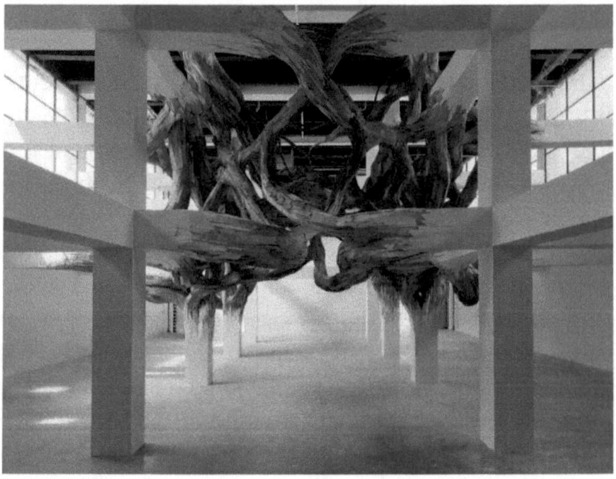

Fig. 1 Baitogogo, a masterpiece of Henrique Oliveira, in Palais de Tokyo, Paris

the TB quality. On the other hand, the connectivity of the trabecular bone network, which can be estimated, for instance, through the Euler-Poincaré characteristic, *EPC*, and the Young modulus of elasticity, E, have shown to be of major importance to describe the mechanical behavior of the structure. On the other hand, the trabecular bone forms a network that is not a regular lattice of straight lines as a truss, by the contrary, nature has chosen a sinuous structural design presenting a highly connected network of bones with rod and plate aspects. Figure 1 is a picture of a masterpiece of Henrique Oliveira[1], a Brazilian artist, that nicely resemble the contrast between a straight grid and a tortuous trabecular structure.

Recently the tortuosity [38], τ, which reflects the network sinuosity degree of a connected path, has been investigated as a geometrical parameter that also affects the mechanical behavior of the trabecular bone structure. In fact, there are several ways to define tortuosity, τ, according to the specific field of application [10]. Nevertheless, the simplest mathematical definition is the ratio of the geodesic length between two points in a connected region to the Euclidian distance connecting these two points. This definition implies that the tortuosity is such that $\tau \geq 1$. In a porous medium the tortuosity of the pore space is quite relevant for the fluid flow and permeability. On the other hand, when modeling the trabecular bone as a two phase porous medium, one question that may arise is how the tortuosity of the trabecular network influences the mechanical competence of the structure.

In [5] a study was conducted, based on the Biot-Allard model, showing the angle dependence of tortuosity and elasticity influence on the anisotropic cancellous bone structure using audiofrequencies in air-filled bovine bone replicas produced by stereolithography 3D printing. In [31] it has been shown that, based on Fourier transform and finite element methods, the normalized stress-strain behavior of a single collagen fiber is influenced by fiber tortuosity. This effect of tortuosity on the

[1] http://palaisdetokyo.com/fr/exposition/exposition-monographique/Henrique-Oliveira.

stress-strain behavior can be accounted for by the relationship between fiber tortuosity and the source of fiber stress during straining. The resulting stress in a fiber during an uniaxial pull is the result of two components. The first source component is the stress generated from increasing the bond lengths between the backbones of the polymer chains. The second source component is the stress generated from decreasing the overall tortuosity of the fiber. Nevertheless, the influence of tortuosity on the elasticity of the trabecular bone itself is not yet fully understood.

Currently a debate has been conducted about the influence of aging to the distribution of vertical and horizontal trabeculae; some studies have shown that trabeculae aligned in the direction of most frequent stress play an important role to the bone structural strength [12, 15]. In particular, it has been observed that with aging the human vertebral bone looses mass and trabecular elements, i. e., losses connectivity, resulting in a weaker bone structure leading to a higher fracture risk. Bone density is the main determinant of bone strength, but the microstructure of the trabecular bone is also important to the mechanical behavior of the structure [13, 30]. The reduction and slender of osteoporotic horizontal trabeculae turn the vertical ones more susceptible to buckling under compression forces, which is no longer reinforced by the horizontal struts. However, how the trabeculae characteristics may influence the bone strength is still a matter of current interest [17].

The first imaged-based studies concerning the estimation of trabecular bone network tortuosity were presented in [38–40], which reveal a high linear correlation between the trabecular network tortuosity in the main stress direction, that can be assumed as vertical, and the trabecular volume fraction (BV/TV), connectivity (EPC) and Young modulus of elasticity (E). This indicates that tortuosity is an important feature of the bone quality and plays a role on its resistance to load. However, due to the connectivity of the TB network, the tortuosity along other horizontal directions may as well influences E in the main stress direction, as load-bearing paths are relevant to spread out applied stress and this is one of the investigation concerns addressed in this paper.

Due to the high coefficients obtained in the linear correlation analysis among these four fundamental parameters, by means of the principal component analysis (PCA) a mechanical competence parameter (MCP) was defined in [41], merging the four previous ones, with the intent of grading the trabecular bone structural fragility. The study was initially done using 15 *ex vivo* distal radius samples obtained by μCT. Here, to further investigate the consistence of the MCP and its potentiality as a parameter to grade the TB fragility, we compute the MCP to two additional cohorts: one also from distal radius obtained *in vivo* by magnetic resonance imaging (MRI) and the second one, from L3 lumbar vertebrae obtained by μCT. The elasticity study was performed in two different ways: simulation by finite element method (FEM) for the first two sample's set and by actual mechanical test for the third one. These analyses are important because verify tortuosity and MCP consistences, as they will be applied to different image acquisition methods and resolutions, and for two different Young modulus estimation techniques.

The paper is organized as follows: Section 2 presents the materials and methods involved and includes a brief explanation on the parameters of interest, namely:

TB volume fraction, Euler-Poincaré characteristic, tortuosity and Young modulus of elasticity. Section 3 provide all the estimates, correlations and principal component analysis and Sect. 4 presents some discussions, while Sect. 5 provide the conclusions.

2 Material and Methods

This section presents the three cohorts that comprise the set of image samples used in our study and briefly explain the concepts and principal aspects concerning the four representative parameters explored in this work, namely, BV/TV, EPC, τ and E.

2.1 Cohort Samples

To further investigate the potentiality of the MCP, the present work considers three different sets of trabecular bone 3D image samples: two sets from distal radius, one of them containing 15 *ex vivo* μCT samples, and the other one containing 103 *in vivo* MRI samples; the third one containing 29 *ex vivo* μCT L3 vertebral samples. The final isotropic resolutions are 34 μm to the μCT and 90 μm to the MRI images, and the main analyzed direction was the axial one (craniocaudal to the vertebrae and distal-proximal to the radius).

The μCT distal radius samples, with lateral size 12 mm, were harvested with a mean distance of 9.75 mm from the distal extremity, and volumes of interest (VOI) were selected with sizes which vary according to the material's clinical analysis. They were imaged with the scanner microCT-20 (Scanco Medical, Brüttisellen, Switzerland) and, to the noise removal, the μCT 3D images were filtered with a Gaussian 3D filter. In each case, the grayscale histogram of the filtered images has two peaks, corresponding to marrow and bone; so, they were binarized using a global threshold equal to the minimum between the two peaks. The 15 image sets have 239 slices each, with 2D ROIs 212 × 212, 237 × 237, 242 × 242, 252 × 252 e 257 × 257 pixels; the 10 other samples have 268 × 268 pixels. Additional details concerning to the sample's preparation and acquisition protocols are described in [27].

A set of 29 μCT vertebral samples were supplied by the Department of Forensic Medicine, Jagiellonian University Medical College. The specimens were taken from female individuals without metabolic bone disease or vertebral fractures. Mean and standard deviation of the individuals age were equal to 57 ± 17 years, respectively. Immediately after dissection, all soft tissue was cleaned out and the samples were placed in containers filled with ethanol. An X-tek Benchtop CT160Xi high-resolution CT scanner (Nikon Metrology, Tring, UK) was used to scan the vertebral bodies. The images were segmented into bone and marrow cavity phases with a global thresholding method. The segmentation threshold was selected automatically based on the MaxEntropy algorithm [26], such that the information entropy consistent with a two-phase model be maximal. The final 3D binarized images have size that vary from 770 until 1088 pixels in x, from 605 until 876 pixels in y and from 413 until 713 slices (z direction), being the size average $950 \times 750 \times 600$.

The elasticity study with these vertebral samples was performed by mechanical test. An MTS Mini Bionix 858.02 loading system with a combined force/torque transducer with range of 25 kN/100 N.m was used to perform the compression tests. The specimens were located between two stiff steel plates which were firmly mounted to the force/torque transduced and to an upper jaw of the loading system. Prior to mechanical testing each probed specimen was glued with a self-curing denture base acrylic resin between two polycarbonate sheets at its endplate surfaces. This procedure was chosen to create two surfaces which will be as parallel as possible above each endplate to transmit the compressive load from the loading system to each specimen in an uniform way. The polycarbonate sheets were removed from the vertebra endplates before the testing. Each vertebra was loaded in compression with a loading rate of 5 mm/min to a certain level of engineering deformation (at most 30 % of the original height of the specimen). The compressive force was monitored during the test with sample rate of 20 Hz. All data that were measured during the compression tests were transformed to plots of applied force and displacement for each specimen. Compliance of the loading system was measured as well, so, during the post-processing, it was possible to gain a true relation between an applied force and deformation of a vertebra body. The stiffness in the linear part of a loading path for each specimen was evaluated and the Young modulus, E, was defined as the ratio of the product of the stiffness and the vertebral height to the mean cross section area of the vertebral body.

A set of 103 MRI radius samples were considered from the distal metaphysis and from a group including healthy subjects and a mix of disease stages. The MRI acquisitions were performed in a 3 Tesla system and scanned in 3D using a T1-weighted gradient echo sequence (TE/TR/a=5 ms/16 ms/25 Âº). The MRI images were acquired with a nominal isotropic resolution of 180 μm. MR image processing and analysis were performed with MATLAB R2012a (The MathWorks, Inc., Natick, MA). The image preparation steps consisted of an initial segmentation using a rectangular region of interest, image intensities homogeneity correction, interpolation and binarization. All the steps were applied as in [2], with the exemption of the interpolation, which was performed by applying a 3D non-local upsampling algorithm, achieving final resolution of 90 μm [29]. It has 65 samples with 80 slices, 10 with 120 and, the other ones, vary from 30 until 200 slices, predominantly between 50 and 100. Each 2D image has laterals dimensions varying from 38 up to 206 pixels, predominantly around 70×100 pixels.

Finite element method simulations were conducted to estimate Young modulus in all the 103 distal radius samples as well as for the 15 μCT distal radius samples. For that, a mesh was created based on the 3D trabecular bone images using an optimized algorithm [1] implemented in Matlab R2011a, which converts each voxel to an hexahedron element (brick element). Compression stress-strain tests were numerically simulated by a finite element linear-elastic-isotropic analysis performed in Ansys v11.0 (Ansys Inc., Southpointe, PA). The bulk material properties were set to $E_{bulk} = 10GPa$, a common value assumed to compact bone, and Poisson's coefficient $\nu = 0.3$. A deformation of 1 % of the edge length was imposed in all the distal radius compression simulations. Computational cost of the simulations was approximately of 5 h per sample on a computer workstation (Quad Core at 2.83 GHz and 8 GB of RAM). After applying the homogenization theory [23], apparent Young modulus results were obtained.

In general, most of the papers published in scientific journals are based on the authors' own set of image samples of subjects and upon them the studies are carried on. Nevertheless, as a normal rule, the set of samples are not made available to the research community and most of the times are not even made available under request. Although all the methods and equipments to get the samples are very well described in the material and methods section, there is a lack of freedom for other researchers to access the image database to work with them. The availability of image sample data would let other researchers to actually see the samples, to reproduce the computations presented in the papers, validating by themselves the algorithms and checking results that were published and, above all, allowing the use of the set of samples to further research that can be carried out either as complementary to the original paper or promoting new developments. In this regard, the image samples that are the basis of our study are *free data samples* made available upon request.

The computations of BV/TV, CEP and τ values were done using *OsteoImage*, a computer program developed by one of the authors especially to TB image analyses. The statistical analyses were performed with the free software RGui [34] and the 3D image reconstructions were done with ImageJ (http://rsbweb.nih.gov/ij/).

2.2 Volume Fraction

The TB volume fraction, BV/TV, represents the quantity of TB content present in the sample volume and is obtained by the ratio:

$$BV/TV = \frac{V_{trab}}{V_{total}}, \tag{1}$$

where V_{trab} is the trabecular volume and V_{total} is the total sample volume. From a 3D binary image sample, the TB volume fraction may be computed using the number of voxels representing the trabecular bone and the total volume is the number of voxels of the whole sample.

2.3 Euler-Poincaré Characteristic

The trabecular network connectivity can be inferred by the Euler-Poincaré characteristic, EPC, which can be estimated by automatic counting of isolated parts, I,

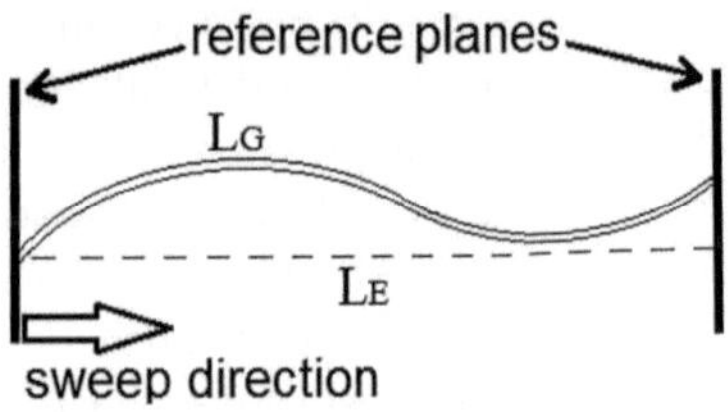

Fig. 2 A filamentous object between reference planes

redundant connections, C, and closed cavities, H [47]:

$$EPC = I - C + H. \tag{2}$$

As the trabeculae have no closed cavities [18] and the number of isolated parts is approximately 1 in a well structured sample, the EPC value should be negative and the lower the value the higher the connectivity [8]; in this case, the connectivity is estimated by its modulus. A positive EPC value indicates that the sample has more isolated parts than connections, and, therefore, the EPC indicates that its structure has lost much of its connectedness.

As EPC is a zero-dimensional measure, it needs to be estimated by a three-dimensional test; for practical purposes, a couple of parallel 2D images can be used, forming a disector [21, 35, 43, 47], and the EPC can be estimated for each one of them inside the volume of interest. In general, the EPC is given normalized by its volume size, EPC_V. The algorithm to compute the EPC can be seen in [36].

2.4 *Tortuosity*

The tortuosity, τ, characterizes how much an object departures from being straight and this concept has been extended to the trabecular bone network. Geometrically, it is defined as

$$\tau = \frac{L_G}{L_E}, \tag{3}$$

where L_G is the geodesic distance between two connected points, say a and b, of the trabecular network without passing across other phases (marrow cavity); and L_E is the Euclidean distance between these points, which will be considered here as the distance between two parallel reference planes (see Fig 2) [50]. This approach allows to classify as tortuous, $\tau \geq 1$, any filamentous structure that is not perpendicular to the reference planes.

Gommes et al. [19] proposed a geodesic reconstruction (GR) algorithm that can be applied on binary images to estimate the geodesic length. This algorithm was implemented in a previous work [38] and was used to the solid phase of the bone samples, sweeping the image along the reference plane direction, reconstructing the trabecular bone network voxel by voxel. The number of GR necessary to recover all the trabeculae of an image depends on their sinuosities, exceeding the number of analyzed slices considered as the Euclidean distance; the equality occurs only in the case of a structure completely perpendicular to the sweeping direction.

During the GR process, the algorithm computes and stores the Euclidean, L_E, and the geodesic, L_G, lengths. A distribution of Euclidean and geodesic lengths is generated. Taking the geodesic distance average, $\langle L_G \rangle$ at each Euclidean distance, the tortuosity can be estimated as the slope of the best fit line of points $(L_E, \langle L_G \rangle)$. This algorithm can be applied directly to 3D binarized μCT or MRI images. More details of the algorithm implementation can be found in [38, 40].

2.5 *Elasticity*

The elasticity is an important property of a material because it reflects its stiffness and flexibility when subject to load. Imposing an uniaxial strain ε to the sample, it is related with the stress σ as follows

$$\sigma = E\varepsilon, \tag{4}$$

where E is the Young modulus of elasticity. Usually, σ is obtained from the sample reaction force, divided by the area where it is being applied on. Rigorously, the trabecular structure is not isotropic [22, 44, 45], hence E is not a scalar, but a symmetric tensor; nevertheless, considering the complexity of modeling a porous structure, an isotropic model can be reasonably assumed [1, 14].

The 3D trabecular bone images were meshed to the elastic simulation using an optimized algorithm [1] implemented in Matlab R2011a (The MathWorks Inc., Natick, MA) which converts each voxel to an hexahedron element (brick element). Compression stress-strain test in each space direction was numerically simulated by a finite element linear-elastic-isotropic analysis performed in Ansys v11.0 (Ansys Inc., Southpointe, PA). The bulk material properties were set to $E_{bulk} = 10GPa$, a common value assumed to compact bone, and Poisson's coefficient $\nu = 0.3$. A deformation of 1 % of the edge length was imposed in all the compression simulations. Computational cost of the simulations was approximately of 5 h per sample on a computer workstation (Quad Core at 2.83 GHz and 8 GB of RAM). After applying the homogenization theory [23], apparent Young modulus results were obtained in each spatial direction (E_x, E_y, E_z).

3 Results

The trabecular volume fraction, the volumetric Euler-Poincaré characteristic, the tortuosity and the Young modulus of elasticity of the three cohort samples were obtained by the procedures stated in the previous section and their values can be found in [3].

Table 1 Tortuosity and E data of the MRI and μCT samples; $\langle\cdot\rangle \pm SD$ is the mean $\pm$ the standard deviation

	MRI	μCT
$\langle\tau_x\rangle \pm$ SD	1.5685 ± 0.15	1.7090 ± 0.19
$\langle\tau_y\rangle \pm$ SD	1.7459 ± 0.23	1.5283 ± 0.07
$\langle\tau_z\rangle \pm$ SD	1.3810 ± 0.14	1.2959 ± 0.07
$\langle E_x\rangle \pm$ SD	112.76 ± 140.42	34.8178 ± 28.87
$\langle E_y\rangle \pm$ SD	143.78 ± 168.27	33.7153 ± 22.05
$\langle E_z\rangle \pm$ SD	466.49 ± 343.26	173.9920 ± 112.81

Table 2 Linear correlation coefficients and p-values for Young modulus of elasticity and tortuosity in x, y and z directions, for the μCT samples

	E_x	E_y	E_z
τ_{+x}	−0.54 (0.0383)	−0.65 (9.0E-03)	−0.72 (2.6E-03)
τ_{+y}	−0.54 (0.0393)	−0.79 (4.7E-04)	−0.65 (8.3E-03)
τ_{+z}	−0.53 (0.0401)	−0.51 (0.0495)	−0.75 (1.2E-03)

Table 3 Linear correlation coefficients and p-values for Young modulus of elasticity and tortuosity in x, y and z directions, for the MRI samples

	E_x	E_y	E_z
τ_{+x}	−0.57 (3.2E-10)	−0.62 (4.1E-12)	−0.69 (5.5E-16)
τ_{+y}	−0.58 (1.4E-10)	−0.53 (9.5E-09)	−0.58 (2.0E-10)
τ_{+z}	−0.43 (6.3E-06)	−0.47 (4.0E-07)	−0.65 (1.3E-13)

3.1 Influence of Trabecular Tortuosity on Elasticity

Table 1 presents the mean and standard deviation (SD) that were obtained for the distal radius μCT and MRI trabecular bone cohorts. Firstly, by a simple inspection of the data in Table 1, it is observed that in the z direction τ has the lowest mean and SD, and the E has the highest value ones, in both groups. This corresponds to the distal-proximal direction, which is normally the direction that is more frequently submitted to tensile and compressive forces, when compared to the x and y ones, corresponding to the horizontal sweeping directions. This evidence is an indication that the trabeculae get aligned to turn the structure stronger, which is in agreement with the very well known fact that the trabecular bone aligns in the direction which it is more frequently mechanically demanded [20, 45, 49].

To further investigate the tortuosity influence on the trabecular bone strength, a linear correlation study was performed including the whole data and the results are provided in Tables 2 and 3.

The linear correlation coefficients between τ and E in the horizontal x, y, and vertical z directions reveal a strong influence of tortuosity's increase to the decrease in bone stiffness. Bone mass loss occurs due mainly to an unbalance between bone formation and bone resorption, and marrow cavity sizes and quantities in certain parts of the trabecular bone are closely related to bone remodeling, being directly

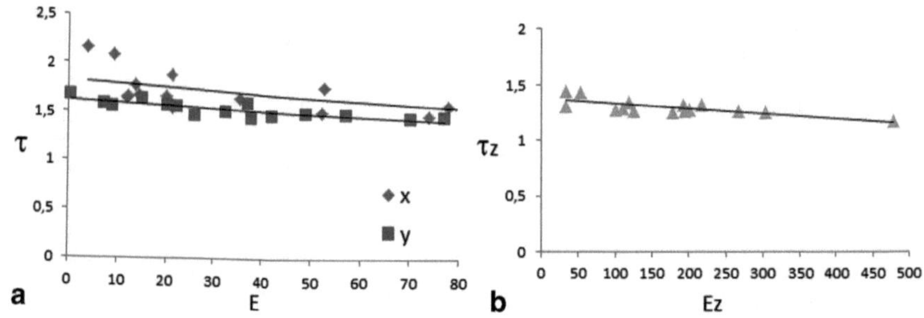

Fig. 3 Linear relationship between E, in MPa, and τ, in the **a** x and y directions and **b** z direction

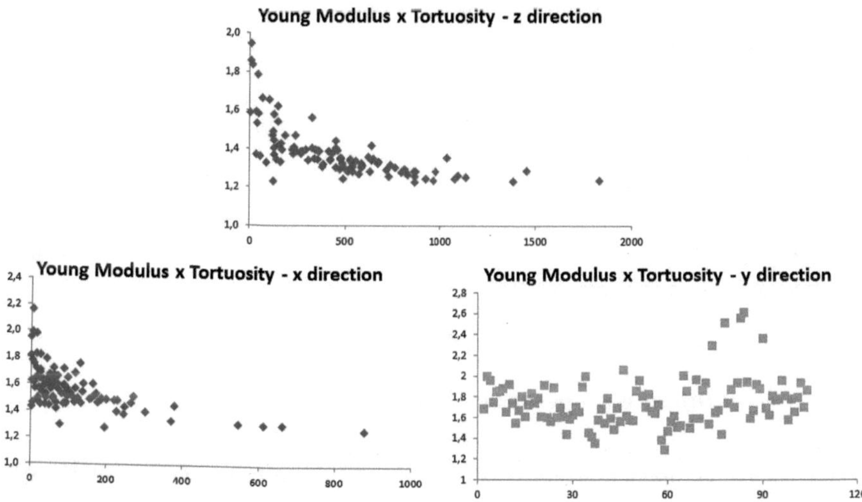

Fig. 4 Linear relationship between E, in MPa, and τ, in the x, y and z directions, for the MRI samples. The inversely proportional relationship between E and τ is remarkable in the z and x directions

proportional to the osteoclasts/osteoblasts activities [4]. The resorption of the horizontal ties occurs primarily [7], turning marrow cavities bigger and, consequently, as the geodesic length depends on the trabecular elements that remain connected, this length gets also bigger, increasing the network tortuosity as seen in any direction. With the bone mass loss, the structure gets weaker, changing its resistance to load, which is reflected in the Young modulus decrease. Figures 3 and 4 illustrate the linear relationship between the two parameters and, in the first case, the best fit line corroborates to their agreement.

Furthermore, it is worthwhile noticing the strong linear correlation between E in the vertical direction z and the tortuosities in horizontal directions x or y. This reveals the relevance of the horizontal ties to the load-bearing of forces in the distal-proximal direction, and enforces the role that the trabecular sideways connectivity play to the bone microarchitecture structural strength [39, 40]. This fact justifies the

Table 4 Linear correlation coefficients (p-value < 0.001) between BV/TV, E, EPC_V and τ to the 15 μCT radius samples

	BV/TV	E	EPC_V
E	0.87	1	
EPC_V	−0.82	−0.73	1
τ	−0.76	−0.75	0.71

Table 5 Linear correlation coefficients (p-value < 0.001) between BV/TV, E, EPC_V and τ to the 103 MRI radius samples

	BV/TV	E	EPC_V
E	0.83	1	
EPC_V	−0.86	−0.83	1
τ	−0.76	−0.65	0.58

Table 6 Linear correlation coefficients (p-value < 0.001) between BV/TV, E, EPC_V and τ to the 29 μCT vertebral samples

	BV/TV	E	EPC_V
E	0.90	1	
EPC_V	−0.86	−0.70	1
τ	−0.77	−0.55	0.71

use of the tortuosity and connectivity simply in z-direction to estimate the mechanical competence parameter given in [41].

3.2 *Mechanical Competence Parameter*

The principal component analysis (PCA) is a technique to reduce a complex data set to a lower dimension to reveal the sometimes hidden, simplified structure that often underlie it. The variable reduction is applicable only when there is a strong correlation between them [25].

The number of principal components (PC) obtained is the same as the number of variables, but the representative PCs are those which present the major fraction over the total variance. The general form of a PC, which relates n variables is:

$$C_1 = b_{11}x_1 + b_{12}x_2 + ... + b_{1n}x_n, \tag{5}$$

where C_1 is the first principal component and b_{1i} is the weight for the variable x_i.

When the PCA is applied to the four trabecular bone parameters considered in this study, the PCA merges morphometrical, geometrical and mechanical information about the trabecular bone structure into a unique parameter.

The linear correlation analysis of the parameters BV/TV, EPC_V, τ and E, for the three cohorts are shown in the Tables 4, 5 and 6.

It is worth noticing that the correlation coefficients between the parameters do not present significant differences among the groups. Although the three cohorts differ with respect to TB sites, by the acquisition methods and resolutions, and also by the techniques to estimate the Young modulus, the results are in complete agreement.

Since the linear correlation coefficients are notably high, this assures that a principal component analysis can be performed among the samples belonging to each one of the three cohorts. In fact, the variance to the first principal component was actually far higher, varying from 3.1 to 3.3, in the three cases. Therefore, this guarantees that these four parameters can be merged into a single new parameter.

Following the definition of the mechanical competence parameter (*MCP*) [41] as the first principal component, for each cohort we have

$$MCP_{\mu CTr} = 0.52 \times BV/TV - 0.49 \times EPC_V + 0.51 \times E - 0.48 \times \tau, \tag{6}$$

to the distal radius μCT,

$$MCP_{MRIr} = 0.53 \times BV/TV - 0.50 \times EPC_V + 0.51 \times E - 0.45 \times \tau, \tag{7}$$

to the distal radius MRI, and

$$MCP_{\mu CTv} = 0.55 \times BV/TV - 0.48 \times EPC_V + 0.50 \times E - 0.47 \times \tau, \tag{8}$$

to the vertebral μCT one.

One can see that the corresponding *MCP* coefficients in the three cases are very close to each other: BV/TV is the biggest one, indicating its high weight in the sample's classification; E has the second one, followed by EPC_V and τ, respectively, but all four weighted parameters have almost equal importance in the *MCP* composition.

The *MCP* values to each cohort can be normalized to fit them into the range between 0 and 1; where 0 has been attributed to the worst value and 1 to the best structural case within the cohort, i. e., taking into account the four fundamental parameters, by evaluating

$$MCP_N = \frac{MCP_k - MCP_{min}}{MCP_{max} - MCP_{min}}, \tag{9}$$

where MCP_k corresponds to the *MCP* value of sample k, MCP_{min} and MCP_{max} are the minimum and maximum *MCP* values within the cohort under analysis. Figure 5 shows, for each cohort, the pictures of the trabecular bone structure for the worst (left column) and best (right column) MCP_N.

According to the results, in each cohort, the sample with $MCP_N = 0$ has the worst combination of the four parameters, that is: low bone content (BV/TV), low connectivity (high EPC_V value), high tortuosity τ and low stiffness (E). The sample with $MCP_N = 1$ has an opposite behavior, representing the best structured sample.

Based on the MCP_N a color spectrum may be generated to visually identify the grade of the samples and classify new ones. Figure 6 shows the MCP_N color spectrum (see eBook version) of the μCT distal radius cohort.

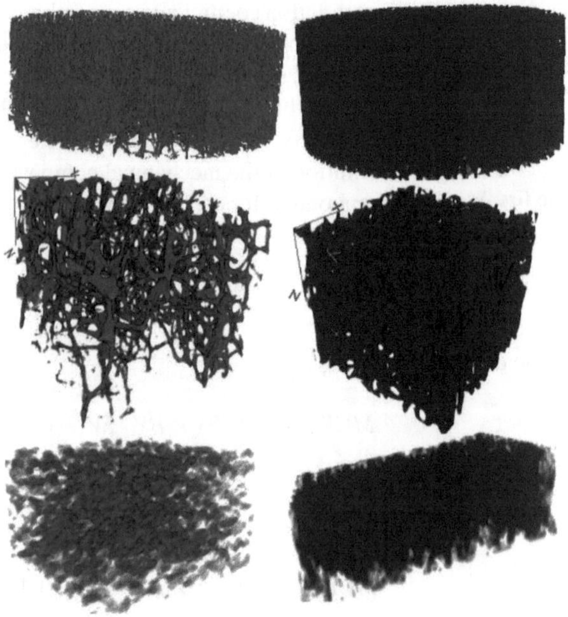

Fig. 5 The *left column* shows the worst and the *right* the best structured samples of each one of the three cohorts: μCT *in vitro* vertebrae in the first row, μCT *in vitro* distal radius in *second row*, and the MRI *in vivo* distal radius in the *third row*

In the literature the Young modulus has been many times used as the main reference to explain the bone mechanical competence [11, 18, 24, 28, 32]. Its higher correlation coefficient obtained with BV/TV is the reason for that, nevertheless, the inclusion of other parameters increase this correlation. In fact, adding EPC_V and τ to the analysis, have shown an increased of r^2 up to 5 %. In other words, the stepwise analysis considering the three parameters, BV/TV, EPC_V and τ explains E evolving from 75 % up to 84 % for the cohorts. One can see that the variability is high meaning that the Young modulus carries around 20 % of the exceeding mechanical competence information, what justifies its consideration on the MCP construction.

4 Discussion

The tortuosity measures the network sinuosity degree compared to a straight one and was recently proposed and investigated as a trabecular bone parameter that correlates very well with trabecular connectivity, volume fraction and Young modulus of elasticity in the z direction, with impacts on the trabecular bone mechanical competence [41]. In this paper the influence of trabecular bone tortuosity to the structural stiffness was shown through the Young modulus of elasticity. The studies were done in the three principal space directions, x, y and z, and used two cohorts: one with 15 μCT *ex vivo* images and the other one with 103 MRI images of *in vivo* distal radius trabecular bone.

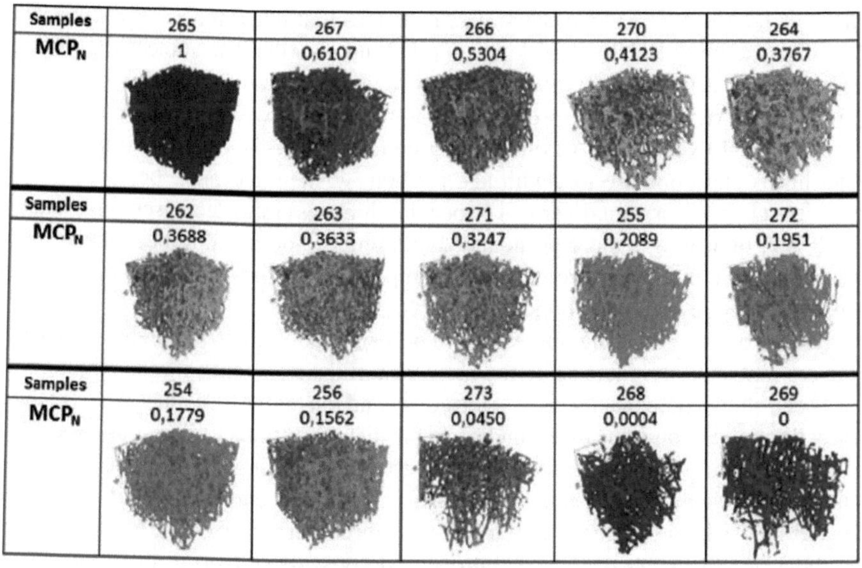

Fig. 6 MCP_N color spectrum (see eBook version) of the μCT distal radius samples where *blue* means better and *red* means worse

In a simulated study where the trabecular structure formed a lattice of orthogonal struts, with 48 vertical and 96 horizontal trabeculae, it has been shown that the removal of just a single center vertical trabecula that is aligned to the direction of load, corresponding to around 2 % of them, causes a decrease of ~ 10 % in the apparent elastic modulus, while the removal of just one center horizontal trabecula, which is perpendicular to the load direction, a little over 1 % was noticed [17]. Of course, if additional horizontal trabeculae loose their connectivity, load-bearing path is also lost providing an over stress on the neighbor vertical trabeculae. This fact shows the importance of the horizontal trabeculae to the structural strength of the bone.

In a very recent review [9] the age-related evolution of the trabecular and cortical bone microstructure of vertebral, femoral neck, distal radius and tibia bodies were discussed and three major processes that lead to bone loss were pointed out: first and most outstanding process is the bone mass loss, mainly caused by trabecular thinning, degradation of the trabecular microstructure and loss of trabecular elements. Second, it is caused by the increase of cortical porosity, which leads to cortical bone loss, and third caused by continuous resorption of the endocortical surface. Also recently a more detailed work has been done on morphological aspects of 3D vertebral trabeculae microstructure, with special attention to the behavior of the vertical and horizontal trabeculae [46]. Here vertical is understood as the natural direction of the gravitational force on the column, which corresponds to the direction of most frequent stress. In the paper, the authors provide an algorithm to segment the trabecular network into vertical and horizontal trabeculae and provide a set of interesting results of age-related changes that occur for vertical trabecular volume fraction (vBV/TV), thickness (Tb.Th), number (Tb.N), connectivity density (Conn.D), structural model index (SMI) and degree of anisotropy (DA), based on *ex vivo* lumbar vertebrae of 40 women and 39 men with an even distribution ranging from 20 to 90 years old. An outstanding conclusion of their study is that vertical and horizontal bone are lost with age for both women and men, being faster for women, and the horizontal/vertical trabecular thickness ratio decreases significantly with age, indicating a more pronounced thinning of horizontal trabeculae. Vertical and horizontal trabeculae are structurally important and their thinning or disruption compromise the trabecular bone strength [15, 16].

The trabeculae thinning, increasing in porosity and diminishing connectivity are factors that cause an increase in the network tortuosity, weakening the structure. It has been shown here that the lowest tortuosity and the highest E values occur in the z direction for all cohorts, corresponding to the distal-proximal radius or craniocaudal directions. This result is a good indication that the trabeculae alignment influences the bone mechanical competence, increasing its resistance to load. Additionally, the moderate linear correlation between E in the z-direction (vertical) and the tortuosities in the x and y directions (horizontal ones), do provide support to the influence of the horizontal tortuosity to the trabecular strength in the vertical direction. This is a somewhat expected result as in mechanical engineering load-bearing structures are build with redundant load paths to provide a safer distribution of forces.

It has to be pointed out that the tortuosity technique used in this paper estimates the bulk trabecular tortuosity in each direction according to the sweeping plane direction and not specifically considering only the vertical or horizontal trabeculae as defined in [46]. In fact, as the trabeculae form a complex network, the influence of loading in one direction gets spread to the other ones. Thus, the results presented here have shown that the influence of the horizontal tortuosities (τ_{+x}, τ_{+y}) on the vertical E is not as strong as the vertical tortuosity (τ_{+z}) on the distal radius, this is in agreement with the achievements given in [15, 16, 46] that the vertebra vertical trabeculae are mainly responsible for the compressive bone strength.

5 Conclusion

Osteoporosis has become a health problem to the aging population and an economic burden worldwide to the public and private health care systems. Bone mass loss causes irreversible damages to the bone microarchitecture which likely leads to fragility fractures.

In this paper we have shown that the mechanical competence parameter *MCP* is suitable to grade the trabecular bone fragility, resuming four important parameters that characterizes the TB quality, namely: volume fraction, connectivity, tortuosity and Young modulus. The *MCP* was investigated for three cohorts from different trabecular bone sites and image resolutions from *in vivo* and *ex vivo* subjects, showing full agreement between them. On the other hand, it has been shown that the tortuosity related to the horizontal sweeping directions influences the TB structural strength providing loading paths to distribute stress mainly driven on vertical trabeculae.

To simplify a direct and intuitive way to observe the trabecular bone structural quality, a normalized MCP_N has been set ranging in the interval $[0, 1]$, making easier the grading of the trabecular bone fragility among samples within a cohort and between different cohorts. A color spectrum has been generated to easy visualization of the trabecular bone fragility grading of a sample. The risk of fracture is quite complex to be well defined, as it depends on several parameters, including exogenous aspects. Of course, the MCP_N is not a fracture risk parameter, but it can help to identify trabecular bone fragility. The results presented here encourage the search of the MCP_N normality pattern based on a cohort of healthy subjects as well as similar ones for osteopenic and osteoporotic populations.

Acknowledgements We would like to thank Dr. K. Arcaro for several preliminary discussions and especially Dr. Z. Tabor for kindly let us make use of his μCT image samples and data. W. L. Roque thank the University for its competence in dealing with the redistribution process.

References

1. Alberich-Bayarri A, Marti-Bonmati L, Perez MA, Lerma JJ, Moratal D (2010) Finite element modeling for a morphometric and mechanical characterization of trabecular bone from high resolution magnetic resonance imaging. In: Moratal D (ed) Finite element analysis. InTechOpen, pp 195–208
2. Alberich-Bayarri A, Marti-Bonmati L, Pérez MA, Sanz-Requena R, Lerma-Garrido JJ, García-Martí G, Moratal D (2010) Assessment of 2D and 3D fractal dimension measurements of trabecular bone from high-spatial resolution magnetic resonance images at 3 tesla. Med Phys 37:4930–4937
3. Arcaro K (2013) Caracterização Geométrica e Topológica da Competência Mecânica no Estudo da Estrutura Trabecular. DSc. Thesis (in Portuguese). Graduate Program in Applied Mathematics, Federal University of Rio Grande do Sul, Porto Alegre, Brazil, July 2013
4. Argenta MA, Gebert AP, Filho ES, Felizari BA, Hecke MB (2011) Methodology for numerical simulation of trabecular bone structures mechanical behavior. CMES 79(3):159–182
5. Aygün H, Attenborough K, Postema M, Lauriks W, Langton CM (2009) Predictions of angle dependent tortuosity and elasticity effects on sound propagation in cancellous bone. J Acoust Soc Am 126:3286–3290
6. Boutroy S, Van Rietbergen B, Sornay-Rendu E, Munoz F, Bouxsein ML, Delmas PD (2008) Finite element analysis based on in vivo HR-pQCT images of the distal radius is associated with wrist fracture in postmenopausal women. J Bone Miner Res 23(3):392–399
7. Carbonare D, Giannini S (2004) Bone microarchitecture as an important determinant of bone strength. J Endocrinol Invest 27:99–105
8. Chappard D, Basle MF, Legrand E, Audran M (2008) Trabecular bone microarchitecture: a review. Morphologie 92:162–170
9. Chen H, Zhou X, Fujita H, Onozuka M, Kubo K-Y (2013) Age-related changes in trabecular and cortical bone microstructure. Int J Endocrinol 2013:213234
10. Clennell MB (1997) Tortuosity: a guide through the maze. In: Lovell MA, Harvey PK (eds) Developments in Petrophysics, vol 122. Geological Society, London, pp 299–344
11. Cohen A, Dempster DW, Müller R, Guo XE, Nickolas TL, Liu XS, Zhang XH, Wirth AJ, van Lenthe GH, Kohler T, McMahon DJ, Zhou H, Rubin MR, Bilezikian JP, Lappe JM, Recker RR,

Shane E (2010) Assessment of trabecular and cortical architecture and mechanical competence of bone by high-resolution peripheral computed tomography: comparison with transiliac bone biopsy. Osteoporos Int 21:263–273
12. Dempster DW (2003) Bone microarchitecture and strength. Osteoporos Int 14(Suppl 5):S54–S56
13. Ebbesen EN, Thomsen JS, Beck-Nielsen H, Nepper-Rasmussen HJ, Mosekilde L (1999) Lumbar vertebral body compressive strength evaluated by dual-energy x-ray absorptiometry, quantitative computed tomography, and ashing. Bone 25:713–724
14. Edwards WB, Troy KL (2012) Finite element prediction of surface strain and fracture strength at the distal radius. Med Eng Phys 34:290–298
15. Fields AJ, Lee GL, Liu XS, Jekir MG, Guo XE, Keaveny TM (2011) Influence of vertical trabeculae on the compressive strength of the human vertebra. J Bone Miner Res 26:263–269
16. Fields AJ, Nawathe S, Eswaran SK, Jekir MG, Adams MF, Papadopoulos P, Keaveny TM (2012) Vertebral fragility and structural redundancy. J Bone Miner Res 27:2152–2158
17. Gefen A (2009) Finite element modeling of the microarchitecture of cancellous bone: techniques and applications. In Leondes CT (ed) Biomechanics system technology: muscular skeletal systems, vol 4, pp 73–112. World Scientific, Singapore (chapter 3)
18. Gomberg BR, Saha PK, Song HK, Hwang SN, Wehrli FW (2000) Topological analysis of trabecular bone MR images. IEEE T Med Imaging 19(3):166–174
19. Gommes CJ, Bons A-J, Blacher S, Dunsmuir JH, Tsou AH (2009) Practical methods for measuring the tortuosity of porous materials from binary or gray-tone tomographic reconstructions. AIChE J 55(8):2000–2012
20. Gong H, Zhu D, Gao J, Lv L, Zhang X (2010) An adaptation model for trabecular bone at different mechanical levels. Biomed Eng Online 9:32
21. Gundersen HJG, Boyce RW, Nyengaard JR, Odgaard A (1993) The Conneuler: unbiased estimation of the connectivity using physical disectors under projection. Bone 14:217–222
22. Hambli R, Bettamer A, Allaoui S (2012) Finite element prediction of proximal femur fracture pattern based on orthotropic behaviour law coupled to quasi-brittle damage. Med Eng Phys 34:202–210
23. Hollister SJ, Fyhrie DP, Jepsen KJ, Goldstein SA (1991) Application of homogenization theory to the study of trabecular bone mechanics. J Biomech 24:825–839
24. Homminga J, Mccreadie BR, Weinans H, Huiskes R (2002) The dependence of the elastic properties of osteoporotic cancellous bone on volume fraction and fabric. J Biomech 36:1461–1467
25. Jolliffe IT (2002) Principal component analysis, 2nd edn. Springer, Berlin
26. Kapur JN, Sahoo PK, Wong ACK (1985) A new method for gray-level picture thresholding using the entropy of the histogram. Graph Mod Im Proc 29:273–285
27. Laib A, Beuf O, Issever A, Newitt DC, Majumdar S (2001) Direct measures of trabecular bone architecture from MR images. Adv Exp Med Biol 496:37–46 (Springer US, chapter 5)
28. Liu XS, Sajda P, Saha PK, Wehrli FW, Bevill G, Keaveny TM, Guo XE (2008) Complete volumetric decomposition of individual trabecular plates and rods and its morphological correlations with anisotropic elastic moduli in human trabecular bone. J Bone Miner Res 23(2):223–235
29. Manjón JV, Coupé P, Buades A, Fonov V, Louis Collins D, Robles M (2010) Non-local MRI upsampling. Med Image Anal 14:784–792
30. Mosekilde L (1993) Vertebral structure and strength in vivo and in vitro. Calcif Tissue Int 53(Suppl 1):S121–S126
31. Ohmura J (2011) Effects of elastic modulus on single fiber uniaxial deformation. Undergraduate Honors Thesis, The Ohio State University, 41pp
32. Parkinson IH, Badiei A, Stauber M, Codrington J, Müller R, Fazzalari NL (2012) Vertebral body bone strength: the contribution of individual trabecular element morphology. Osteoporos Int 23:1957–1965
33. Portero-Muzy NR, Chavassieux PM, Milton D, Duboeuf F, Delmas PD, Meunier PJ (2007) Euler strut-cavity, a new histomorphometric parameter of connectivity reflects bone strength and speed of sound in trabecular bone from human os calcis. Calcified Tissue Int 81:92–98

34. R Development Core Team (2010) R: a language and environment for statistical computing. R Foundation for Statistical Computing, Vienna, Austria, 2010. ISBN 3-900051-07-0
35. Roberts N, Reed M, Nesbitt G (1997) Estimation of the connectivity of a synthetic porous medium. J Microsc 187:110–118
36. Roque WL, de Souza ACA, Barbieri DX (2009) The euler-poincaré characteristic applied to identify low bone density from vertebral tomographic images. Rev Bras Reumatol 49:140–152
37. Roque WL, Arcaro K, Tabor Z (2010) An investigation of the mechanical competence of the trabecular bone. In: Dvorkin E, Goldschmit M, Storti M (eds) Mecánica computacional, vol XXIX, pp 2001–2009. AMCA, Buenos Aires
38. Roque WL, Arcaro K, Freytag I (2011) Tortuosidade da rede do osso trabecular a partir da reconstrução geodésica de imagens binárias tridimensionais. Anais do XI Workshop de Informática Médica, pp 1708–1717
39. Roque WL, Arcaro K, Alberich-Bayarri A (2012) Tortuosity and elasticity study of distal radius trabecular bone. In: Rocha A, Calvo-Manzano JA, Reis LP, Cota MP (eds) (2012) Actas de la 7ª Conferencia Ibérica de Sistemas y Tecnologías de Información, vol 1. AISTI - UPM, 2012.
40. Roque WL, Arcaro K, Lanfredi RB (2012) Tortuosidade e conectividade da rede trabecular do rádio distal a partir de imagens micro-tomográficas. Rev Bras Eng Bio 28:116–123
41. Roque WL, Arcaro K, Alberich-Bayarri A (2013) Mechanical competence of bone: a new parameter to grade trabecular bone fragility from tortuosity and elasticity. IEEE T Bio-Med Eng 60:1363–1370
42. Saha PK, Xu Y, Duan H, Heiner A, Liang G (2010) Volumetric topological analysis: a novel approach for trabecular bone classification on the continuum between plates and rods. IEEE T Med Imaging 29(11):1821–1838
43. Sterio DC (1984) The unbiased estimation of number and sizes of arbitrary particles using the disector. J Microsc 134:127–136
44. Tabor Z (2007) Estimating structural properties of trabecular bone from gray-level low-resolution images. Med Eng Phys 29:110–119
45. Tabor Z (2009) On the equivalence of two methods of determining fabric tensor. Med Eng Phys 31:1313–1322
46. Thomsen JS, Niklassen AS, Ebbesen EN, Brüel A (2013) Age-related changes of vertical and horizontal lumbar vertebral trabecular 3d bone microstructure is different in women and men. Bone 57:47–55
47. Vogel HJ, Kretzschmar A (1996) Topological characterization of pore space in soil—sample preparation and digital image-processing. Geoderma 73:23–38
48. Wesarg S, Erdt M, Kafchitsas Ks, Khan MF (2010) Direct visualization of regions with lowered bone mineral density in dual-energy CT images of vertebrae. In: Summers RM, Bram van Ginneken MD (eds) Medical Imaging 2011: Computer-Aided Diagnosis. SPIE Proceedings, 2010
49. Wolff J (1986) The law of bone remodeling. Springer-Verlag, Berlin (translation of the german 1892 edition) edition
50. Wua YS, van Vliet LJ, Frijlink HW, Maarschalka KV (2006) The determination of relative path length as a measure for tortuosity in compacts using image analysis. Eur J Pharm Sci 28:433–440

Influence of Beam Hardening Artifact in Bone Interface Contact Evaluation by 3D X-ray Microtomography

I. Lima, M. Marquezan, M. M. G. Souza, E. F. Sant'Anna and R. T. Lopes

Abstract Trabecular bone screws are commonly used for fixation of fractures in order to increase holding power in the fine sponge bone. The success of skeletal anchorage using mini screws is related to their stability in the bone tissue. Factors that influence the immediate stability of metal implants are related to the design of the device to the quantity and quality of bone and to insertion technique. The present work studied bone interface contact parameter by x-ray microtomography. The results identified the importance of evaluating the metallic artifact around the mini screws, which can be assessed by different pixel size dilation image processing. It can be noted a correlation pattern between beam hardening artifact correction and bone interface contact measurements.

1 Introduction

X-ray computed (micro)tomography ((μ)CT) is a diagnostic method used to obtain the knowledge of X-ray absorption in the interior of structures. For that purpose, the photons transmitted after interaction of the X-ray beam with the object are recorded in a detector. During this procedure, a series of projections at various angles around the object is collected and with an adequate number of projections it is possible to obtain cross-sectional views of the examined object (Fig. 1). So, the more directions from which the measurements are made, the more arrangements of objects can be distinguished.

The CT basic physical principle of X-ray attenuation is based on Lambert- Beer's law of absorption, which is related to the attenuation coefficient. Therefore, it is possible to describe how the materials attenuate the X-ray beam. The interactions responsible for this attenuation are mainly Compton scattering (proportional 1/E) and photoelectric absorption. The contribution of the last effect depends on the effective atomic number Z and it is particularly important when low energies are employed (Z^3/E^3).

I. Lima (✉) · M. Marquezan · M. M. G. Souza · E. F. Sant'Anna · R. T. Lopes
Federal University of Rio de Janeiro, Ilha do Fundão, Rio de Janeiro, Brazil
e-mail: inaya@lin.ufrj.br

J. M. R. S. Tavares, R. Natal Jorge (eds.), *Developments in Medical Image Processing and Computational Vision,* Lecture Notes in Computational Vision and Biomechanics 19,
DOI 10.1007/978-3-319-13407-9_12

Fig. 1 CT attenuation principle scheme

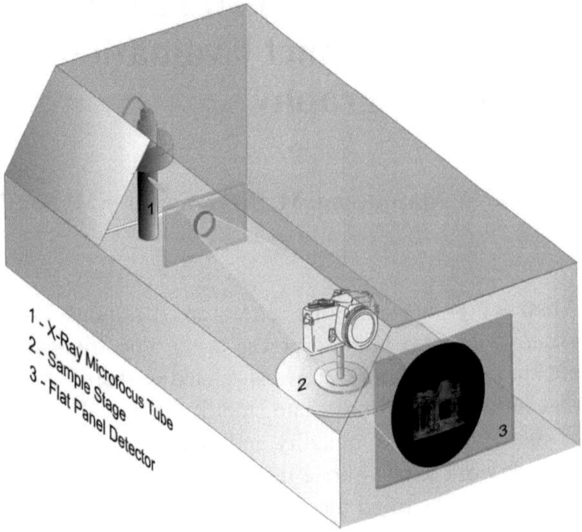

Beer's law assumes a narrow X-ray beam and a monochromatic radiation. In practice, CT images are obtained with the assumption that some particular effective energy characterizes the X-ray beam as a whole and the attenuation coefficients are discretized into several element volumes. Measurements of this coefficient of numerous ray projections provide sufficient data to solve multiple equations for attenuation parameter. However, the assumption that the X-ray beam is monochromatic, according to the common models, is not realistic because the relationship between the intensity and photon flux is described by a spectral function. In Eq. (1) it is possible to observe the general relationship between the incident energy $I_o(E)$ and the object attenuation parameter μ (x,y,z;E).

$$I_d(x,y) = \int_0^{E_{max}} \eta(E) I_0(E)\, exp\left(-\int \mu(x,y,z;E)\, dz\right) dE \tag{1}$$

In Eq. (1) the range of integration over z covers the entire scanned object. This is the key equation for X-ray imaging via projection radiography in which I_d(x,y) is the projection image of μ(x,y,z;E) and η(E) represents the quantum efficiency of the detector at energy E.

In this sense, the more absorbent the object is, the fewer the X-ray photons detected. Because low energy X-rays are more efficiently attenuated than high energy X-rays, the distribution of energies is slanted toward higher energies, which lead to a beam hardening artifact. In other words, beam-hardening results from the preferential absorption of low-energy photons from the beam.

A major effect of beam hardening is the enhancement of the image edges. This is one of the most difficult image artifacts of CT because quantitative measurements are highly influenced by this problem due to its relation with the attenuation coefficient. In addition the same material can result in different gray levels depending on the surrounding material, which is known as the environmental density artifact, such as bone implant. Figure 2 shows examples of μCT images of several kinds of materials illustrating the mentioned beam hardening effect.

Cormack and Hounsfield received the Noble prize in 1979 for their work with CT and since then their theory is widely used although enormous amount of computation is generally required to generate CT images. Since then CT became one of the most important of all X-ray procedures worldwide.

Over the years, CT scan has been applied in the medical area with success, however, due to the relative low resolution (in the order of mm) of these images, new efforts were made to achieve better image quality. Therefore, X-ray micro-computed tomography (μCT) systems were developed with a resolution down to 1 μm using an assembly of X-ray sources and detectors to achieve that goal. These systems are commonly called industrial scanners, and are intended for the analysis of inanimate objects. They are a little different from medical equipment in some aspects. In medical CT, the X-ray source is linked to the detector, which is located at the other side of the patient. Together, source and detector are rotated around, and translate along, the patient. Unfortunately this design can promote the appearance of an artifact caused by the patient motion, with a negative effect on the image quality. Figure 3 illustrates an example of μCT radius images without (a) and with (b) patient movement. Theoretically, this motion artifact can be reduced by a faster scanning time, tube alignment or post processing of the scan. This issue does not exist in industrial systems because in this case the X-ray source and the detector remain fixed while the object is translated along its z axis to perform the scan.

Requirements for image quality improvement (adequate spatial and contrast resolutions) in the clinical sphere have led to higher patient doses, which eventually becomes a limiting factor in examinations and quality control management. Because industrial μCT does not examine living subjects, the energy of the X-ray source is high, enabling the inspection of dense materials. Furthermore, the X-ray focal spot is reduced in order to increase resolution. In fact, the improvement in the system resolution due to X-ray tube filament is assigned to the brightness factor, which is equal to the electron flux density emitted by the filament in a certain solid angle. However, obtaining small diameters requires special features, since the X-ray spot size is limited by the amount of heat generated at the anode. Therefore, good target high atomic number materials, such as titanium and tungsten are required. The smaller the X-ray spot size the greater the specific heat power for the focus area, leading to establish limits to the capacity of the target. So, the accuracy of high resolution in CT/μCT is strongly influenced by the spatial stability of the X-ray focal spot. The disadvantage of μCT scanner materials is generally the limited size of the samples, which cannot exceed some centimeters.

In this sense; Eq. (1) has to be modified because the construction of a linear model for measurements is needed. By using this model idealized measurements can be expressed as certain averages of attenuation coefficient. While the choice of coordinates is arbitrary, having a fixed reference frame is crucial for any tomography method. By convention the slices are defined by fixing the last coordinate. In this context, Eq. (1) can be rewritten more simply (Eq. 2), where L represents the trajectory of

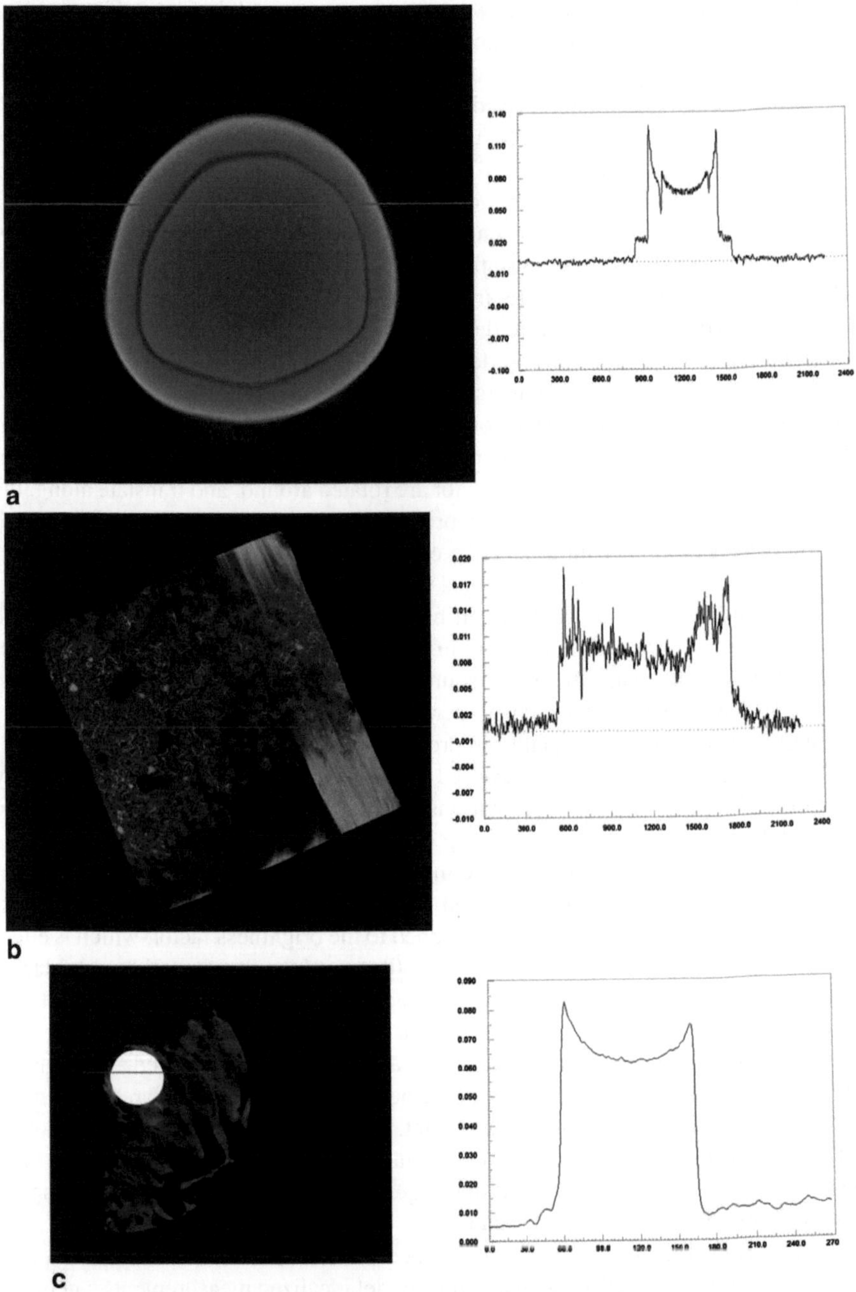

Fig. 2 Beam hardening contribution in μCT images

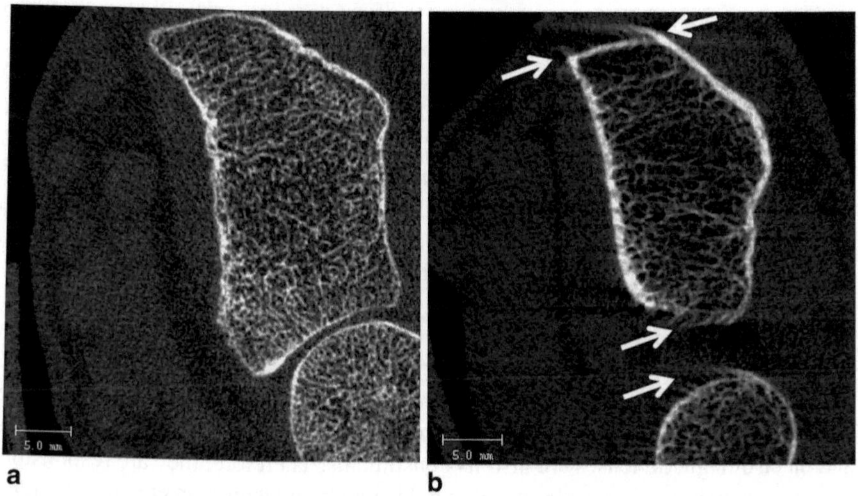

Fig. 3 Illustration of μCT radius image without **a** and with **b** patient movement. *The arrows* show the movement artifact

the radiation through the object, dl is its distance increment along L. Also in (2), we have the term $ln(\frac{I_0}{I_d})$, which is called ray sums and represents the contribution of all μ along the radiation path.

$$ln\left(\frac{I_0}{I_d}\right) = ln\left[e^{-\int \mu(x,y)dl}\right] \rightarrow \ln\left(\frac{I_0}{I}\right) = \int_L \mu(x,y)dl = P(x,y) \qquad (2)$$

A set of ray sums over a given angle, parallel to the beam radiation, forms the projection term P. Each projection is acquired with the object (X-ray tube-detector system) rotated by an angle φ relative to the original position. So, it is possible to obtain a projection for each angle φ.

The information from transmitted X-rays is processed by a computer in order to obtain the CT/μCT images. In order to achieve this goal the theory of image reconstruction from projections is applied. In general words, the attenuation coefficient in each point (x,y) of the scanned object can be found from the projections using the inverse of the Radon transform. There are a number of alternatives to perform the reconstruction, such as the direct Fourier method or iterative approach. Currently, the most used reconstruction algorithms are based on the direct reconstruction method called filtered backprojection algorithm, which is mainly a combination of filtering and a good numerical stability. Basically, the function of the filter used describes a low pass filter that can be used to globally balance the noise and spatial resolution in the reconstruction results. The filtered back projection issue was first described in the 60s but the key theory on CT filtering reconstruction was presented on the 70s and implemented by Hounsfield, who is acknowledged as the inventor of the CT technique. A great evolution in μCT reconstruction theory was achieved when using a series of X-ray cone beam projections directly into 3D density distribution. Cone beam CT is a 3D extension of 2D fan beam CT and has the advantage of the reduction of data collection time, which is particularly important when moving structures are scanned.

The 3D data set of the scanned object is obtained by stacking contiguous 2D images. Here, the source trajectory is a circle and each horizontal row of the detector is ramp-filtered as if it was a projection of a 2D object. Then, the filtered projection data are back projected along the original rays and the middle slice is reconstructed exactly. The 2D algorithms reconstruct a slice of the scanned object. But, if volumetric data knowledge is required, the complete procedure must be performed slice by slice. Description of μCT reconstruction algorithms can be largely found in the literature.

In order to record the transmitted X-ray beam, a detection system must be used. The use of image intensifier (II) with a charge coupled device (CCD) can be found in many old CT systems. The II are closed vacuum tubes amplifying image signals. They are made of glass, aluminum or non-ferromagnetic metal, which allows the flow of electrons from the photocathode to the anode. Input and output phosphorus and electromagnetic lenses are also its constituents. Therefore, they are responsible for the conversion of X-ray photons into light signals and their diameter are generally about 23–57 cm. The function of the input phosphor is to absorb the X-rays and emit light radiation. It is typically made of cesium iodide activated with sodium screen, but can also be made of zinc-cadmium activated with copper. However the first option is better because the crystals are vertically oriented, which helps to channel the light. The electronic signal from the II is captured by the CCD and then sent to a TV monitor resulting in a representation of the radiographic image in real time. In fact, the digitalization can be performed through CCD or by direct capture of the X-ray detector with a flat panel detector.

The CCD cameras are in general composed of amorphous Si with a scintillation layer, which is basically cesium iodide. Silicon has a low X-ray absorption coefficient, which leads to a small number of photons detected by the CCD. This results in a significant quantum noise. In order to decrease this noise, it is possible to increase the dose of radiation or the quantum detection efficiency. As increasing the dose is undesirable, priority is given to increasing the quantum efficiency of radiation detectors. The quantum efficiency of the detector system can be increased by adding a scintillation layer above the CCD. X-rays are absorbed by this layer, which has a high absorption coefficient, and then converted into visible light (wavelength or near-visible).

The flat panel detectors are based on flat-screen arrangement of amorphous silicon photodiodes and thin transistors in combination with scintillators CsI (Tl) devices. They replace the image intensifier and video camera, recording the image sequences in real time. The transition of II to flat panel is facilitated by the advantages they offer, such as images without distortion, excellent contrasts, large dynamic range and high sensitivity to X-rays

μCT emerged as a non-destructive method of analysis [11], to investigate the interface between bone and screws. Trabecular bone screws are commonly used for fixation of fractures in order to increase holding power in the fine trabecular bone. The holding strength of a screw is directly linked with bone quality, which is a very important issue in clinical healthcare [1].

In the medical area, titanium screws are used for fixation of fractures in order to increase holding power in the fine trabecular bone. In Orthodontics, in the last 2 decades, fixations screws were modified to be used as anchorage devices. These screws are called miniscrews or mini-implants. They are widespread in clinical practice because they allow tooth movement in three dimensions with minimal effect on other teeth.

The success of miniscrews is related to primary stability, which is defined as the absence of mobility in the bone bed after mini-implant placement [5] and depends on the mechanical engagement of an implant with the bone socket [2]. If the initial mechanical retention of the MI is not observed, a larger miniscrew should be used or the insertion site should be modified [3]. On the other hand, exaggerated tension during insertion may result in heating and damage to the bone tissue, including ischemia and necrosis, or even fracture of mini-implant [10].

After primary stability is achieved, the healing process starts and, due to osseointegration, the implant gains secondary stability [14]. Osseointegration is a direct structural and functional connection between ordered, living bone and the surface of a load-carrying implant. There is a direct bone-to-metal interface without interposition of non-bone tissue [9].

The contact surface of the bone to mini-implant, called bone to implant contact (BIC), has traditionally been assessed by histological techniques [4, 6, 10, 13]. The histological technique presents some disadvantages: it requires the destruction of the sample for making the histological slides; the analysis depends on the subjectivity of the operator; and it is necessary to evaluate lots of cross sections to obtain a global view of the sample.

The great advantage of μCT in dental area is the non-destructive nature of the technique as well as that it obtains information of the entire sample volume. However, one of the biggest challenges of the μCT BIC evaluation is to avoid the beam-hardening artifact presented in the reconstructed images, caused by the metal of the screws. In this context, the objective of this study was to evaluate BIC parameter of mini screws inserted into bone blocks by μCT.

2 Materials and Methods

Bovine samples (Fig. 4) (Bos taurus, Angus lineage) were removed from pelvic bones immediately after the animals were slaughtered with the use of a trephine bur (8 mm ø x 20 mm long, Sin Implants, São Paulo, Brazil) adapted to a low speed motor handpiece (Beltec LB100, Araraquara, Brazil), under irrigation.

The samples received implantation of a conical solid miniscrew, made of Ti-6Al-4 V alloy (INP®, São Paulo, Brazil), with 1.4 mm diameter and 6 mm long, and after that they were immersed in sterile physiological solution and stored frozen (– 20 °C). In order to perform the μCT, the samples were removed from the freeze, defrosted at room temperature ant then scanned.

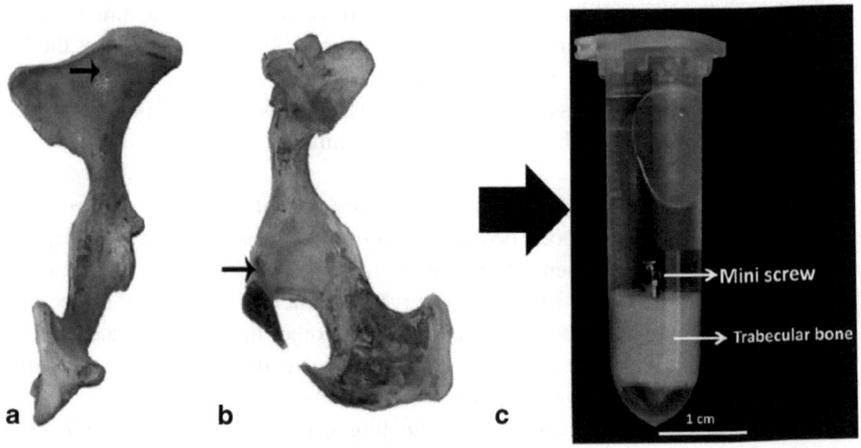

Fig. 4 Bovine samples: Macroscopic view of the right half of the pelvic bone. **a** Caudal view: *the arrow* indicates the gluteus iliac wing bone. **b** Medial view: *the arrow* indicates the caudal portion of the pubic bone

The images (Fig. 4c) were acquired in a high resolution system (Bruker/Skyscan μCT, model 1173, Kontich, Belgium, software version 1.6) at a pixel resolution of 9.3 μm, using a 1 mm thick aluminum filter, 80 kV, 90 μA, and exposure time of 800 ms. A flat panel detector with a matrix of 2240 × 2240 pixels was used. The samples were kept in 2 ml Eppendorf tubes containing saline solution during acquisition to avoid dehydration. The μCT images were reconstructed (NRecon software, InstaRecon, Inc. Champaign, IL, USA, version 1.6.4.1) and evaluated in the CT-Analyzer software (version 1.10, Bruker/Skyscan μCT, Kontich, Belgium).

After the scanning, quantitative evaluations were performed directly in 3D. The volume of interest (VOI) corresponded to a 3.4 mm diameter cylinder surrounding the mini screw, which means 1 mm beyond the mini screw (Fig. 5). In this particular study only the regional changes on trabecular microarchitecture were evaluated. In total, 366 slices were analyzed, which is equivalent to a cylinder volume equal to 15 mm^3.

In this study, the intersection surface between the trabecular bone and the mini-screw (IS) and the bone surface (BS) was calculated to evaluate BIC parameter. For that purpose, after the reconstruction procedure, μCT data were segmented with a global threshold. However, the metal artifact surrounding the mini-implant must be identified and take into account when BIC evaluation is performed. In this step, different values of pixel size dilation distant from the mini-implant interface were studied. 2D and 3D morphological operation approaches involving dilatation of pixels/voxels from the surface were used. All the steps were performed by using round kernel operation with many radius values (2, 4, 6, 8, 10 and 12). BIC evaluation was also performed without any morphological operation in order to compare the impact of this approach.

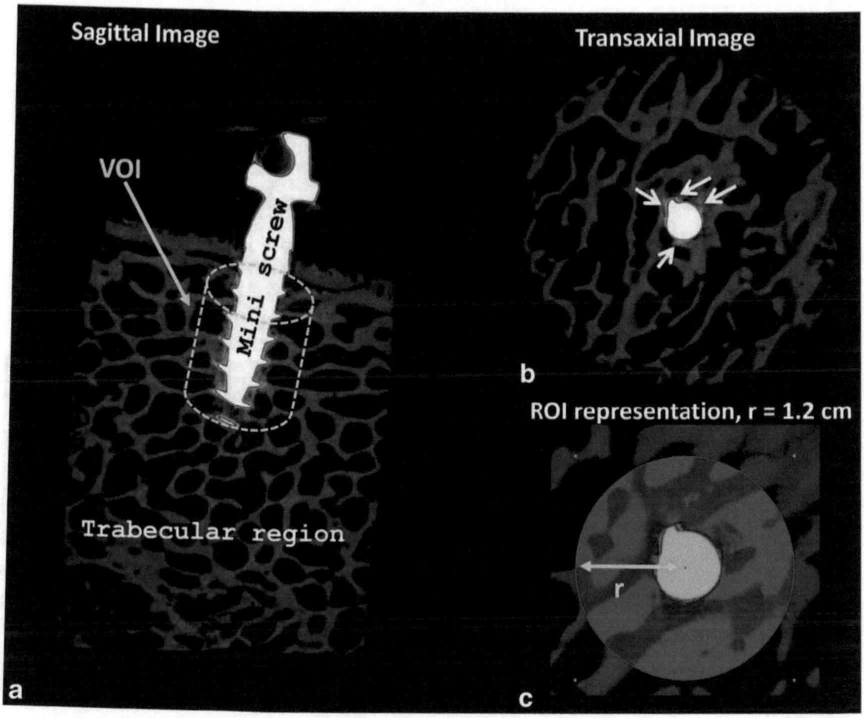

Fig. 5 μCT cross-sections of bone implant contact **a** sagittal view, **b** transaxial view, **c** better detail of beam hardening effect

3 Results

Cortical bone is dense and has a solid structure whereas trabecula has a honeycomb organization and is believed to distribute and dissipate the energy from articular contact loads. Although about 80 % of the total skeletal mass is cortical bone, trabecular bone has a much greater surface area than cortical [15]. In this study, only the region surrounding the trabeculae was evaluated. The possibility of using μCT, a non-invasive and non-destructive technique for the evaluation of the bone-implant interface was explored.

Although μCT provides a good quality data for bone and implant interface investigation, beam hardening artifact corrections must be taken into account. This issue is caused by the non-linear relation between the attenuation values and the measurement values of the projection. Like all medical and industrial X-ray beams, μCT uses a polyenergetic X-ray spectrum (X-ray attenuation coefficients are energy dependent). After passing through a given thickness of an object, lower energy X-rays are attenuated to a greater extent than higher energy X-rays are. As the X-ray beam propagates through a thickness of materials, the shape of the spectrum becomes skewed toward higher energies. In this sense, beam hardening phenomenon

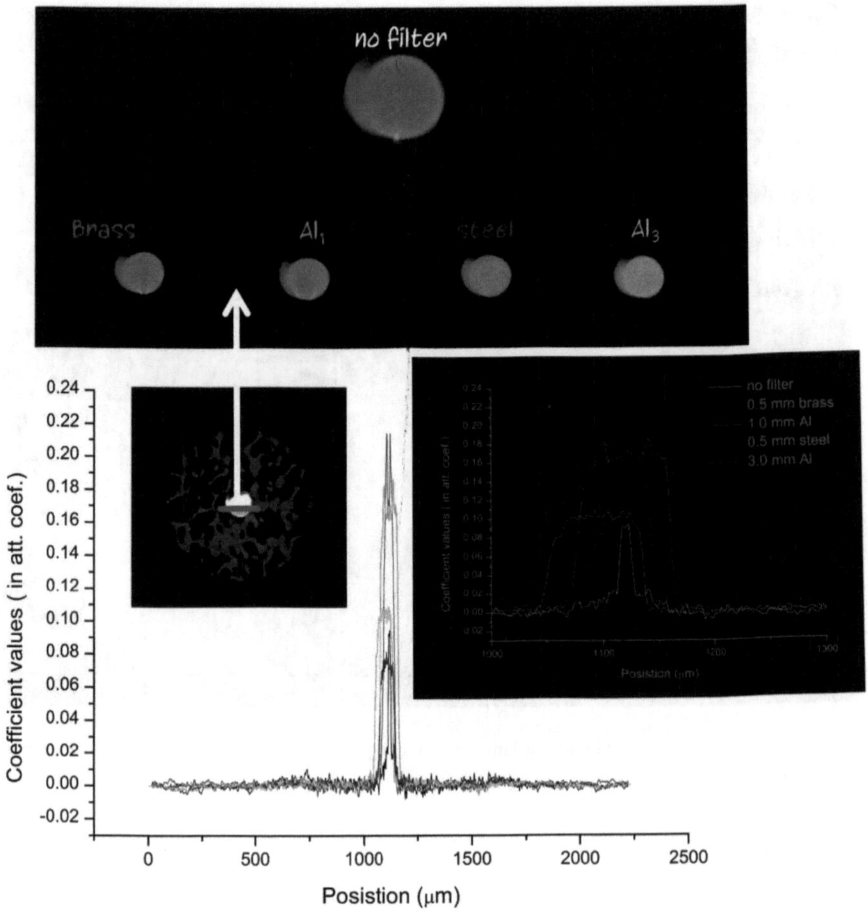

Fig. 6 Beam hardening contribution in different metallic filters applications. Note in the reconstruction slices of mini-screws and they corresponding profile along the arrow line

induces artifacts in μCT because rays from some projection angles are hardened to a differing extent than rays from other angles, which mixed up the reconstruction algorithms. This phenomenon leads to an image error, which reduces the image quality in CT/μCT measurements. In fact, these issues clearly indicate serious impact on quantitative μCT measurements. In this study, in order to avoid this issue a combination of two approaches was used. The scans were acquired over 360° and an aluminum filter of 1.0 mm of thickness placed at the exit window of the X-ray tube was used in this scan step. Figure 6 shows μCT profiles obtained with different kind of materials. It is possible to note that the metallic filter affects the effective energy and in consequence the attenuation coefficient. Note in the slices reconstructions the reduced artefacts compared to no filter μCT slice reconstructed image.

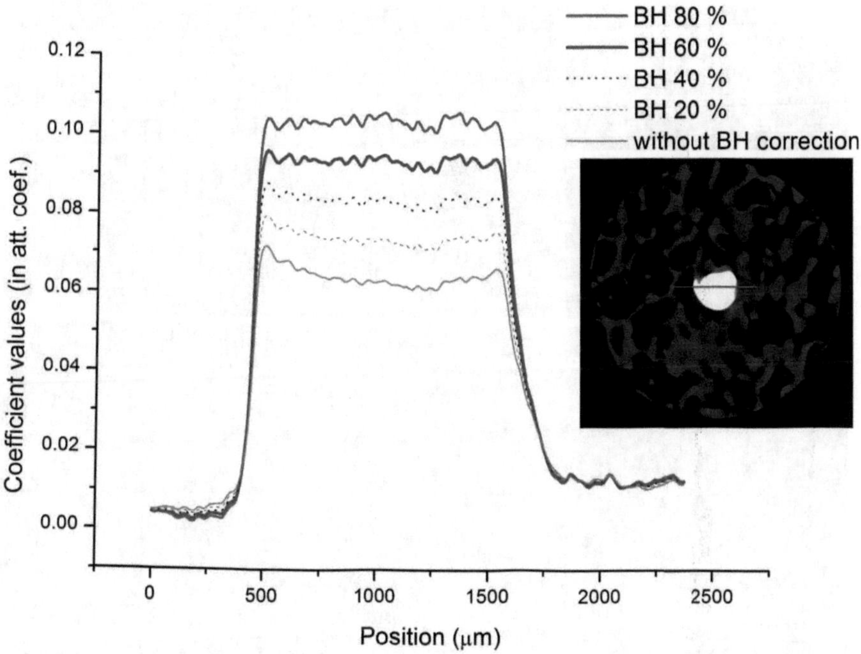

Fig. 7 Typical μCT signal profile through the center of the bone implant sample: different beam hardening correction depth values of 360° scanning

Another attitude was taken during the reconstruction progression. A few reconstruction parameters can be adjusted on the reconstruction software and one of them is the beam hardening correction. This option compensates the problem by a linear transformation in which several correction (0, ..., 100) depths can be selected according to the object density. Bone and metal can be easily distinguished in Fig. 7. It is also possible to see the difference between the profiles along the arrow line with and without beam hardening correction through the center of the sample. Fine-tuning function was used in order to obtain the optimum depth correction value.

In order to evaluate BIC the ratio between the intersection surfaces (IS) of the mini-screw and the trabecular bone was calculated. Traditionally, the contact surface of the bone tissue with the screw, called BIC was studied through, histological techniques [4]. Alternatively, the μCT emerged as a non-destructive method of analysis. However, some important differences are observed between the two techniques. In the first one, 2D images are evaluated while in the second one we have the possibility of accessing all the 3D data. Furthermore, due to artifacts created by the metal in μCT, a small image strip adjacent to the bone tissue mini-implant should be disregarded during the analysis. Due to these facts, a new index of analysis can be created when μCT is used: the osteointegration volume/total volume of the implant, which is effective for predicting the mechanical attachment of implants to the bone [8]. In this study, we believe that it would be more appropriate to call the index "bone implant

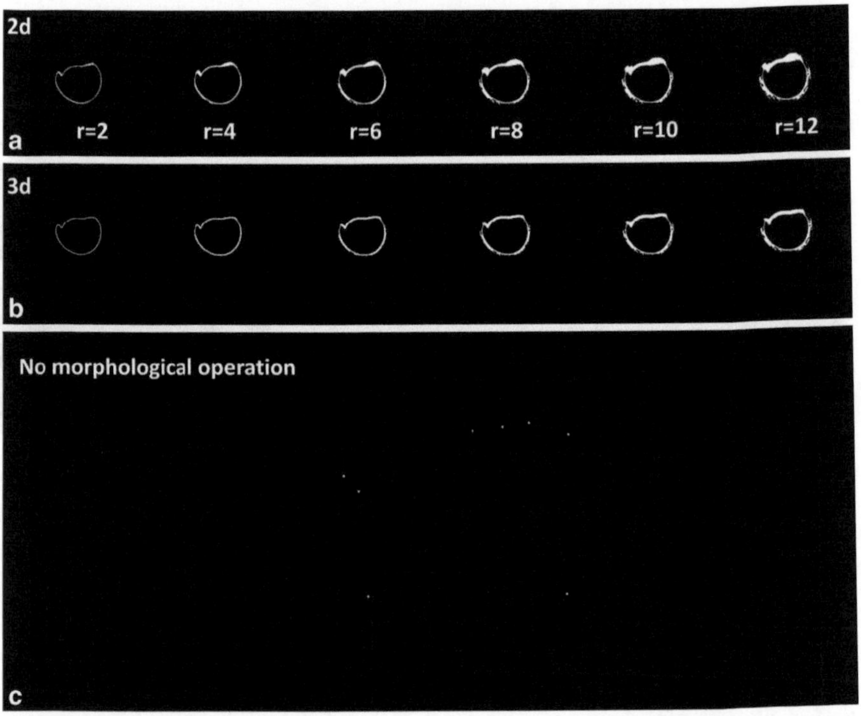

Fig. 8 μCT transaxial binary images used at intersection between bone and implant surface (IS) with different pixel(a)/voxel(b) values of dilation. It is possible to see what happens when no image processing analyzis is performed **a.** r represents the values of the round kernel radius of the dilation morphological operation

intersection volume/total volume", because there was no osteointegration area itself since the installation of the mini-implant was performed in ex vivo tissue, with no healing periods.

However, one of the biggest challenges of the BIC evaluation by μCT is to avoid the beam hardening artifact presented in the reconstructed images, which are caused by the metal of the screws. For that purpose, some image processing analyzes can be performed. In this study, morphological operation on binary images was used in order to remove pixels/voxels near to the implant surface. The procedure was applied directly in 2D/3D with round kernel operator. In Fig. 5b this effect can be observed, represented by the white arrows. Figure 8 shows the influence of the dilation procedure for calculating the IS parameter. It is also possible to visualize the difference when no morphological operation is applied. The mathematical results of this procedure are presented in table 1.

In this way, BIC values were calculated based on a cylindrical VOI that eliminates the closest pixels/voxels near the implant surface in order to avoid metal-induced artifacts and assumes that the presence of bone in this VOI is a predictor of actual BIC.

Table 1 μCT BIC results: different pixel/voxels sizes of round kernel dilation in order to avoid metal-induced artifact

Radius size dilatation (r)	Pixel dilatation		Voxel dilatation	
	IS (mm)	BIC (%)	IS (mm)	BIC (%)
2	14.42	81.6	17.68	91.3
4	14.23	80.5	13.74	77.7
6	13.86	78.4	13.00	73.5
8	13.65	77.2	12.66	71.6
10	13.50	76.4	12.32	69.7
12	13.48	76.3	12.00	67.9
No Morphological operation	0.053			0.30

The specific metallic content of an implant may affect the severity of artifacts on CT images. Titanium alloy hardware causes the least obtrusive artifact of CT imaging, whereas stainless steel implants cause significant beam attenuation and artifact. Knowledge of the composition of the implanted material at the time of the CT examination may be helpful, as technical parameters may be then adjusted to minimize artifacts and to spare the patient from excess radiation.

The composition of the dental implant and mini-implant is very similar. Both are composed by titanium alloys, so the data of this study can be useful in dental implant studies.

The present study focused the evaluation of BIC by μCT and identified that it is important to investigate the metallic artifact around the mini screws, which can be assessed by different pixel size dilation showing a correlation pattern between beam hardening artifact correction and BIC measurements.

4 Conclusion

3D X-ray microtomograhy is a new reality approach employed in the quantitative assessment of orthodontic mini-implants. Apart from its great potentiality, beam hardening corrections is required in order to obtain a diagnostic image quality. The results show that beam hardening artifact affects bone interface contact evaluation by X-ray microtomography. A strong relation between the voxels disposed near the surface of the miniscrews and BIC assessment was found.

Acknowledgments The authors would like to thanks CNPQ and FAPERJ for financial support.

References

1. Fyhrie DP (2005) Summary-measuring 'bone quality'. J Musculoskelet Neuronal Interact 5:318–320
2. Cehreli MC, Kaarasoy D, Akca K, Eckert SE (2009) Meta-analysis of methods used to assess implant stability. Int J Oral Maxillofac Implants 24 (6):1015–1032
3. Garfinkle JS, Cunnigham LL Jr, Beeman CS, Kluemper GT, Hicks EP, Kim MO (2008) Evaluation of orthodontic mini-implant anchorage in premolar extraction therapy in adolescents. Am J Orthod Dentofac 133(5):642–153
4. Gedrange T, Hietschold, V, Mai R, Wolf P, Nicklisch M, Harzer W (2005) An evaluation of resonance frequency analysis for the determination of the primary stability of orthodontic palatal implants. A study in human cadavers. Clin Oral Implants Res 16:425–431
5. Javed F, Romanos GE (2010) The role of primary stability for succesful immediate loading of dental implants. J Dent 38(8):612–620
6. Kim S, Choi B, Li J, Kim H, Ko C (2008) Peri-implant bone reactions at delayed and immediately loaded implants: an experimental study. Oral Maxillofacial Surgery 105:144–148
7. Kim SH, Lee SJ, Cho IS, Kim SK (2009) Rotational resistance of surface-treated mini-implants angle. Orthodontist 79(5):899–907
8. Liu S, Broucek J, Virdi AS, Sumner DR (2012) Limitation of using micro-computed tomography to predict implant contact and mechanical fixation. J Microsc 245:34–42
9. Mavrogenis AF, Dimitriou R, Parvizi J, Babis GC (2009) Bioloy of implant osseointegration. J Musculoskelet Neuronal Interact 92(2):61–71
10. Park Y, Yi K, Jung Y (2005) Correlation between microtomography and histomorphometry for assessment of implant osseointegration. Clin Oral Impl 16:156–160
11. Sennerby L, Wennerberg A, Pasop F (2001) A new microtomographic technique for non-invasive evaluation of the bone structure around implants. Clin Oral Impl Res 12:91–94
12. Verna LC, Melsen B (2009) Immediate loading of orthodontic mini-implants: a histomorphometric evaluation of tissue reaction. Eur J Orthod 31:21–29
13. Weiss P, Obadia L, Magne D, Bourges X, Rau C, Weitkamp T, Khairoun I, Bouler JM, Chappard D, Gauthier O, Daculsi G (2003) Synchrotron X-ray microtomography (on micron scale) provides three-dimensional imaging representation of bone ingrowth in calcium phosphate biomaterials. Biomaterials 24:4591–4601
14. Wilmes B, Rademacher D, Olthog G, Drescher D (2006) Parameters affecting primary stability of orthodontic mini-implants. J Orofac Orhtopedics 67(3):162–174
15. Zhao L, Xu Z, Yang Z, Wei X, Tang T, Zhao Z (2009) Orthodontic mini-implant stability in different healing times before loading: a microscopic computerized tomographic and biomechanical analysis. Oral Surg Oral Med Oral Pathol Oral Radiol Endod 108:196–202

Anisotropy Estimation of Trabecular Bone in Gray-Scale: Comparison Between Cone Beam and Micro Computed Tomography Data

Rodrigo Moreno, Magnus Borga, Eva Klintström, Torkel Brismar and Örjan Smedby

Abstract Measurement of anisotropy of trabecular bone has clinical relevance in osteoporosis. In this study, anisotropy measurements of 15 trabecular bone biopsies from the radius estimated by different fabric tensors on images acquired through cone beam computed tomography (CBCT) and micro computed tomography (micro-CT) were compared. The results show that the generalized mean intercept length (MIL) tensor performs better than the global gray-scale structure tensor, especially when the von Mises-Fisher kernel is applied. Also, the generalized MIL tensor yields consistent results between the two scanners. These results suggest that this tensor is appropriate for estimating anisotropy in images acquired in vivo through CBCT.

R. Moreno (✉) · E. Klintström · Ö. Smedby
Department of Radiology and Department of Medical and Health Sciences, Linköping University, Linköping, Sweden

Center for Medical Image Science and Visualization (CMIV), Linköping University, Linköping, Sweden

Linköping University, Campus US, 581 85 Linköping, Sweden
e-mail: rodrigo.moreno@liu.se

M. Borga
Department of Biomedical Engineering, Linköping University, Linköping, Sweden

Center for Medical Image Science and Visualization (CMIV), Linköping University, Linköping, Sweden
e-mail: magnus.borga@liu.se

E. Klintström
e-mail: eva.klintstrom@lio.se

T. Brismar
Department of Radiology, Karolinska University Hospital at Huddinge, Huddinge, Sweden
e-mail: torkel.brismar@gmail.com

Ö. Smedby
e-mail: orjan.smedby@liu.se

J. M. R. S. Tavares, R. Natal Jorge (eds.), *Developments in Medical Image Processing and Computational Vision*, Lecture Notes in Computational Vision and Biomechanics 19,
DOI 10.1007/978-3-319-13407-9_13

1 Introduction

Fabric tensors aim at modeling through tensors both orientation and anisotropy of trabecular bone. Many methods have been proposed for computing fabric tensors from segmented images, including boundary-, volume-, texture-based and alternative methods (cf. [21] for a complete review). However, due to large bias generated by partial volume effects, these methods are usually not applicable to images acquired in vivo, where the resolution of the images is in the range of the trabecular thickness. Recently, different methods have been proposed to deal with this problem. In general, these methods directly compute the fabric tensor on the gray-scale image, avoiding in that way the problematic segmentation step.

Different imaging modalities can be used to generate 3D images of trabecular bone in vivo, including different magnetic resonance imaging (MRI) protocols and computed tomography (CT) modalities. The main disadvantages of MRI are that it requires long acquisition times that can easily lead to motion-related artifacts and that the obtained resolution with this technique is worse compared to the one obtained through CT in vivo [8]. Regarding CT modalities, cone beam CT (CBCT) [16, 22] and high-resolution peripheral quantitative CT (HR-pQCT) [1, 5] are two promising CT techniques for in vivo imaging. Although these techniques are not appropriate to all skeletal sites, their use is appealing since they can attain higher resolutions and lower doses than standard clinical CT scanners. CBCT has the extra advantages with respect to HR-pQCT that it is available in most hospitals in the western world, since it is used in clinical practice in dentistry wards, and, on top of that, the scanning time is shorter (30s vs. 3min), so it is less prone to motion artifacts than HR-pQCT.

As already mentioned, there are many methods available for computing tensors describing anisotropy in gray-scale [21]. A strategy for choosing the most appropriate method is to assess how similar the tensors computed from a modality for in vivo imaging (e.g., CBCT) are with respect to the ones computed from the reference imaging modality (micro-CT) for the same specimens. This was actually the strategy that we follow in this chapter.

From the clinical point of view, it seems more relevant to track changes in anisotropy than in the orientation of trabecular bone under treatment, since osteoporosis can have more effect on its anisotropy than on its orientation [13, 23]. Thus, the aim of the present study was to compare anisotropy measurements from different fabric tensors computed on images acquired through cone beam computed tomography (CBCT) to the same tensors computed on images acquired through micro computed tomography (micro-CT).

Due to its flexibility, we have chosen in this study our previously proposed generalized mean intercept length (MIL) tensor [18] (GMIL) with different kernels and, due to its simplicity, the global gray-scale structure tensor (GST) [25]. This chapter is an extended version of the work in [20].

The chapter is organized as follows. Section 2 presents the material and methods used in this study. Section 3 shows comparisons between using GMIL and GST in both CBCT and micro-CT data. Finally, Sect. 4 discusses the results and outlines our current ongoing research.

2 Material and Methods

2.1 *Material*

The samples in this study consisted of 15 bone biopsies from the radius of human cadavers donated to medical research. The biopsies were approximately cubic with a side of 10 mm. Each cube included a portion of cortical bone on one side to facilitate orientation. The bone samples were placed in a test tube filled with water and the tube was placed in the centre of a paraffin cylinder, with a diameter of approximately 10 cm, representing soft tissue to simulate measurements in vivo. After imaging, a cube, approximately 8 mm in side, with only trabecular bone was digitally extracted from each dataset for analysis.

2.2 *Image Acquisition and Reconstruction*

The specimens were examined both with CBCT and with micro-CT. The CBCT data were acquired with a 3D Accuitomo FPD 80 (J. Morita Mfg. Corp., Kyoto, Japan) with a current of 8 mA and a tube voltage of 85 kV. The obtained resolution was 80 micrometers isotropic. The micro-CT data were acquired with a μ CT 40 (SCANCO Medical AG, Bassersdorf, Switzerland) with a tube voltage of 70 kVp. The voxels have an isotropic resolution of 20 microns. Figure 1 shows slices and volume renderings of one of the imaged specimens.

2.3 *Methods*

The tensors were computed through the generalized MIL tensor (GMIL) and the GST.

2.3.1 GMIL Tensor

Basically, the GMIL tensor is computed in three steps. The mirrored extended Gaussian image (EGI) [12] is computed from a robust estimation of the gradient. Second, the EGI is convolved with a kernel in order to obtain an orientation distribution function (ODF). Finally, a second-order fabric tensor is computed from the ODF. More formally, the generalized MIL tensor is computed as:

$$\mathsf{MIL} = \int_{\Omega} \frac{v\,v^T}{C(v)^2}\, d\Omega, \tag{1}$$

where v are vectors on the unitary sphere Ω, and C is given by:

$$C = H * E, \tag{2}$$

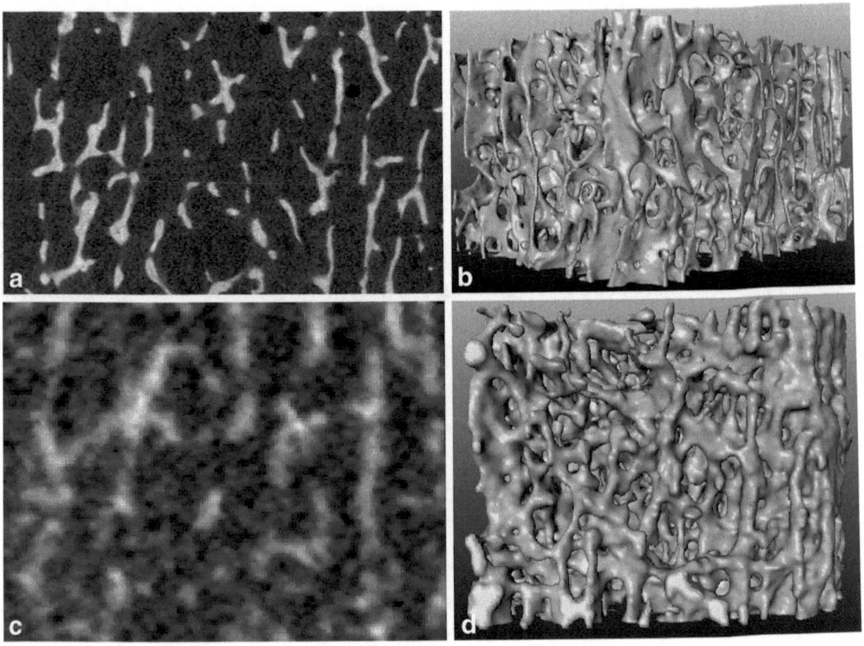

Fig. 1 Slices (*left*) and volume renderings (*right*) of one of the imaged specimens. Top: images acquired through micro-CT. Bottom: images acquired through CBCT

that is, the angular convolution ($*$) of a kernel H with the mirrored EGI E. Thanks to the Funk-Hecke theorem [3, 9], this convolution can be performed efficiently in the spherical harmonics domain when the kernel is positive and rotationally symmetric with respect to the north pole.

One of the advantages of the GMIL tensor is that different kernels can be used in order to improve the results. In this study, the half-cosine (HC) and von Mises-Fisher (vMF) kernels have been applied to the images. The HC has been selected since it makes equivalent the generalized and the original MIL tensor. The HC is given by:

$$H(\phi) = \begin{cases} \cos(\phi), & \text{if} \phi \leq \pi/2 \\ 0, & \text{otherwise,} \end{cases} \tag{3}$$

with ϕ being the polar angle in spherical coordinates. Moreover, the vMF kernel, which is given by [14]:

$$H(\phi) = \frac{\kappa}{4\pi \sinh(\kappa)} e^{\kappa \cos(\phi)}, \tag{4}$$

has been selected since it has a parameter κ that can be used to control its smoothing action. In particular, the smoothing effect is reduced as the values of κ are increased [18].

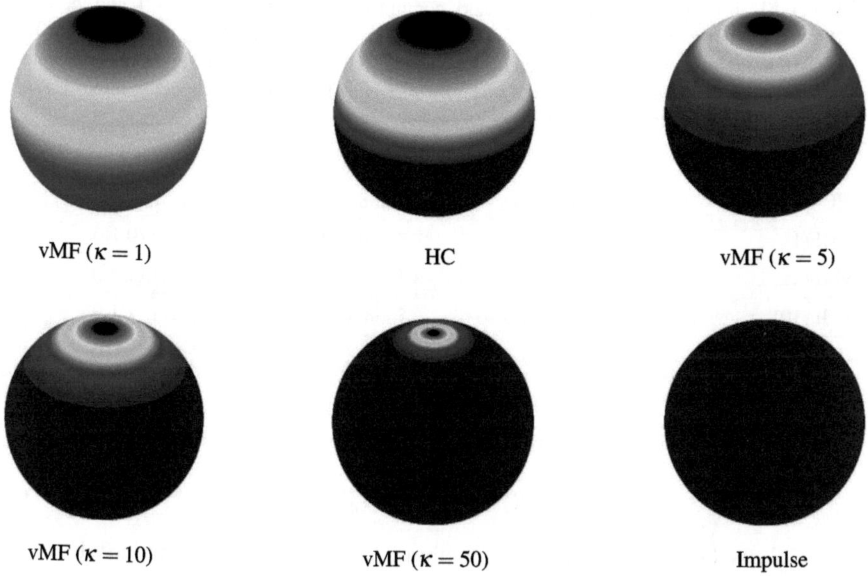

Fig. 2 Graphical representation of some kernels from the broadest to the narrowest, where zero and the largest values are depicted in blue and red respectively. Notice that the impulse kernel has been depicted as a single red dot in the north pole of the sphere

Figure 2 shows different kernels that can be used with the GMIL tensor. As already mentioned, these kernels must be positive and symmetric with respect to the north pole. As shown in the figure, the HC kernel is too broad (it covers half of the sphere), which can result in excessive smoothing. On the contrary, the impulse kernel is the sharpest possible kernel. As shown in [18], the GST makes use of the impulse kernel. In turn, the size of the smoothing effect of the vMF kernel can be controlled through the parameter κ. As shown in the figure, vMF is broader than the HC for small values of κ and it converges to the impulse kernel in the limit when $\kappa \to \infty$.

2.3.2 GST Tensor

On the other hand, the GST computes the fabric tensor by adding up the outer product of the local gradients with themselves [25], that is:

$$\mathsf{GST} = \int_{p \in I} \nabla I_p \nabla I_p^T \, dI, \tag{5}$$

where I is the image and ∇I_p is the gradient.

Notice that GST related to the well-known local structure tensor (ST) which has been used in the computer vision community since 1980s [4]. There are different methods for computing ST, including quadrature filters [7], higher-order derivatives

Table 1 Mean (SD) of E1' for fabric tensors computed on CBCT and micro-CT and the mean difference (SD) between both values. HC and vMF refer to the generalized MIL tensor, with the HC, and vMF kernels respectively. Parameter κ for vMF is shown in parenthesis. Positive and negative values of the difference mean over- and under estimations of CBCT with respect to micro-CT. All values have been multiplied by 100

Tensor	micro-CT	CBCT	Difference
HC	44.65 (1.54)	42.38 (0.90)	2.25 (0.84)
vMF(1)	34.12 (0.29)	34.70 (0.18)	0.42 (0.15)
vMF(5)	51.55 (3.56)	47.07 (2.17)	4.51 (1.82)
vMF(10)	58.98 (4.63)	53.90 (3.21)	5.11 (2.13)
GST	45.69 (1.58)	44.79 (1.58)	0.90 (2.09)

[15] or tensor voting [19]. However, the most used ST is given by:

$$\mathsf{ST}_\sigma(p) = G_\sigma * \nabla I_p \nabla I_p{}^T \tag{6}$$

where G_σ is a Gaussian weighting function with zero mean and standard deviation σ. In fact, ST becomes the GST when $\sigma \to \infty$. The main advantage of this structure tensor is that it is easy to code.

3 Results

As already mentioned, the focus in this chapter is the estimation of anisotropy. As a matter of fact, both the GMIL (and therefore the MIL tensor) and the GST tensors yield the same orientation information, since they have the same eigenvectors (cf. [18] for a detailed proof). This means that only the eigenvalues of the tensors are of interest for the purposes of this chapter.

The following three values have been computed for each tensor:

$$E1' = E1/(E1 + E2 + E3)$$
$$E2' = E2/E1,$$
$$E3' = E3/E1,$$

where E1, E2 and E3 are the largest, intermediate and smallest eigenvalues of the tensor. These three values have been selected since they are directly related to the shape of the tensor.

Tables 1–3 show the mean and standard deviation of E1', E2' and E3' computed on micro-CT and CBCT for the tested methods, and the mean difference and standard deviation between micro-CT and CBCT. As a general trend, the tested methods tend to overestimate E1' and underestimate E2' and E3' in CBCT. As shown, the best performance is obtained by vMF with κ =1 with small differences between tensors computed in both modalities. However, the tensors computed with this broad kernel are almost isotropic (cf. Tables 2 and 3), which makes it not suitable for detecting

Table 2 Mean (SD) of E2' for fabric tensors computed on CBCT and micro-CT and the mean difference (SD) between both values. HC and vMF refer to the generalized MIL tensor, with the HC, and vMF kernels respectively. Parameter κ for vMF is shown in parenthesis. Positive and negative values of the difference mean over- and under estimations of CBCT with respect to micro-CT. All values have been multiplied by 100

Tensor	micro-CT	CBCT	Difference
HC	65.94 (5.85)	71.50 (3.53)	−6.11 (2.19)
vMF(1)	93.70 (1.69)	95.27 (1.02)	−1.84 (0.73)
vMF(5)	52.13 (9.54)	61.63 (6.53)	−8.48 (3.09)
vMF(10)	39.41 (9.74)	48.31 (7.75)	−8.96 (4.43)
GST	80.71 (10.66)	78.58 (7.66)	2.24 (7.41)

Table 3 Mean (SD) of E3' for fabric tensors computed on CBCT and micro-CT and the mean difference (SD) between both values. HC and vMF refer to the generalized MIL tensor, with the HC, and vMF kernels respectively. Parameter κ for vMF is shown in parenthesis. Positive and negative values of the difference mean over- and under estimations of CBCT with respect to micro-CT. All values have been multiplied by 100

Tensor	micro-CT	CBCT	Difference
HC	58.29 (2.93)	65.18 (2.20)	−5.58 (2.98)
vMF(1)	91.09 (1.01)	92.92 (0.67)	−1.59 (0.89)
vMF(5)	42.72 (5.11)	51.20 (3.71)	−9.55 (4.49)
vMF(10)	31.17 (4.94)	37.81 (3.91)	−6.64 (2.70)
GST	38.71 (4.90)	44.96 (3.78)	−6.31 (4.40)

Table 4 Correlations between CBCT and micro-CT of E1', E2' and E3' of different fabric tensors. HC and vMF refer to the generalized MIL tensor, with the HC, and vMF kernels respectively. Parameter κ for vMF is shown in parenthesis. 95 % confidence intervals are shown in parentheses

Tensor	E1'	E2'	E3'
HC	0.90 (0.73;0.97)	0.91 (0.76;0.97)	0.67 (0.23;0.88)
vMF(1)	0.90 (0.72;0.97)	0.90 (0.73;0.97)	0.70 (0.29;0.89)
vMF(5)	0.91 (0.75;0.97)	0.91 (0.75;0.97)	0.80 (0.48;0.93)
vMF(10)	0.92 (0.76;0.97)	0.90 (0.72;0.97)	0.84 (0.57;0.94)
GST	0.51 (0.00;0.81)	0.71 (0.33;0.90)	0.51 (0.00;0.81)

anisotropies in trabecular bone. It is also worthwhile to notice that the standard deviation of the differences increases with narrower kernels, such as GST. This means that a mild smoothing effect from middle range kernels such as vMF with κ=10, have a positive effect in the estimation of fabric tensors, since the differences between micro-CT and CBCT are reduced while keeping the anisotropy of the tensors.

Table 4 shows the correlations between the measurements obtained on CBCT and micro-CT. Also, Fig. 1 (left) shows the corresponding correlation plots for E1', E2' and E3' for HC, vMF (with $\kappa = 10$) and GST. It can be seen that the best correlations are yielded by vMF with different values of κ, and GST has a poor performance.

Figure 3 (right) shows correlation plots of the three eigenvalues normalized by the sum of them for the same three methods. As shown in this figure, the tensors yielded by the three methods have different shapes. First, vMF with $\kappa = 10$ generates the most anisotropic tensors with larger differences between E1 and E2 than HC and GST. Second, HC generates the most isotropic tensors with smaller differences between values of E1, E2 and E3 than the other tensors. Finally, unlike GST, both HC and vMF generate tensors that are close to be orthotropic, that is, E2 $\approx$ E3. This is in line with the common assumption of orthotropy for trabecular bone [28].

Figures 4–6 show Bland-Altman plots for the generalized MIL tensor with the HC and vMF (with $\kappa = 10$) kernels and the GST. As seen in these figures, GST yields wider limits of agreement, i.e., larger discrepancies between CBCT and micro-CT, than HC and vMF, in particular for E2' and E3'. One of the advantages of using the vMF kernel is that its parameter can be adjusted in order to improve the correlations between CBCT and micro-CT. Figure 7 shows the evolution of the correlations between CBCT and micro-CT with the parameter κ of the generalized MIL tensor with the vMF kernel. From this figure, E1' and E2' attain their maxima at $\kappa = 10$, $\kappa = 5$ respectively, while E3' asymptotically approaches a correlation of 0.875 when $\kappa \rightarrow \infty$. Since the three measurements determine the shape of the tensor, we suggest to choose the value of κ that maximizes the three correlations, that is, that maximizes (E1'+E2'+E3')/3. In our case, such a value is $\kappa = 10$, as is also shown in Fig. 7.

4 Discussion

We have compared in this chapter the anisotropy of different fabric tensors estimated on images acquired through CBCT and micro-CT of 15 trabecular bone biopsies from the radius. The results presented in the previous section show strong correlations between micro-CT and CBCT for the generalized MIL tensor with HC and vMF kernels, especially with $\kappa = 10$. In addition, good agreements between measurements in CBCT and the reference micro-CT have been shown through Bland-Altman plots for HC, vMF with $\kappa = 10$ and GST. An interesting result is that the GST yields clearly lower correlation values than the generalized MIL tensor using either HC or vMF kernels. We have shown that the GST can be seen as a variant of the generalized MIL tensor where the impulse kernel is applied instead of the HC [18].

In this line, the results from the previous section suggest that the use of broader smoothing kernels such as HC or vMF has a positive effect for increasing the correlation of the tensors computed on images acquired through suitable scanners for in vivo with the ones that can be computed from images acquired in vitro. Although the three tested methods yield tensors that share their eigenvectors, their eigenvalues are different, as shown in Fig. 3, which is a natural consequence of using different smoothing kernels. Moreover, the high correlations reported for HC and vMF enable

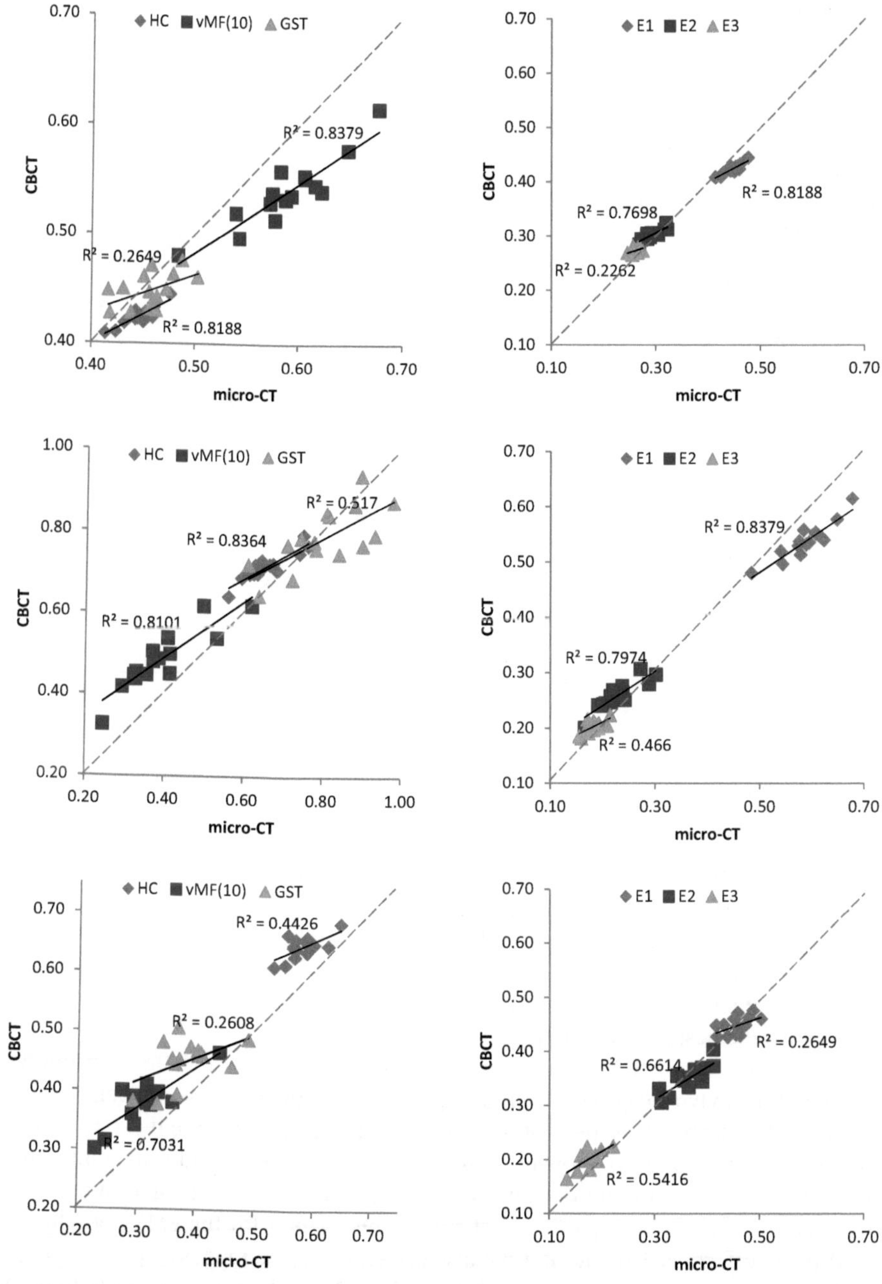

Fig. 3 *Left*: correlation plots for E1' (top), E2' (*middle*) and E3' (*bottom*) between CBCT and micro-CT for HC, vMF (κ = 10) and GST. *Right*: correlation plots for HC (*top*), vMF (κ = 10) (*middle*) and GST (*bottom*) between CBCT and micro-CT for the three eigenvalues normalized by the sum of them

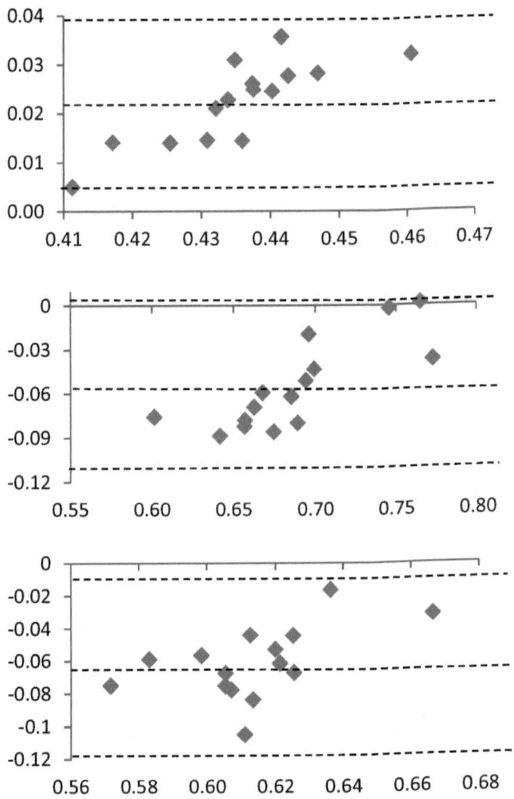

Fig. 4 Bland-Altman plots for E1' (*top*), E2' (*middle*) and E3' (*bottom*) between CBCT and micro-CT for HC. The vertical and horizontal axes show the measurements on micro-CT minus those computed on CBCT, and the mean between them respectively. The mean difference and the mean difference ±1.96 SD are included as a reference in dotted lines

to eliminate of the systematic errors reported in Tables 1–3 and in the Bland-Altman plots for these two types of fabric tensors.

Another interesting observation is that vMF yielded better results than the standard HC. This means that κ can be used to tune the smoothing in such a way that the results are correlated with in vitro measurements. For the imaged specimens, a value of κ = 10 yielded the best correlation results.

The results presented in this chapter suggest that advanced fabric tensors are suitable for in vivo imaging, which opens the door to their use in clinical practice. In particular, the results show that the generalized MIL tensor is the most promising option for use in vivo. As shown in this chapter, this method is advantageous since it has the possibility to improve its performance by changing the smoothing kernel by a more appropriate one, as it was shown in this chapter for the vMF kernel.

A poor performance of the GST has also been reported in images acquired through multi-slice computed tomography (MSCT) [26]. The authors of that study hypothesized that such a bad performance could be due to voxel anisotropy obtained from MSCT. However, the results from the current study suggest that the problems of the GST are more structural, since they are also present in CBCT with isotropic voxels.

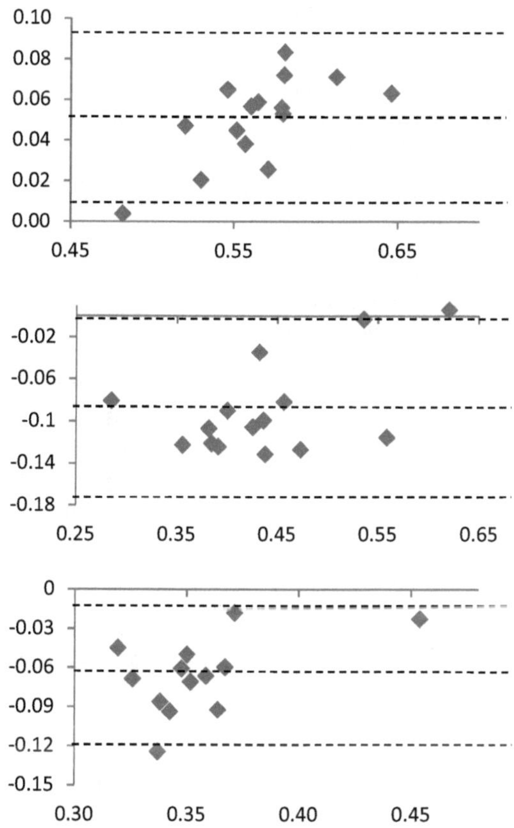

Fig. 5 Bland-Altman plots for E1' (*top*), E2' (*middle*) and E3' (*bottom*) between CBCT and micro-CT for vMF with $\kappa = 10$. The vertical and horizontal axes show the measurements on micro-CT minus those computed on CBCT, and the mean between them respectively. The mean difference and the mean difference ± 1.96 SD are included as a reference in dotted lines

Thus, the problems of GST seem more related to the applied kernel (the impulse kernel) than to the voxel anisotropy of the images.

Ongoing research includes performing comparisons in different skeletal sites, different degrees of osteoporosis and comparing the results with images acquired through HR-pQCT and micro-MRI [6, 11]. Furthermore, relationships between fabric and elasticity tensors will be explored. The MIL tensor has extensively been used for predicting elasticity tensors in trabecular bone [2, 10, 27]. However, since the GMIL with the vMF kernel has a better performance than the MIL tensor for reproducing in vitro measurements, we want to investigate whether or not the GMIL tensor can also be used to increase the accuracy of the MIL tensor for predicting the elastic properties of trabecular bone.

In the same line, we have recently hypothesized that trabecular termini (i.e., free ended trabeculae [24]) should not be considered for computing fabric tensors since contribution of termini to the mechanical competence of trabecular bone is rather limited [17]. Thus, it is worthwhile to assess the power of fabric tensors that disregard termini for predicting elasticity.

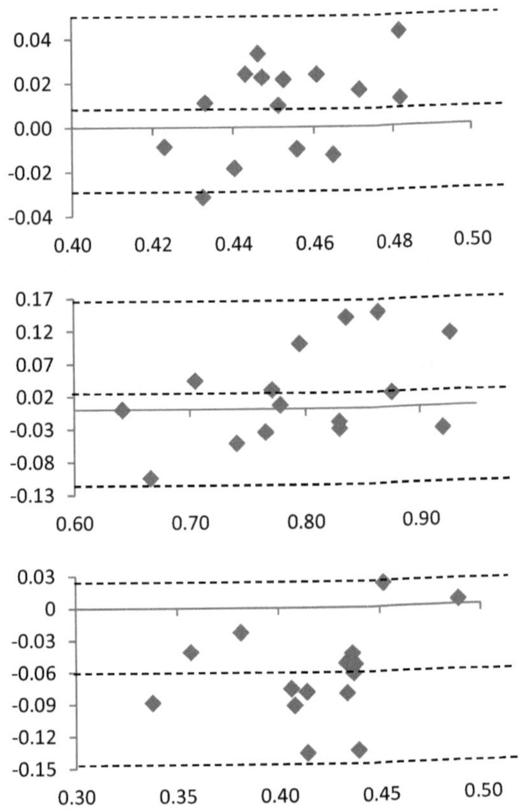

Fig. 6 Bland-Altman plots for E1' (*top*), E2' (*middle*) and E3' (*bottom*) between CBCT and micro-CT for GST. The vertical and horizontal axes show the measurements on micro-CT minus those computed on CBCT, and the mean between them respectively. The mean difference and the mean difference ±1.96 SD are included as a reference in dotted lines

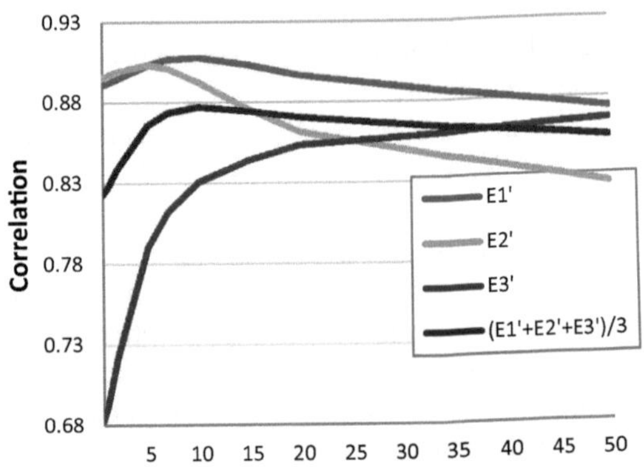

Fig. 7 Evolution of the correlations between CBCT and micro-CT with the parameter κ of the generalized MIL tensor with the vMF kernel

Acknowledgements We thank Andres Laib from SCANCO Medical AG for providing the micro-CT data of the specimens. The authors declare no conflict of interest.

References

1. Burghardt A, Link T, Majumdar S (2011) High-resolution computed tomography for clinical imaging of bone microarchitecture. Clin Orthop Relat Res 469(8):2179–2193
2. Cowin S (1985) The relationship between the elasticity tensor and the fabric tensor. Mech Mater 4(2):137–147
3. Driscoll JR, Healy DM (1994) Computing Fourier transforms and convolutions on the 2-sphere. Adv Appl Math 15(2):202–250
4. Förstner W (1986) A feature based correspondence algorithm for image matching. Int Arch Photogramm Remote Sens 26:150–166
5. Geusens P, Chapurlat R, Schett G, Ghasem-Zadeh A, Seeman E, de Jong J, van den Bergh J (2014) High-resolution in vivo imaging of bone and joints: a window to microarchitecture. Nat Rev Rheumatol. 10(5):304–313
6. Gomberg B, Wehrli F, Vasilić B, Weening R, Saha P, Song H, Wright A (2004) Reproducibility and error sources of μ-MRI-based trabecular bone structural parameters of the distal radius and tibia. Bone 35(1):266–276
7. Granlund GH, Knutsson H (1995) Signal processing for computer vision. Kluwer Academic, Dordrecht
8. Griffith J, Genant H (2012) New advances in imaging osteoporosis and its complications. Endocr 42:39–51
9. Groemer H (1996) Geometric applications of Fourier series and spherical harmonics. Cambridge University Press
10. Gross T, Pahr D, Zysset P (2013) Morphology-elasticity relationships using decreasing fabric information of human trabecular bone from three major anatomical locations. Biomech Model Mechanobiol 12(4):793–800
11. Hipp J, Jansujwicz A, Simmons C, Snyder B (1996) Trabecular bone morphology from micro-magnetic resonance imaging. J Bone Miner Res 11(2):286–297
12. Horn BKP (1984) Extended Gaussian images. Proc IEEE 72(12):1671–1686
13. Huiskes R (2000) If bone is the answer, then what is the question? J Anat 197:145–156
14. Jupp PE, Mardia KV (1989) A unified view of the theory of directional statistics, 1975–1988. Int Stat Rev 57(3):261–294
15. Köthe U, Felsberg M (2005) Riesz-transforms versus derivatives: on the relationship between the boundary tensor and the energy tensor. In: Scale Space and PDE Methods in Computer Vision, Hofgeismar Germany. LNCS 3459:179–191
16. Monje A, Monje F, Gonzalez-Garcia R, Galindo-Moreno P, Rodriguez-Salvanes F, Wang H (2014) Comparison between microcomputed tomography and cone-beam computed tomography radiologic bone to assess atrophic posterior maxilla density and microarchitecture. Cli Oral Implants Res 25(6):723–728
17. Moreno R, Smedby Ö (2014) Volume-based fabric tensors through lattice-Boltzmann simulations. In: Proceedings International Conference on Pattern Recognition (ICPR), Stockholm Sweden, pp 3179–3184
18. Moreno R, Borga M, Smedby Ö (2012) Generalizing the mean intercept length tensor for gray-level images. Med Phys 39(7):4599–4612
19. Moreno R, Pizarro L, Burgeth B, Weickert J, Garcia MA, Puig D (2012) Adaptation of tensor voting to image structure estimation. In: Laidlaw D, Vilanovaeds A (eds) New developments in the visualization and processing of tensor fields. Springer. pp 29–50
20. Moreno R, Borga M, Smedby Ö (2013) Correlations between fabric tensors computed on cone beam and micro computed tomography images. In: Tavares J, Natal-Jorge R (eds) Computational vision and medical image processing (VIPIMAGE). CRC Press (2013), pp 393–398
21. Moreno R, Borga M, Smedby Ö (2014) Techniques for computing fabric tensors: a review. In: Burgeth B, Vilanova A, Westin CF (eds) Visualization and processing of tensors and higher order descriptors for multi-valued data. Springer, pp 271–292

22. Mulder L, van Rietbergen B, Noordhoek NJ, Ito K (2012) Determination of vertebral and femoral trabecular morphology and stiffness using a flat-panel C-arm-based CT approach. Bone 50(1):200–208
23. Odgaard A, Kabel J, van Rietbergen B, Dalstra M, Huiskes R (1997) Fabric and elastic principal directions of cancellous bone are closely related. J Biomech 30(5):487–495
24. Tabor Z (2005) Novel algorithm detecting trabecular termini in μCT and MRI images. Bone 37(3):395–403
25. Tabor Z, Rokita E (2007) Quantifying anisotropy of trabecular bone from gray-level images. Bone 40(4):966–972
26. Tabor Z, Petryniak R, Latała Z, Konopka T (2013) The potential of multi-slice computed tomography based quantification of the structural anisotropy of vertebral trabecular bone. Med Eng Phys 35(1):7–15
27. Zysset PK (2003) A review of morphology-elasticity relationships in human trabecular bone: theories and experiments. J Biomech 36(10):1469–1485
28. Zysset PK, Goulet RW, Hollister SJ (1998) A global relationship between trabecular bone morphology and homogenized elastic properties. J Biomech Eng 120(5):640–646

Fractured Bone Identification from CT Images, Fragment Separation and Fracture Zone Detection

Félix Paulano, Juan J. Jiménez and Rubén Pulido

Abstract The automation of the detection of fractured bone tissue would allow to save time in medicine. In many cases, specialists need to manually revise 2D and 3D CT images and detect bone fragments and fracture regions in order to check a fracture. The identification of bone fragments from CT images allows to remove image noise and undesirable parts and thus improves image visualization. In addition, the utilization of models reconstructed from CT images of patients allows to customize the simulation, since the result of the identification can be used to perform a reconstruction that provides a 3D model of the patient anatomy. The detection of fracture zones increases the information provided to specialists and enables the simulation of some medical procedures, such as fracture reduction. In this paper, the main issues to be considered in order to identify bone tissue and the additional problems that arise if the bone is fractured are described. The identification of fractured bone includes not only bone tissue segmentation, but also bone fragments labelling and fracture region detection. Moreover, some fragments can appear together after the segmentation process, hence additional processing can be required to separate them. After that, currently proposed approaches to identify fractured bone are analysed and classified. The most recently proposed methods to segment healthy bone are also reviewed in order to justify that the techniques used for this type of bone are not always suitable for fractured bone. Finally, the aspects to be improved in the described methods are outlined and future work is identified.

F. Paulano (✉) · J. J. Jiménez · R. Pulido
University of Jaén, Campus Las Lagunillas s/n, Jaén, Spain
e-mail: fpaulano@ujaen.es

J. J. Jiménez
e-mail: juanjo@ujaen.es

R. Pulido
e-mail: rpulido@ujaen.es

J. M. R. S. Tavares, R. Natal Jorge (eds.), *Developments in Medical Image Processing and Computational Vision,* Lecture Notes in Computational Vision and Biomechanics 19,
DOI 10.1007/978-3-319-13407-9_14

1 Introduction

The automatic identification of bone tissue from computed tomographies (CT images) is a helpful procedure in medical visualization and simulation. Nowadays, the specialist has to manually revise 2D and 3D CT images to detect bone fragments and fracture regions to check a fracture in many cases. The segmentation of bone fragments removes image noise and undesirable parts and therefore improves image visualization. Advances in the visualization of medical images are rewarding because they prevent the specialists reviewing 2D and 3D images manually and thus they enable time saving. In medical simulation, the result of the segmentation can be used to perform a reconstruction that provides a 3D model of the patient anatomy which can be utilized to customize the simulation. These generated models are also useful to provide additional information during the intervention. On the other hand, the detection of fracture zones increases the information provided to specialists and enables the simulation of some medical procedures, such as bone fracture reduction.

In the literature, many methods have been proposed to segment healthy bone. Most of these methods are focused on a specific bone or require previous learning. These constraints do not allow to apply them to the segmentation of fractured bone, since the shape of the bone fragments is often unpredictable, especially in fractures caused by trauma. On the other hand, the identification of fractured bone adds some additional tasks. Specifically, it requires to label fragments and, in some cases, to separate wrongly joined fragments. Moreover, some applications also require to detect bone regions. Thus, specific methods are needed in order to identify fractured bones from CT images. In addition, each type of fracture has different features, hence there are necessary different methods in order to identify bone fragments in all type of fractures. In this paper, the main aspects to be considered to identify healthy and fractured bone are described. This allows to check what techniques applied in healthy bone segmentation may or may not be used to identify fractured bone. Moreover, the identification of fractured bone includes not only bone tissue segmentation, but also bone fragment labelling and fracture region detection, hence these processes are also analysed. After the segmentation process, several bone fragments can appear together as only one. Therefore, some additional processing can be required. Once all these issues are analysed, currently proposed approaches to segment healthy bone, identify fractured bone, separate bone fragments and detect fracture zones are revised and classified. This enables the outline of the aspects to be improved and the identification of future work.

In the next section, the main issues for both healthy and fractured bone detection are discussed. This includes the special aspects to be considered in each type of bone fracture. Then, we describe and classify previous work related to the segmentation of healthy and fractured bone. In the case of fractured bone, the approaches used to label fragments, to separate wrongly joined fragments and to detect fracture regions are also classified. Finally, this review allows to know the strengths and weakness of each approach and thus the issues that remain unsolved.

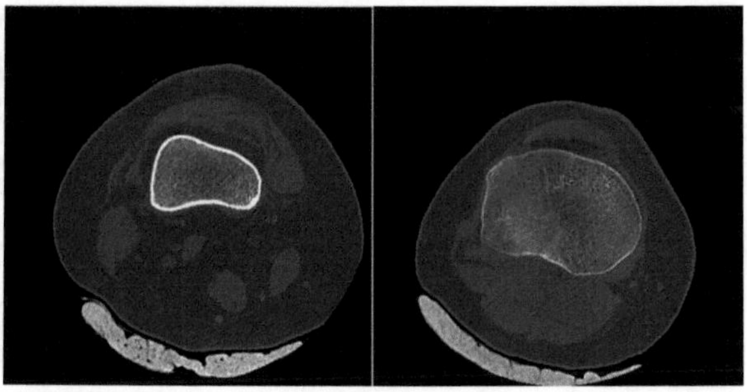

Fig. 1 Two CT images belonging to the same patient dataset. The intensity values of the cortical zone are different in the diaphysis (*left*) and the epiphysis (*right*). The cortical area is much thinner in the epiphysis (*right*)

2 Issues for Bone Detection

2.1 Healthy Bone

The segmentation of bone tissue from CT images is a complex process. It is difficult to find a solution that works in all cases. In a bone, there are two very distinct zones: cortical and trabecular tissue. Cortical tissue is very dense and it can be found in the outer part of the bone. Trabecular tissue is mainly in the inner part of the bone. This type of tissue is more heterogeneous and it has less intensity in a CT image. In addition, the intensity value for the same tissue differs between slices. This happens with both cortical and trabecular tissues. For instance, intensity values on the diaphysis and the epiphysis are different in a long bone (Fig. 1). Near the joints, the cortical zone is very thin. This zone even disappears in the area closest to the join. Therefore, the transition of the intensity values near the joints generally appears to be fuzzy and some areas within the bone may have similar intensity than the soft tissue surrounding the bone. This may cause incomplete segmentation or overgrowing [14].

2.2 Fractured Bone

Fractured bone tissue is more difficult to identify because it has some additional features to be considered. Due to the fact that bone fragments may have arbitrary shape and can belong to any bone in a nearby area, it is necessary to label all the fragments during the segmentation process. In some cases, this labelling requires expert knowledge. In addition, a priori knowledge can not be easily used because it is uncommon to find two identical fractures and therefore it is difficult to predict the shape of the bone fragments, specially in comminuted fractures. On the other hand, bone fragments are not completely surrounded by cortical tissue, since they have areas on the edges without cortical tissue due to the fracture. Finally, proximity between fragments and the resolution of the CT image may cause that different fragments appear together as one in the image. For this reason, smoothing filters

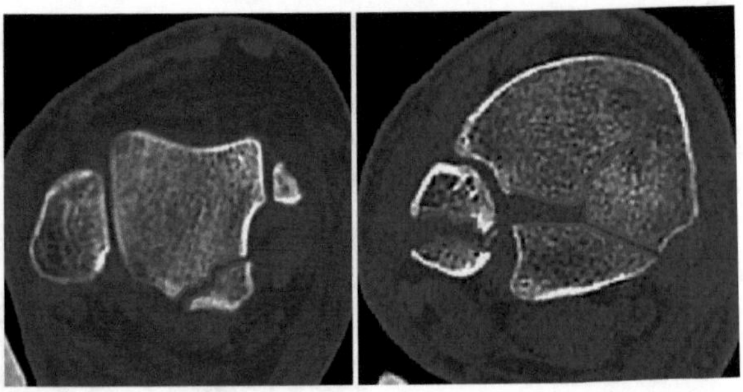

Fig. 2 CT slices that represent some different simple bone fractures. Fracture lines are marked in *red*

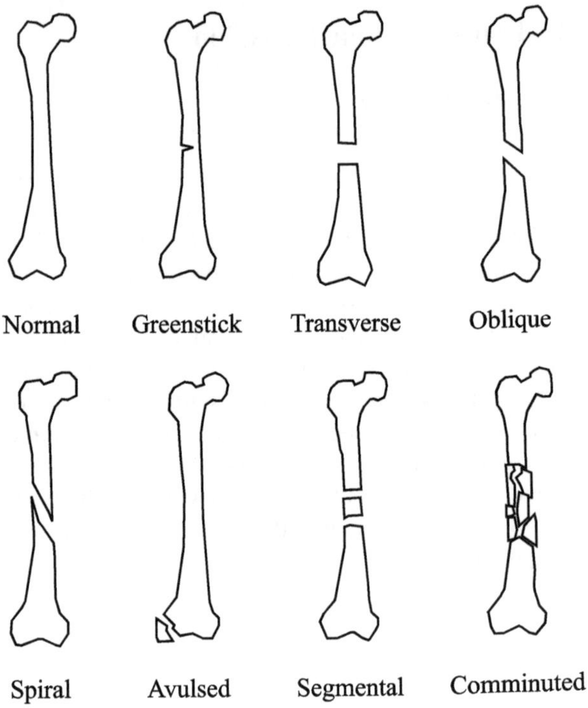

Fig. 3 Fractured bones classified by their fracture lines

should be used with caution. This type of filters can deform the shape of bone fragments and fracture zones or even remove small bone fragments. In some cases, it is necessary to detect the fracture zone of each fragment after its segmentation. The fracture zone is the area of the bone where the fracture occurs and is composed of trabecular tissue (Fig. 2). In situations in which bone fragments appear connected, it is difficult to accurately identify the fractured zone of each fragment. Therefore, post-processing can be necessary to delimit fracture zones in these situations.

The method applied in fractured bone identification depends on the fracture type. Based on the fracture line, a fracture can be classified as (Fig. 3): greenstick, transverse, oblique, spiral, avulsed, segmental and comminuted [7]. In a greenstick

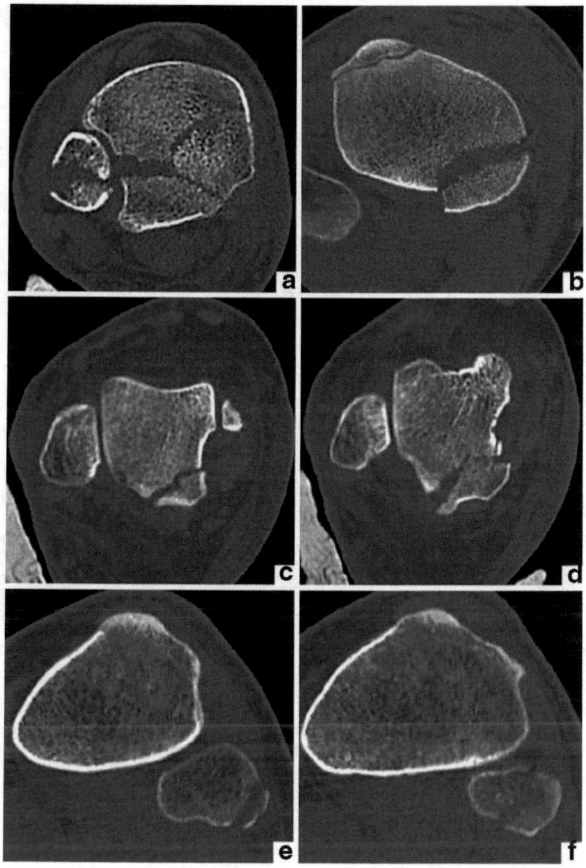

Fig. 4 CT images that represent different simple fractures. (**a**) contains, among others, a greenstick fracture, since the bone is not completely broken. The remaining images contain simple fractures with (**b**) and without (**c**, **d**, **e**, **f**) bone displacement

fracture (Fig. 4a) there are no fragments because the bone is not completely broken. Thus, labelling is not necessary. Since the fracture barely changes the shape of the bone, segmentation methods that are based on previous knowledge are available. Nevertheless, the edges of the fracture zone, composed of trabecular tissue, may require special processing. The detection of the fracture zone is specially complicated since the bone is not completely broken and trabecular tissue is very heterogeneous. Therefore, the fracture zone can be fuzzy in the CT image.

Transverse, oblique and spiral fractures (Fig. 4b, c, d, e, and f) can be similarly treated during the segmentation. Despite of having different fracture lines, these types of fracture generate two fragments with similar shape. Labelling is necessary, but expert knowledge is not required. Segmentation methods that can be applied depend on whether or not there is displacement. If there is no displacement (Fig. 4c, d, e, and f), they can be processed as a greenstick fracture but considering that there are two fragments. These two fragments can be completely joined, hence an additional processing to separate them may be required. In order to detect fracture zones, the same issues applicable to greenstick fractures should be considered. In the case

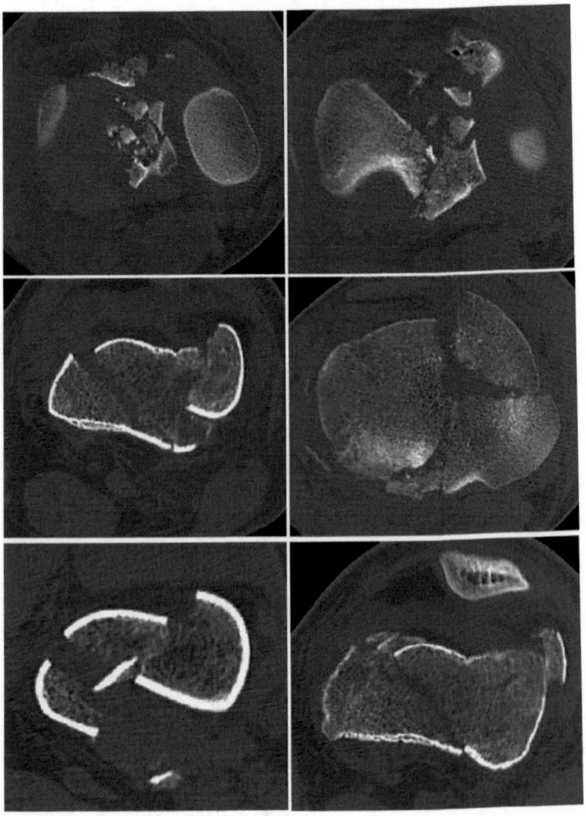

Fig. 5 CT images representing highly comminuted bone fractures

that there is displacement (Fig. 4b), the probability that both fragments are jointly segmented decreases and methods based on prior knowledge are almost discarded. In return, the fracture zone is easier to be identified. Avulsed fractures normally occur near a join thus the fracture zone is composed almost exclusively by trabecular tissue and the boundaries of the fragments are weak. This complicates the identification of the fracture zone because practically the entire fragment is surrounded by trabecular tissue. Segmental fractures are simple fractures that generate three bone fragments. Therefore, they can be treated as transverse or oblique fractures but considering that there are two distinct fracture regions. Comminuted fractures (Fig. 5) add some additional constraints, hence this is the type of fracture that is more complicated to be segmented. Comminuted fractures usually generate small fragments and bone may be deformed due to the fracture. This is because comminuted fractures are usually associated with crush injuries. In most cases, some fragments overlap in the CT image and require additional processing to be separated. Labelling is necessary and expert knowledge is strongly required to identify fragments. The detection of fracture zones is complicated in this case. Due to the complexity of the fracture, several fracture zones are generated. Since the relationship between fragments in this type of fractures is many-to-many, it can be necessary not only to identify fracture zones, but also to delimit which part of the fracture zone corresponds to each fragment. As mentioned before, some fragments can overlap due to the fracture and therefore post-processing and expert knowledge can be required to accurately identify fracture zones.

3 Currently Proposed Approaches

3.1 *Healthy Bone*

In recent years, many approaches have been proposed in order to segment bone tissue from CT images. Most of these methods are focused on the segmentation of a specific area. In [25] authors combine region growing, active contours and region competition to segment carpal bones. An expectation maximization algorithm has been utilized to segment phalanx bones [23]. The method requires a previously generated CT atlas. In [18], 3D region growing is used to segment the inferior maxillary bone from CT images. In order to fill holes in the segmented surface, a morphological operation of closing is used. Then, 3D ray casting is applied to segment the internal region of the bone by determining which points are inside of the outer shell. The segmented voxels are classified as cortical or trabecular bone using a fuzzy c-means algorithm. To improve the result, an adapted median filter allows to remove outliers. A 3D region growing method has also been used to segment bone tissue in [32]. Both the seeds and the threshold are calculated automatically. Since they use an unique threshold, some areas of bone are not segmented and they propose a method to fill them. This segmentation approach has been tested to segment skull and spine bones. A novel active contour model is utilized to segment bone tissue in [28]. The statistical texture method has also been proposed to segment mandible bones from CT images [19]. In [17] authors use a 3D deformable balloon model to segment the vertebral bodies semi-automatically. Graph cuts have also been used to segment vertebrae [2]. Previously, seeds are automatically placed using the matched filter and vertebrae are identified with a statistical method based on an adaptive threshold. Cortical and trabecular bone are then separated by using a local adaptive region growing method. In [15], Willmore flow is integrated into the level set method to segment the spinal vertebrae. Graph cuts have also been employed to segment the hip bone [16]. Most of these approaches can not be applied to the segmentation of fractured bone tissue because they take advantage of the prior knowledge of the shape of the bones.

Statistical methods are frequently used to segment bone tissue [3]. In this case, they use a generative model to classify pixels into cortical bone or another tissue. A learned model is constructed by modeling probability functions using Gaussian mixture models. Then, the learned model allows to assign a probability to each pixel and a maximum a-posteriori probability rule enables a crisp classification. In [12], a genetic algorithm is used to search the better procedure to segment bone tissue and to separate cortical and trabecular tissue. For that, the genetic algorithm requires previous expert information. Despite the results obtained, learning based methods can not be easily used to segment fractured bones because previous learning is not available in most cases.

Several methods are based on the fact that the shape and the anatomy of the bone are known [31]. In this work, an adaptive threshold method is utilized to segment bone tissue. However, the method can not be applied to segment bone fractures because it is based on the supposition that bone fragments are completely surrounded by cortical tissue, and this is not always true in the case of a fracture. All the revised works for segmenting healthy bone from CT images are summarized in Table 1.

3.2 *Fractured Bone*

The methods applied to the segmentation of healthy bone could not be suitable for segmenting fractured bone. This is because, as seen in the previous section, fractured bone has different features. Moreover, the identification of fracture bone requires to carry out additional steps, such as labelling the fragments or splitting wrongly joined fragments. Currently proposed methods to perform these steps are described below.

3.2.1 Fragment Segmentation and Labelling

There are several papers that are focused on the identification of fractured bone. With this aim, threshold-based methods are used in most cases. The most basic threshold-based method consist in defining an intensity interval that corresponds to bone tissue and calculating the pixels in the image that belong to this interval [24]. The intensity interval can be defined manually or can be calculated from the information provided by the image. On the other hand, the interval can be used in the hole stack or can be defined for each slice. The second option is usually the most successful because, as seen in Sect. 2, intensity values differ between slices. Several works propose to use thresholding to segment fractured bone. In [20], ulna, radius and carpus are segmented to simulate a virtual corrective osteotomy. Therefore, the segmentation is performed on non-fractured bones and then the segmented bones are virtually cut. In order to separate bone from other tissues, an user-defined threshold is used. In [27], the area where the bones are located is detected using a threshold-based method. Then, they present manual and semi-automatic tools for interactively segmenting bone fragments. This toolkit includes separation, merge and hole filling tools to generate individually segmented fragments from the result of the threshold-based segmentation. Thus, the method achieves accuracy at the expense of requiring a lot of user intervention. A global fixed threshold method has been utilized in [26] to detect the trabecular bone fracture zone. Due to the difference of intensity values between slices, it is difficult to set a threshold that fits all the slices.

Region growing is a threshold-based method that allows to limit the segmentation to a specific area [8]. To that end, the algorithm requires to place seeds before starting

Table 1 Summary of the works for identifying healthy bone which are described in this paper

Authors	Requirements	Interaction	Methods	Evaluation set	Achievements
Sebastian et al. (2003)	–	Specify parameters	Region growing, active contours and region competition	Carpus	Combine the advantages of all the methods used
Mastmeyer et al. (2006)	–	Set seeds and markers	3D deformable balloon model	Vertebrae	Vertebra separation
Battiato et al. (2007)	A learned model	Set the threshold	Gaussian mixture models	Knee	Cortical tissue pixels classification
Ramme et al. (2009)	CT atlas	Place landmarks	Expectation maximization	Phalanxes	Semi-automatic segmentation
Moreno et al. (2010)	–	Set the seed point	3D region growing	Inferior maxilar	Bone tissue classification
Zhao et al. (2010)	–	–	3D region growing	Skull	Threshold and seeds automatically selected
Aslan et al. (2010)	–	–	Graph cuts and region growing	Vertebrae	Automatic cortical and trabecular tissue classification
Zhang et al. (2010)	–	–	Adaptive thresholding	Calcaneus and vertebra	Automatic segmentation
Truc et al. (2011)	–	–	Active contours	Knee and heart	Bone contours extraction from CT and MRI images
Nassef et al. (2011)	–	–	Statistical texture	Mandible	Identification of different bone tissues
Janc et al. (2011)	Expert bone identification	–	Genetic algorithm	Mandible, skull and knee	Cortical and trabecular tissues separation
Lim et al. (2013)	–	Set initial contours	Level set	Vertebrae	Deal with missing information
Malan et al. (2013)	Previous manual segmentation	–	Graph cuts	Hip	Detailed tissue classification

All the works require CT images as input

the segmentation. The selection of the seed points can be performed manually or automatically. The manual placement of the seeds enables the labelling of the different bone fragments. Moreover, the algorithm also needs to define an intensity interval. As in the previous case, the interval can be defined globally or for each slice. Once the seeds have been placed and the interval has been defined, the algorithm check all their neighbouring pixels. If the intensity of a neighbouring pixel is outside of the defined interval, it is discarded. Otherwise, the pixel is included in the segmented area and its adjacent pixels are studied. The algorithm stops when there are no pixels to study. The result of the algorithm can differ depending on the criteria used to accept or discard pixels. The basic algorithm accepts a pixel if its intensity is inside the interval. This approach allows to detect small bone features but image noise can also be segmented. However, noise can be mostly reduced using smoothing filters. Therefore, this approach can be suitable for segmenting fractured bone. Other approaches decide to accept or discard a pixel based on the intensity value of its neighbours. The simplest option is to accept a pixel if all its neighbours have intensity values inside the interval. Another option is to use a criteria based on statistical values calculated from the neighbouring pixels. In this case, small features could be discarded. Thus, this variation could not be suitable for segmenting fractured bone.

Region growing based methods are the best used for segmenting fractured bone. A semi-automatic threshold-based method and region growing have been utilized to extract bone contours from CT scans in [10]. Before that, thresholding is applied to obtain the area where bone tissue is located. Then, redundant contours are removed using an absolute and a relative spatial criterion. To improve the result, smoothing algorithms are applied and close contours are joined. In [11], authors use an interactive method to segment complex humeral bone fractures. In a first step, the method calculates a sheetness measure in order to extract the cortical layer of the fragments. Then, a semi-automatic region growing is performed on the obtained 3D sheetness data. Voxels with a sheetness measure less than a threshold are labeled as belonging to cortical bone fragments. Region growing is performed using a wave propagation strategy in order to reduce memory consumption and increase computation speed. Seed points and the sheetness threshold are interactively selected by the user. The placement of the seed is used to label the bone fragments, hence this process is repeated until all the fragments have been labelled. In [9], authors also use a sheetness-based method to segment fractured pelvic bones. In order to identify cortical tissue, a local adaptive thresholding method, based on the sheetness measure and a weight factor, is utilized. In order to segment trabecular tissue, a region growing method, based on the previous cortical bone segmentation, is applied using an adaptive threshold. In [14], authors present a multi-region segmentation approach to identify pelvic fractures. The seed points are automatically established by searching in the image pixels that have an intensity value higher than a threshold. Once a seed is found, its region is propagated to avoid finding another seed inside it. After that, a region growing algorithm propagates all regions in turns. In each cycle of propagation, the gray values of the fronts are set to be equal and reduced by the threshold iteratively. To that end, the threshold value is determined in an iterative process.

Table 2 Summary of the works to identify fractured bone which are described in this paper. The bone fragments are labelled in all cases

Authors	Requirements	Interaction	Methods	Evaluation set	Achievements
Neubauer et al. (2005)	–	Define the threshold	Thresholding	Ulna, radius and carpus	Semi-automatic bone fragments separation
Pettersson et al. (2006)	Prototypes	Generate the prototype	Morphon non-rigid registration	Hip	Automatic segmentation
Gelaude et al. (2006)	–	Customization	Thresholding and region growing	Pelvis and humerus	Contours adaptation
Harders et al. (2007)	–	Set seed points	Region growing	Humerus	Labelling is performed during segmentation
Fornaro et al. (2010)	–	Set seed points	Adaptive thresholding and region growing	Acetabulum	Automatic detection of incorrect bone fragment separation
Tomazevic et al. (2010)	–	Interactive tools	Thresholding	Articulations	Accurate segmentation
Tassani et al. (2012)	Prototypes	Prototype generation	Global thresholding	Femur and tibia	Fracture zone detection
Lee et al. (2012)	–	Region combination and separation	Region growing	Pelvis	Automatic definition of thresholds and seeds

All the works also require CT scans as input.

Other proposed method to segment fractured bone is based on registration [22]. In order to automatically segment fractured hip bones, they use an extension of the non-rigid Morphon registration [13]. The proposed method registers each bone fragment with a prototype. The method is limited to simple fractures, since it requires a prototype for registering each bone fragment. The main disadvantage of this method is that it requires prototypes of the fractured parts, hence it is limited to the specific fractures defined by the prototypes. Other segmentation methods [1] could be tested in order to segment fractured bone tissue. Table 2 summarizes all the revised methods for identifying fractured bones.

3.2.2 Fragment Separation

The proximity between fragments and the resolution of the medical images can cause that several bone fragments appear together after the segmentation procedure.

In that case, these bone fragments must be separated. Current works usually propose methods not only to identify bone fragments, but also to separate wrongly joined fragments.

Some proposed methods allow to separate bone fragments manually. These methods achieve accuracy at the expense of requiring a lot of user intervention. In [11], authors use a manual procedure to separate erroneously connected fragments. To that end, the user can draw a cut line onto the surface of the bone fragments to define a set of separation voxels. Then, these set is grown parallel to the screen and extruded along the viewing vector. After that, the segmentation process is repeated to determine if the connection still exists. This manual procedure takes about five minutes. In [27], authors present a tool to separate bone fragments in a 3D model. For this purpose, the user must position seed points on different fracture locations and the tool calculates the fracture line in between. If there is no fragment line visible, a cut tool can be used.

Manual tasks take a long time, hence other methods try to split bone fragments as automatically as possible. A semi-automatic watershed-based method has been used to separate erroneously joined bone fragments resulted from a threshold-based segmentation [20]. The proposed method needs that the user selects a voxel located on the boundary between the two fragments. Then, a watershed based segmentation algorithm performs the separation. This method achieves good results, but manual corrections need to be performed in case of inaccuracies. In [9], authors propose to apply a 3D connected component algorithm to separate bone fragments in simple cases. Moreover, the algorithm also allows to reject small fragments and remove false positive labelled structures. In order to deal with fractures in which the boundary of the bone is weak, they propose to use graph cuts. For that, seeds have to be added by the user to each bone fragment. They also introduce an optimized Ransac algorithm to detect fracture gap planes and thus to identify incorrect bone fragment separation. With the aim of refining the segmentation in zones with low bone density, they use another graph cut based approach. Another proposed solution consists in performing a re-segmentation [14]. If the proposed multi-region segmentation fails, authors provide a manual region combination algorithm that allows to blend the wrongly-segmented regions, and a region re-segmentation that enables the separation of the incompletely-segmented objects. Region combination allows to combine several fragments into one interactively. The user needs to select the fragments one by one and the algorithm combines them into one. The region re-segmentation consists in applying the multi-region segmentation algorithm to a specific region defined by the user. The initial threshold is set higher than usual in order to ensure that the two regions are detected. The target threshold does not change during the growing process. These two algorithms, region combination and region re-segmentation, can be executed repeatedly until all the bone fragments are accurately separated. All the revised works to separate wrongly joined bone fragments are summarized in Table 3.

Table 3 Summary of the works to separate erroneously joined fragments which are described in this paper

Authors	Requirements	Interaction	Methods	Evaluation set	Achievements
Neubauer et al. (2005)	–	Select a voxel located between the fragments	Watershed	Ulna, radius and carpus	Some cases are resolved by selecting a voxel on the border
Harders et al. (2007)	–	Draw a cut line	Interactive method	Humerus	All cases are separated drawing a line
Fornaro et al. (2010)	–	Set seeds	3D connected components labelling and graph cuts	Acetabulum	Detect incorrect bone fragments separation automatically
Tomazevic et al. (2010)	–	Set seed points and a cut tool	Interactive method	Articulations	Accurate separation of bone fragments
Lee et al. (2012)	–	Interactive region combination and separation	Region re-segmentation	Pelvis	User only has to specify the region of interest

3.2.3 Fracture Zone Identification

Sometimes, it is useful to perform the identification of the fractured area. For instance, the simulation of a fracture reduction and the virtual analysis of the fracture can require to previously calculate this area. Therefore, some approaches have been proposed to calculate the fractured area after the segmentation of bone fragments.

Statistical based approaches have been proposed to identify fractured zones [29]. In this work, authors semi-automatically reconstruct highly fragmented bone fractures. Before performing the fracture reduction, they need to separate intact and fractured zones of each bone fragment. For that purpose, they propose to use a mixture model consisting of two Gaussian probability distributions to perform a binary classification. They choose a threshold that enables the classification of intact-surface intensities and minimizes the type I classification errors. Thus, this threshold allows to separate fractured and intact surfaces. After classifying all points, the fractured surface is the largest continuous region of fractured surface points. In [33], an extension of the previous method that improves fragment alignment in highly fragmented bone fractures has been presented. In order to separate fractured and intact surfaces, they use a two-class Bayesian classifier based on the intensity values previously mapped on the surface vertices.

Other proposals take advantage of the specific shape of a particular type of bone. In [30], authors present an approach to semi-automatically perform the reduction of cylindrical bones. In order to identify vertices of the fractured area, they check the normal orientation of each vertex and compare it with the bone axis. This method does not work when fracture lines are almost parallel to the bone axis.

Curvature analysis has also been used to identify fractured surfaces [21]. In this work, authors present a procedure to virtually reduce proximal femoral fractures. In order to obtain fracture lines in each slice, they use curvature analysis. For that purpose, a 3D curvature image is generated. To begin with, 0 or 1 values are assigned to each voxel depending on the voxel position: 1 is assigned if the voxel is inside the fragment region and 0 is assigned if it is outside. After that, the surface voxels are defined as 1-value voxels adjacent to 0-value voxels. The 3D curvature image is generated by setting K_{abs} to each voxel belonging to the fracture surface and 0 to the rest of voxels, where $K_{abs} = |k_1| + |k_2|$. k_1 and k_2 are the maximum and the minimum curvature respectively, and are obtained from K and H

$$K = \frac{h_{xx}h_{yy} - h_{xy}^2}{(1 + h_x^2 + h_y^2)^2} \tag{1}$$

$$H = \frac{(1 + h_x^2)h_{yy} + (1 + h_y^2)h_{xx} - 2h_x h_y h_{xy}}{2(1 + h_x^2 + h_y^2)^{3/2}} \tag{2}$$

where $h(x, y)$ is a quadratic function fitted to 3D points generated from the surface voxels. Once the 3D curvature image is generated, an interactive line-tracking software allows to extract the fracture zone from the generated 3D curvature image.

In [26], authors perform a comparison with healthy models in order to identify trabecular tissue in fractured zones. To that end, authors compare the fractured region of interest in both pre-failure and post-failure slices. These regions are identified as disconnected trabecular tissue in the slice. If the regions of interest of both slices overlap less that a predefined threshold, the region is classified as broken. The threshold is determined by minimizing the root mean square error (RMSE) between resulted values and values manually calculated

$$RMSE = \sqrt{\frac{\sum_i (a_{i(x)} - v_i)^2}{n}} \tag{3}$$

where $a_{i(x)}$ and v_i are the calculated and the visually obtained values respectively and n is the number of analysed cases. Finally, they apply a median filter to remove the generated noise.

Interactive methods have also been proposed to identify fracture surfaces in order to be used in virtual craniofacial reconstruction [4, 6, 5]. In these works, fracture contours are extracted interactively from segmented bone fragments. With that aim, user has to select points belonging to the fractured area and then a contour tracing algorithm generates the rest of the points. Once the fracture contours are calculated, the 3D surface is generated by collating the contours extracted from each slice. Table 4 summarizes all the analysed works to detect fracture zones.

Table 4 Summary of the works to identify fracture zones which are described in this paper

Authors	Requirements	Interaction	Methods	Evaluation set	Achiev ements
Winkelbach et al. (2003)	Cylindrical bones	–	Comparison of normal vectors	Femur	Automatic identification in cylindrical bones
Willis et al. (2007), Zhou et al. (2009)	–	Set threshold and subdivide fractured zones	Gaussian mixture models and Bayesian classifiers	Tibia	Identification of fracture zones in comminuted fractures
Bhandarkar et al. (2007) Chowdhury et al. (2009)	–	Select points belonging to the fractured zone	Contour tracing algorithms	Mandible	User only has to select the end points of the fracture contour in each slice
Okada et al. (2009)	–	Extract fracture lines	Curvature analysis	Femur	The 3D curvature image eases the interaction
Tassani et al. (2012)	A healthy model	Visually check values to set the threshold	Comparison with healthy models	Femur and tibia	Interaction is only required to define the threshold

4 Discussion

The previous revision allows us to made a classification of the methods used to identify both healthy and fractured bone (Fig. 6). In order to identify fractured bones, it is necessary not only to segment, but also to label the bone fragments. Considering the previous revision, threshold-based methods have been used in most cases. Currently proposed threshold-based methods obtain good results, but they can be improved in some aspects. The selection of threshold intensity values is one of the most challenging procedures. Threshold values are difficult to be determined even manually and each slice may require a different threshold value. In addition, it is particularly difficult to set the threshold to segment bone tissue near the joints. The ideal would be that the threshold values were selected automatically from the information available in the set of slices in all cases. Because of the complexity of the fractures, it is difficult to label bone fragments automatically. This procedure may require expert knowledge, but it must be reduced as possible. Thresholding-based approaches do not label bone fragments, hence fragments have to be labelled after the segmentation process. Other approaches try to solve it by using seeded-based methods. By the time they place the seeds, they identify the bone fragments. Thus, seeds should be placed by an expert in some cases. Ideally, all the bone fragments should be segmented automatically and simple bone fragments should be identified

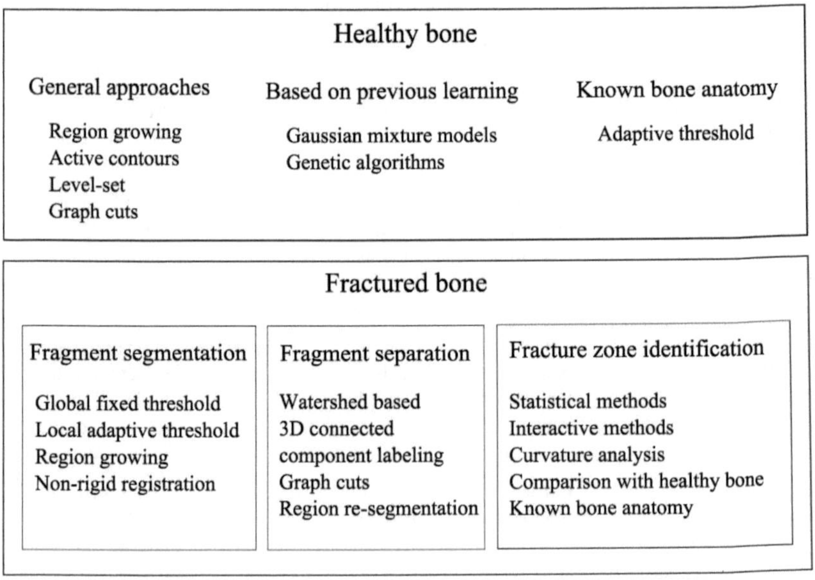

Fig. 6 Schema representing the different approaches currently proposed to identify both healthy and fractured bone

without user intervention. Then, the expert could decide the bone to which each fragment belongs in the most complex cases.

Due to the fracture, two different fragments can be completely joined. This is specially common in fractures caused by crashes. In addition, the image resolution can cause that very close fragments appear joined. These joined fragments are difficult to be separated during the segmentation process, hence current fractured bone identification approaches propose to separate them after the segmentation. New methods that solve this problem in a more automatic way are required. One solution would be to improve the segmentation method, hence no joined fragments are generated. This would be the faster solution, because no additional methods are required. However, the usual resolution of the CT scans makes it very difficult. The alternative is to implement a method that automatically separates wrongly joined fragments resulted from the segmentation. Manual and semi-automatic fragment separation takes a lot time, hence these new methods would be important to enable time saving. On the other hand, the use of higher resolution images, such as μCT, could avoid that fragments appear together in most cases. Nevertheless, this type of images is not always available.

Once all the bone fragments have been identified, some applications, such as fracture reduction or fracture analysis, require to detect fracture zones. Different interactive methods have been proposed to delimit the fracture area. Some of these methods propose to calculate fracture lines in each slice and then join them to generate the fracture area. Following this approach, it is easier to detect and fix anomalies in each slice. In contrast, this type of methods usually requires more time since fracture line detection is performed in each slice and user interaction is needed. Other methods use 3D interactive techniques to identify the fracture zone. These methods are usually faster but the interaction is usually much more complex. Methods based on prior knowledge have also been proposed to identify the fracture zone. These methods are usually faster but are restricted to specific bones and fracture types. In summary, currently proposed methods to detect fracture zones are based on previous knowledge or need user interaction (Fig. 6). Therefore, new methods that calculate fracture zones using the information available in the slice would be useful. In addition, these new methods should be as automatic as possible.

All these shortcomings are summarized in the following points:

- Separate wrongly joined bone fragments after or during the segmentation process without user intervention.
- Select the threshold for each slice automatically from the information available in the CT stack.
- Label the bone fragments with minimal user interaction.
- Detect fracture zones using information from the CT stack as automatically as possible.

5 Conclusion

In this paper, the main issues to be considered when identifying both healthy and fractured bone tissues have been described. Moreover, currently proposed methods for healthy and fractured bone identification have been discussed and classified. This revision has shown that most of the methods applied to the segmentation of healthy bone can not be utilized to identify fractured bone. Moreover, it has allowed to know which algorithms have been applied in order to identify each type of bone and fracture as well as the results obtained. In the case of the identification of fractured bones, emphasis has also been placed in the proposed methods to label bone fragments, separate fragments that have been segmented together incorrectly and detect fracture zones. Finally, the shortcomings of the currently available methods have been revised and identified.

Acknowledgements This work has been partially supported by the Ministerio de Economía y Competitividad and the European Union (via ERDF funds) through the research project TIN2011-25259.

References

1. Allili MS, Ziou D (2007) Automatic colour–texture image segmentation using active contours. Int J Comput Math 84(9):1325–1338
2. Aslan MS, Ali A, Rara H, Farag AA (2010) An automated vertebra identification and segmentation in CT images. In: 2010 IEEE International conference on image processing, IEEE, 233–236

3. Battiato S, Farinella GM, Impoco G, Garretto O, Privitera C (2007) Cortical bone classification by local context analysis. In: Gagalowicz A, Philips W (eds) Computer vision/Computer graphics collaboration techniques, vol. 4418. Springer, Berlin pp 567–578
4. Bhandarkar SM, Chowdhury AS, Tang Y, Yu JC, Tollner EW (2007) Computer vision guided virtual craniofacial reconstruction. Comput Med Imaging Graph J Comput Med Imaging Soc 31(6):418–427
5. Chowdhury AS, Bhandarkar SM, Robinson RW, Yu JC (2009) Virtual craniofacial reconstruction using computer vision, graph theory and geometric constraints. Pattern Recognit Lett 30(10):931–938
6. Chowdhury AS, Bhandarkar SM, Robinson RW, Yu JC (2009) Virtual multi-fracture craniofacial reconstruction using computer vision and graph matching. Comput Med Imaging Graph J Comput Med Imaging Soc 33(5):333–342
7. Egol K, Koval KJ, Zuckerman JD (2010) Handbook of fractures. Lippincott Williams & Wilkins (LWW), Philadelphia
8. Fan J, Zeng G, Body M, Hacid MS (2005) Seeded region growing: an extensive and comparative study. Pattern Recognit Lett 26(8):1139–1156
9. Fornaro J, Székely G, Harders M (2010) Semi-automatic segmentation of fractured pelvic bones for surgical planning. In: Bello F, Cotin S (eds) Biomedical simulation, vol. 5958. Springer, Berlin pp 82–89
10. Gelaude F, Vander Sloten J, Lauwers B (2006) Semi-automated segmentation and visualisation of outer bone cortex from medical images. Comput Meth Biomech Biomed Eng 9(1):65–77
11. Harders M, Barlit A, Gerber C, Hodler J, Székely G (2007) An optimized surgical planning environment for complex proximal humerus fractures. In: MICCAI Workshop on interaction in medical image analysis and visualization
12. Janc K, Tarasiuk J, Bonnet AS, Lipinski P (2011) Semi-automated algorithm for cortical and trabecular bone separation from CT scans. Comput Meth Biomech Biomed Eng 14(1):217–218
13. Knutsson H., Andersson M. (2005) Morphons: segmentation using elastic canvas and paint on priors. In: IEEE International conference on image processing 2005, IEEE, II–1226
14. Lee PY, Lai JY, Hu YS, Huang CY, Tsai YC, Ueng WD (2012) Virtual 3D planning of pelvic fracture reduction and implant placement. Biomed Eng Appl Basis Commun 24(3):245–262
15. Lim PH, Bagci U, Bai L (2013) Introducing Willmore flow into level set segmentation of spinal vertebrae. IEEE Transac Biomed Eng 60(1):115–122
16. Malan DF, Botha CP, Valstar ER (2013) Voxel classification and graph cuts for automated segmentation of pathological periprosthetic hip anatomy. Int J Comput Assist Radiol Surg 8(1):63–74
17. Mastmeyer A, Engelke K, Fuchs C, Kalender WA (2006) A hierarchical 3D segmentation method and the definition of vertebral body coordinate systems for QCT of the lumbar spine. Med Image Anal 10(4):560–577
18. Moreno S, Caicedo SL, Strulovic T, Briceño JC, Briceño F, Gómez S, Hernández M (2010) Inferior maxillary bone tissue classification in 3D CT images. In: Bolc L, Tadeusiewicz R, Chmielewski LJ, Wojciechowski K (eds) Computer vision and graphics, vol. 6375. Springer, Berlin, pp 142–149
19. Nassef TM, Solouma NH, Alkhodary M, Marei MK, Kadah YM (2011) Extraction of human mandible bones from multi-slice computed tomographic data. In: 2011 1st Middle East conference on biomedical engineering, IEEE, 260–263
20. Neubauer A, Bühler K, Wegenkittl R, Rauchberger A, Rieger M (2005) Advanced virtual corrective osteotomy. Int Congr Ser 1281:684–689
21. Okada T, Iwasaki Y, Koyama T, Sugano N, Chen Y, Yonenobu K, Sato Y (2009) Computer-assisted preoperative planning for reduction of proximal femoral fracture using 3-D-CT data. IEEE Transac Biomed Eng 56(3):749–759
22. Pettersson J, Knutsson H, Borga M (2006) Non-rigid registration for automatic fracture segmentation. In: IEEE International conference on image processing, 1185–1188
23. Ramme AJ, DeVries N, Kallemyn NA, Magnotta VA, Grosland NM (2009) Semi-automated phalanx bone segmentation using the expectation maximization algorithm. J Digital Imaging 22(5):483–491

24. Sahoo P, Soltani S, Wong A (1988) A survey of thresholding techniques. Comput Vision Graph Image Process 41(2):233–260
25. Sebastian TB, Tek H, Crisco JJ, Kimia BB (2003) Segmentation of carpal bones from CT images using skeletally coupled deformable models. Med Image Anal 7(1):21–45
26. Tassani S, Matsopoulos GK, Baruffaldi F (2012) 3D identification of trabecular bone fracture zone using an automatic image registration scheme: A validation study. J Biomech 45(11):2035–2040
27. Tomazevic M, Kreuh D, Kristan A, Puketa V, Cimerman M (2010) Preoperative planning program tool in treatment of articular fractures: process of segmentation procedure. In: XII Mediterranean conference on medical and biological engineering and computing 2010, 29, 430–433
28. Truc PTH, Kim TS, Lee S, Lee YK (2011) Homogeneity and density distance-driven activecontours for medical image segmentation. Comput Biol Med 41(5):292–301
29. Willis A, Anderson D, Thomas T, Brown T, Marsh JL (2007) 3D reconstruction of highly fragmented bone fractures. Medical Imaging 2007: Image processing. Proceedings of the SPIE, 6512
30. Winkelbach S, Westphal R, Goesling T (2003) Pose estimation of cylindrical fragments for semi-automatic bone fracture reduction. In: Pattern recognition, Springer, Berlin, pp 566–573
31. Zhang J, Yan CH, Chui CK, Ong SH (2010) Fast segmentation of bone in CT images using 3D adaptive thresholding. Comput Biol Med 40(2):231–236
32. Zhao K, Kang B, Kang Y, Zhao H (2010) Auto-threshold bone segmentation based on CT image and its application on CTA bone-subtraction. In: 2010 Symposium on photonics and optoelectronics, 1–5
33. Zhou B, Willis A, Sui Y, Anderson D, Thomas T, Brown, T (2009) Improving inter-fragmentary alignment for virtual 3D reconstruction of highly fragmented bone fractures. SPIE Medical Imaging, 7259

On Evolutionary Integral Models for Image Restoration

E. Cuesta, A. Durán and M. Kirane

Abstract This paper analyzes evolutionary integral based methods for image restoration. They are multiscale linear models where the restored image evolves according to a Volterra equation, and the diffusion is handled by a convolution kernel. Well-posedness, scale-space properties, and long term behaviour are investigated for the continuous and semi-discrete models. Some numerical experiments are included. They provide different rules to select the kernel, and illustrate the performance of the evolutionary integral model in image denoising and contour detection.

1 Introduction

Mathematical modelling in image processing involves a great variety of tools, [2, 16, 34]. In the case of image denoising, the idea of considering a restored image u as a consequence of an evolution from an initial noisy image u_0, is the basis of the multiscale analysis, [1]. The process is usually described through PDEs models of the form

$$u_t(t,\mathbf{x}) = F(\mathbf{x}, u, \nabla u, \nabla^2 u), \ (t,\mathbf{x}) \in [0,T] \times \Omega,$$

$$u(0,\mathbf{x}) = u_0(\mathbf{x}), \quad \mathbf{x} \in \Omega, \tag{1}$$

$$\frac{\partial u}{\partial n}(t,\mathbf{x}) = 0, \quad (t,\mathbf{x}) \in [0,T] \times \partial\Omega, \tag{2}$$

E. Cuesta (✉) · A. Durán
Department of Applied Mathematics, E.T.S.I. of Telecomunication, University of Valladolid, Valladolid, Spain
e-mail: eduardo@mat.uva.es

A. Durán
e-mail: angel@mac.uva.es

M. Kirane
Laboratoire de Mathématiques, Image et Applications, Université de La Rochelle, Avenue M. Crépeau, 17042 La Rochelle Cedex, France
e-mail: mokhtar.kirane@univ-lr.fr

J. M. R. S. Tavares, R. Natal Jorge (eds.), *Developments in Medical Image Processing and Computational Vision*, Lecture Notes in Computational Vision and Biomechanics 19,
DOI 10.1007/978-3-319-13407-9_15

where ∇u, and $\nabla^2 u$ are, respectively, the gradient and Hessian matrices of u with respect to the space variable $\mathbf{x} = (x, y)$; $\Omega \subset \mathbb{R}^2$ is a bounded domain (typically a square) with boundary $\partial\Omega$; (2) is an homogeneous Neumann boundary condition; u_0 stands for the image to be restored; and F is a second-order differential operator, [1, 2, 27]. The possibilities for F should satisfy basic properties concerning, at least, three aspects of the model: the well-posedness of the continuous problem and discretizations (a way of controlling the stability of the process); the satisfaction of scale-space properties (as a way to have architectural properties of the multiscale analysis, to ensure that the evolved image is a regularized version of the original one or the preservation of important features of the image); finally, the control of this smoothing and also the edge-enhancing in the multiscale process.

In this sense, although the classical Gaussian filtering, with $F(\mathbf{x}, u, \nabla u, \nabla^2 u) = \operatorname{div}(\nabla u)$ in (1), is well-posed, provides stable discretizations and satisfies several scale-space properties, sometimes it is not efficient in the control of the diffusion, mainly because of the oversmoothing effect. In order to overcome this and other drawbacks, the literature stresses two main ideas: a nonlinear control of the diffusion, and the inclusion of anisotropy to make this control local and capable to discriminate discontinuities and edges. Several proposals in this sense can be seen in, e.g. [1–3, 14, 22, 32, 33], and references therein.

More recent is the use of evolutionary integral equations of the form, [25]

$$\begin{aligned} u(t,\mathbf{x}) &= u_0(\mathbf{x}) + \int_0^t k(t-s)Lu(s,\mathbf{x})\,\mathrm{d}s, \quad (t,\mathbf{x}) \in [0,T]\times\Omega, \\ \frac{\partial u}{\partial n}(t,\mathbf{x}) &= 0, \quad (t,\mathbf{x}) \in \partial\Omega\times[0,T], \end{aligned} \tag{3}$$

as models for the multiscale analysis. In (3), $L = \Delta$ stands for the Laplace operator, and $k(t)$ is a convolution kernel. The case $k(t) = 1$ leads to the heat equation, and $k(t) = t$ to the wave equation with zero initial velocity. (A more general context can be seen e.g. in [9, 18, 23]). If $k(t)$ is differentiable, and $k(0) = 0$, then (3) is equivalent to the integro-differential problem

$$\begin{aligned} u_t(t,\mathbf{x}) &= \int_0^t k'(t-s)Lu(s,\mathbf{x})\,\mathrm{d}s, \quad (t,\mathbf{x}) \in [0,T]\times\Omega, \\ u(0,\mathbf{x}) &= u_0(\mathbf{x}), \quad \mathbf{x}\in\Omega, \\ \frac{\partial u}{\partial n}(t,\mathbf{x}) &= 0, \quad (t,\mathbf{x}) \in [0,T]\times\partial\Omega. \end{aligned} \tag{4}$$

In [8, 11] a control of the diffusion based on (4) with

$$k(t) = k_\alpha(t) = t^{\alpha-1}/\Gamma(\alpha), \tag{5}$$

has been proposed, where $\alpha \in (1,2)$, and Γ is the Gamma function. Model (4), (5) interpolates the linear heat equation ($\alpha = 1$), and the linear wave equation ($\alpha = 2$), leading α to take a role of viscosity parameter, a term to control the diffusion of the image through the scales [23]. It is also natural to try to handle the diffusion through a selection of α as function of the image at the scale. In [11] a numerical technique, consisting of discretizing (4), (5) with a possibly different value of α for each pixel of the image is introduced. This procedure is modified in [10] to allow to consider a nonconstant viscosity parameter. This approach forms part of the growing interest in the use of fractional calculus for signal processing problems, see [21] for a review of fractional linear systems and also [12, 31], along with references therein.

The purpose of this paper is going more deeply into the evolutionary integral modelling for image restoration, generalizing [8, 11] in several ways, representing the following novelties:

- Under several non-restrictive hypotheses on the kernel k, the continuous model (3) is proved to satisfy scale-space properties (grey-level shift invariance, reverse-contrast invariance, translational invariance, and conservation of average value). Furthermore, the solution is shown to behave as the constant average value for long times. (Although the application of the evolutionary model (1) to image restoration does not usually require long times of computation, a good behaviour in this sense should always be taken into account).
- The semi-discrete (in space) version of (3) is also studied. Under some hypotheses on the discrete spatial operator, it is proved that the corresponding semi-discrete model also possesses several scale-space properties (grey-level shift invariance, reverse-contrast invariance, and conservation of a semi-discrete average value) as well as the constant behaviour as limit for long times. When the semi-discrete model is considered as an approximation to the continuous one (3), these properties enforce the relation between them.
- From the computational point of view, the freedom to choose the kernel k is strongly emphasized, since it can be used to control several features of the image: restoration, noise removal, or edge detection. Such properties are illustrated here by means of some examples with medical images.

According to these new results, the structure of the paper is as follows. Section 2 is devoted to the analysis of the above mentioned properties of the continuous model (3). These properties are proved for the Laplace operator, although the way how to extend them to more general spatial operators, [13], is described. The study of the semi-discrete (in space) version is carried out in Sect. 3. Finally, Sect. 4 illustrates the performance of the model with numerical examples. Some details about the implementation are explained and the corresponding codes are applied to several images by using different choices of the kernel. Sect. 5 contains some conclusions and future lines of research.

2 Continuous Evolutionary Integral Models

With the purpose of investigating the degree of adaptation of the evolutionary integral approach to the image processing rules, derived here are some properties of the continuous model (3). The following hypotheses on the kernel function k are assumed:

(H1) $k(t) = 0$ if $t \leq 0$, and $k(t) > 0$ if $t > 0$.
(H2) $k(t)$ is piecewise differentiable, of subexponential growth.
(H3) The integral

$$\int_0^{+\infty} k(t)\,\mathrm{d}t,$$

is divergent but $k(t)$ is locally integrable on $(0, +\infty)$.
(H4) $k(t)$ is 2-regular, [25]; this means that there is a constant $c > 0$ such that if $\mathcal{L}(k)(z)$ denotes the Laplace transform of $k(t)$, then

$$\left| z^n \frac{d^n}{dz^n} \mathcal{L}(k)(z) \right| \leq c \left| \mathcal{L}(k)(z) \right|,$$

for all z with $\mathrm{Re}(z) > 0$, and $n = 0, 1, 2$.

2.1 Well-Posedness

A first point of analysis concerns the well-posedness of the problem, which is usually a nontrivial question for some nonlinear models in image processing, [1, 22, 33]. In this case, under the hypotheses (H1)–(H4), results about existence, uniqueness, and regularity of solutions are obtained directly from the general theory of Volterra equations. Let $S(t)$ be the resolvent of (3), that is, the transitional operator such that

$$u(t, \mathbf{x}) = S(t)\, u_0(\mathbf{x}), \quad t \geq 0, \quad \mathbf{x} \in \Omega, \tag{6}$$

is the solution of (3) at $\mathbf{x}$ and time t, with initial condition u_0. It can be proved, see e.g. [25], Theorem 3.1, that u in (6) is C^1_t and there is $M \geq 1$ such that

$$||u(t, \mathbf{x})|| \leq M ||u_0(\mathbf{x})||,$$

$$||u_t(t, \mathbf{x})|| \leq \frac{M}{t} ||u_0(\mathbf{x})||, \quad t > 0.$$

These inequalities introduce the diffusion character of (3), [25].

2.2 Scale-Space Properties

A second group of theoretical properties of the model consists of scale-space properties. They are collected in the following theorem.

Theorem 1 *Let $S(t)$ be the transitional operator defined in (6). Under the hypotheses (H1)–(H4) the following properties hold:*

(P1) *Grey level shift invariance: $S(t)(u_0 + C) = S(t)u_0 + C$, for any constant C, and if $u_0 = 0$, then $S(t)u_0 = 0$.*

(P2) *Reverse contrast invariance: for* $t \geq 0$, $S(t)(-u_0) = -S(t)u_0$.
(P3) *Translational invariance: if* $\tau_{\mathbf{h}}(u_0)(\mathbf{x}) = u_0(\mathbf{x}+\mathbf{h})$, *for* $\mathbf{x}, \mathbf{x}+\mathbf{h} \in \Omega$, *then*

$$S(t)(\tau_{\mathbf{h}} u_0) = \tau_{\mathbf{h}} \left(S(t)u_0\right), \quad t \geq 0.$$

(P4) *Conservation of average value: if* $t > 0$,

$$\frac{1}{A(\Omega)} \int_\Omega u_0(\mathbf{x})\,\mathrm{d}x = \frac{1}{A(\Omega)} \int_\Omega S(t)u_0(\mathbf{x})\,\mathrm{d}x,$$

where $A(\Omega)$ *stands for the area of* Ω.

Proof Hereafter, for the sake of the simplicity of the notation, $u_0(\mathbf{x})$ will be denoted by u_0. Properties (P1)–(P3) are consequence of the uniqueness of solution. It is clear that $S(t)u_0 = 0$ if $u_0 = 0$. On the other hand, if C is a constant, the functions $u_1(t) = S(t)(u_0 + C)$ and $u_1(t) = S(t)(u_0) + C$ are solutions of (3) with initial condition $u_0 + C$; thus, uniqueness proves (P1). The same argument proves (P2). As far as (P3) is concerned, note that

$$\tau_{\mathbf{h}} u_0(\mathbf{x}) + \int_0^t k(t-s)\Delta\tau_{\mathbf{h}} \left(S(t)u_0\right)\,\mathrm{d}s$$
$$= \tau_{\mathbf{h}} u_0(\mathbf{x}) + \int_0^t k(t-s)\tau_{\mathbf{h}}\Delta \left(S(t)u_0\right)\,\mathrm{d}s = \tau_{\mathbf{h}} \left(S(t)u_0\right).$$

Thus, $\tau_{\mathbf{h}} \left(S(t)u_0\right)$ satisfies (3) with initial condition $\tau_{\mathbf{h}} u_0$, and therefore coincides with $S(t)(\tau_{\mathbf{h}} u_0)$. Finally, observe that if

$$I(t) = \int_\Omega u(t,\mathbf{x})\,\mathrm{d}x,$$

then the regularity of the solution implies that $I(t)$ is continuous, for $t \geq 0$, differentiable, for $t > 0$, and

$$\frac{\mathrm{d}}{\mathrm{d}t} I(t) = \int_\Omega u_t(t,\mathbf{x})\,\mathrm{d}x = \int_\Omega \int_0^t k'(t-s)\Delta u(s,\mathbf{x})\,\mathrm{d}s\,\mathrm{d}x$$
$$= \int_0^t k'(t-s)\left(\int_\Omega \Delta u(s,\mathbf{x})\,\mathrm{d}x\right)\mathrm{d}s.$$

Now, the divergence theorem, and the boundary conditions imply that $\frac{\mathrm{d}}{\mathrm{d}t} I(t) = 0$ and therefore I is constant, for all $t \geq 0$. □

2.3 Long Time Behaviour

A final relevant property is the behaviour of the solution as $t \to +\infty$. Assuming, for simplicity, that the square domain is $\Omega = (0,1) \times (0,1)$, and using separation of variables, the solution of (3) can be expressed in the form

$$u(t,\mathbf{x}) = \sum_{l,m} T_{l,m}(t) V_{l,m}(\mathbf{x}), \tag{7}$$

where $\{V_{l,m}\}_{l,m}$ is an orthogonal basis of eigenfunctions of the eigenvalue problem for the Laplace operator

$$\Delta V(\mathbf{x}) = \lambda V(\mathbf{x}), \quad \mathbf{x} \in \Omega,$$
$$\frac{\partial V}{\partial n}(\mathbf{x}) = 0, \quad \mathbf{x} \in \partial\Omega,$$

that has the eigenvalues $\lambda_{l,m} = -(l\pi)^2 - (m\pi)^2$, with a complete, orthogonal system of eigenfunctions, $V_{l,m}(\mathbf{x}) = \cos(l\pi x)\cos(m\pi y)$, for $l, m \in \mathbb{N} \cup \{0\}$. In particular $V_{0,0}(\mathbf{x}) = 1$, $\lambda_{0,0} = 0$. The expansion of the initial condition is, using the orthogonality, of the form

$$u_0(\mathbf{x}) = \sum_{l,m} \gamma_{l,m} V_{l,m}(\mathbf{x}), \quad \gamma_{l,m} = \frac{\int_\Omega u_0(\mathbf{x}) V_{l,m}(\mathbf{x})\,\mathrm{d}\mathbf{x}}{\int_\Omega V_{l,m}^2(\mathbf{x})\,\mathrm{d}x},$$

where in particular $\gamma_{0,0} = (1/A(\Omega)) \int_\Omega u_0(\mathbf{x})\,\mathrm{d}\mathbf{x}$ is the average grey value. The time-dependent components of the expansion (7) satisfy the integro-differential problems

$$T'_{l,m}(t) = \lambda_{l,m} \int_0^t k'(t-s) T_{l,m}(s)\,\mathrm{d}s, \quad t > 0, \quad l, m \in \mathbb{N} \cup \{0\}, \tag{8}$$
$$T_{l,m}(0) = \gamma_{l,m}, \quad T'_{l,m}(0) = 0, \quad l, m \in \mathbb{N} \cup \{0\}$$

that can be written in terms of the Laplace transform

$$z\mathcal{L}\left(T_{l,m}\right)(z) = \gamma_{l,m} + \lambda_{l,m}\mathcal{L}\left(k'\right)(z)\mathcal{L}\left(T_{l,m}\right)(z).$$

This leads to

$$\mathcal{L}\left(T_{l,m}\right)(z) = \frac{\gamma_{l,m}}{z\left(1 - \lambda_{l,m}\mathcal{L}(k)(z)\right)}.$$

Therefore, for $\lambda_{l,m} < 0$, and under the hypotheses (H1)–(H4), as $t \to +\infty$, $T_{l,m}(t) \to 0$ and the solution u behaves like

$$T_{0,0}(t) V_{0,0}(\mathbf{x}) = \gamma_{0,0} = (1/A(\Omega)) \int_\Omega u_0(\mathbf{x})\,\mathrm{d}\mathbf{x}.$$

Remark 1 Extension to more general spatial operators. The previous analysis has been performed by using the Laplacian as spatial operator. The model (3) can be generalized by considering an unbounded, closed, densely defined linear operator L with domain $D(L)$ on some Hilbert space $H(\Omega)$ of functions defined on Ω. Some of the previous properties also hold in this general case. More explicitly, we assume the following:

(h1) L is negative, in the sense that $\langle Lu, u\rangle \leq 0$, where $\langle\cdot,\cdot\rangle$ stands for the inner product in $H(\Omega)$, and $u \in D(L)$.
(h2) L is self-adjoint under Neumann boundary conditions.

(h3) Under Neumann boundary conditions, $\lambda = 0$ is a simple eigenvalue of L with Ker(L) generated by the constant functions.

It can be seen that under hypotheses (H1)–(H3), properties (P1), (P2) and (P4) of Theorem 1 also hold in this case. On the other hand, the satisfaction of property (P3) requires the additional hypothesis of commutation between the operator L and $\tau_{\mathbf{h}}$. Finally, concerning the long-term behaviour, the conclusion above is also satisfied by using the Spectral Theorem (e.g. [5]) for L as follows: there is a spectral family of projections $\{P_\lambda\}_\lambda$ in such a way that

$$u(t,\mathbf{x}) = \int_{-\infty}^{0} \mathrm{d}(P_\lambda u)(t,\mathbf{x}).$$

Then (8) becomes

$$(P_\lambda u)_t(t) = \lambda \int_0^t k'(t-s)(P_\lambda u)\,\mathrm{d}s,$$
$$(P_\lambda u)(0) = P_\lambda u_0.$$

As before, the use of the Laplace transform implies that $(P_\lambda u)(t) \to 0$ as $t \to +\infty$ for any $\lambda < 0$, and therefore

$$u(t,\mathbf{x}) \to P_0 u_0 = \frac{1}{A(\Omega)} \int_\Omega u_0(\mathbf{x})\,\mathrm{d}\mathbf{x}, \quad t \to +\infty.$$

This generalization can be applied, for example, to operators consisting of some fractional powers of the Laplacian, [13].

3 Semi-Discrete Evolutionary Integral Models

A semi-discrete (in space) version of (3) will be now introduced and analyzed. Consider a uniform $M \times M$ pixel mesh of Ω, with length $h > 0$, let $L_h : \mathbb{R}^N \to \mathbb{R}^N$ be a discrete operator on $\mathbb{R}^N, N = M^2$, satisfying the following requirements:

(R1) L_h is symmetric and negative semi-definite.
(R2) $\lambda = 0$ is a simple eigenvalue with the corresponding eigenspace generated by $\mathbf{e} = (1, 1, \ldots, 1)^T \in \mathbb{R}^N$.

Then the semi-discrete evolutionary integral model has the form

$$\mathbf{u}_h(t) = \mathbf{u}_{0,h} + \int_0^t k(t-s)L_h\mathbf{u}_h(s)\,\mathrm{d}s, \quad 0 \le t \le T, \tag{9}$$

where $k(t)$ satisfies (H1)–(H4), $\mathbf{u}_h(t)$ stands for the $N \times 1$ vector-image function at time t at the pixel mesh, $\mathbf{u}_{0,h}$ is the initial data at the grid points. For convenience, $\mathbf{u}_h$ will be sometimes considered as a matrix, in such a way that $(\mathbf{u}_h(t))_{i,j}$ will stand for the component associated to the pixel at the position (i,j) of the mesh, $i, j = 1, \ldots, M$. Neumann boundary conditions are somehow included in L_h, see Remark 4 below.

3.1 Well-Posedness, Scale-Space Properties and Long Time Behaviour

The solution operator for (9) is

$$S_h(t)\mathbf{u}_{0,h} = \mathbf{u}_h(t), \quad t \geq 0. \tag{10}$$

The same theory as in the continuous case guarantees well-posedness of (9), under (H1)–(H4), [25]. On the other hand, some scale-space properties and the long-term behaviour are proved in the following result.

Theorem 2 *Let $S_h(t)$ be the solution operator (10) associated to (9), where L_h satisfies (R1), (R2) above. Then the following properties hold:*

(Q1) *Grey level shift invariance: $S_h(t)(0) = 0$, $\quad S_h(t)(\mathbf{u}_0 + C) = S_h(t)\mathbf{u}_0 + C$, for any constant C.*
(Q2) *Reverse contrast invariance: for $t \geq 0$, $S_h(t)(-\mathbf{u}_0) = -S_h(t)\mathbf{u}_0$.*
(Q3) *Conservation of average value: if $t > 0$ and $(\mathbf{u}_{0,h})_{i,j}$ is the value of $\mathbf{u}_{0,h}$ at the (i,j)th-pixel,*

$$\frac{1}{N}\sum_{i,j=1}^{M} (\mathbf{u}_{0,h})_{i,j} = \frac{1}{N}\sum_{i,j=1}^{M} \left(S_h(t)\mathbf{u}_{0,h}\right)_{i,j}.$$

(Q4) *(Behaviour at $t \to +\infty$). Let $\mathbf{e}$ be given by (R2). Then*

$$\lim_{t\to+\infty} \left(S_h(t)\mathbf{u}_{0,h}\right) = \left(\frac{1}{N}\sum_{i,j=1}^{M} (\mathbf{u}_{0,h})_{i,j}\right)\mathbf{e}.$$

Proof Properties (Q1)–(Q2) are proved in a similar way to those corresponding in Theorem 1. As for property (Q3), consider $\mathbf{u}_h(t) = S_h(t)\mathbf{u}_{0,h}$ and

$$I(t) = \frac{1}{N}\sum_{i,j=1}^{M} \mathbf{u}_h(t)_{i,j}.$$

Differentiating with respect to t, and using (R1), (R2), we have

$$\begin{aligned}
\frac{\mathrm{d}}{\mathrm{d}t} I(t) &= \frac{1}{N}\sum_{i,j=1}^{M} \mathbf{u}_h'(t)_{i,j} = \frac{1}{N}\sum_{i,j=1}^{M} \int_0^t k'(t-s)\,(L_h\mathbf{u}_h(s))_{i,j}\,\mathrm{d}s \\
&= \int_0^t k'(t-s)\left(\frac{1}{N}\sum_{i,j=1}^{M} L_h\mathbf{u}_h(s)_{i,j}\right)\mathrm{d}s = \int_0^t k'(t-s)\langle L_h\mathbf{u}_h(s), \mathbf{e}\rangle\,\mathrm{d}s \\
&= \int_0^t k'(t-s)\langle \mathbf{u}_h(s), L_h^T\mathbf{e}\rangle\,\mathrm{d}s = 0,
\end{aligned}$$

where $\langle \cdot, \cdot \rangle$ denotes the Euclidean product in $\mathbb{R}^N$. Therefore, $I(t)$ is constant. Finally, for the proof of (Q4), note that, according to (R1) and (R2), L_h is diagonalizable, and the eigenvalues $\lambda_1, \ldots, \lambda_N$ are non-positive, with $\lambda_1 = 0$ simple. We can also write

$$L_h = P D_h P^{-1},$$

where $D_h = \mathrm{diag}(\lambda_1, \ldots, \lambda_N)$ stands for the diagonal matrix whose diagonal entries are $\{\lambda_1, \ldots, \lambda_N\}$, and P is orthogonal with the first column given by $(1/M)\mathbf{e}$. (In the representation of the spectrum, the λ_j are repeated according to the geometric multiplicity of the eigenvalues.) By using (H1)–(H4), (9) is equivalent to

$$\begin{aligned} \mathbf{u}_h'(t) &= \int_0^t k'(t-s) L_h \mathbf{u}_h(s)\, \mathrm{d}s, \quad t \in [0, T] \\ \mathbf{u}_h(0) &= \mathbf{u}_{0,h}. \end{aligned} \tag{11}$$

Then, if $\mathbf{v}_h(t) = P^{-1}\mathbf{u}_h(t)$, (11) is transformed into

$$\begin{aligned} \mathbf{v}_h'(t) &= \int_0^t k'(t-s) D_h \mathbf{v}_h(s)\, \mathrm{d}s, \quad t \in [0, T], \\ \mathbf{v}_h(0) &= P^{-1}\mathbf{u}_{0,h}. \end{aligned} \tag{12}$$

The differential system (12) is consequently decoupled and has the form

$$(v_{h,j}')(t) = \lambda_j \int_0^t k'(t-s) v_{h,j}(s)\, \mathrm{d}s, \quad 1 \leq j \leq N,$$

where $\mathbf{v}_h = (v_{h,1}, v_{h,2}, \ldots, v_{h,N})^T$. Now as in the proof of Theorem 1 Property (P4), we have that $v_{h,j}(t) \to 0$ as $t \to +\infty$, for $j = 2, \ldots, N$, and

$$v_{h,1}(t) = v_{h,1}(0) = \left(P^T \mathbf{u}_{0,h}\right)_1 = \frac{1}{M} \sum_{i,j=1}^{M} (u_{0,h})_{i,j}.$$

Therefore, since the first column of P is $\frac{1}{M}\mathbf{e}$,

$$\lim_{t \to +\infty} \mathbf{u}_h(t) = \lim_{t \to +\infty} P\mathbf{v}_h(t) = \left(\frac{1}{N} \sum_{i,j=1}^{M} (\mathbf{u}_{0,h})_{i,j} \right) \mathbf{e}.$$

□

Remark 2 Since Eq. (9) can be written as

$$\mathbf{u}_h(t) = \mathbf{u}_{0,h} + \int_0^t L_h k(t-s) \mathbf{u}_h(s)\, \mathrm{d}s, \quad 0 \leq t \leq T,$$

the following generalization

$$\mathbf{u}_h(t) = \mathbf{u}_{0,h} + \int_0^t L_h D(t-s) \mathbf{u}_h(s)\, \mathrm{d}s, \quad 0 \leq t \leq T, \tag{13}$$

will be considered in Sect. 4. In (13), $D(t)$ is a $N \times N$ diagonal matrix of kernels $D = \mathrm{diag}(k_1, \dots, k_N)$, with each k_j satisfying (H1)–(H4). From a theoretical point of view, Theorem 2 also holds for (13) (the proof does not present relevant difficulties). However, in a computational sense, (13) is more convenient, since it emphasizes the role of the convolution kernel with a 'pixel by pixel' strategy, [11].

Remark 3 We note that translational invariance must be here understood in the grid direction, and with multiple values of the mesh length (see [33]). In this sense, an analogous property to (P3) can also be proved.

Remark 4 When (9) is considered as a semi-discrete approximation to the continuous model (3), the operator L_h will approximate the Laplace operator with Neumann boundary conditions. In this sense, several choices can be mentioned. A typical example is based on the second-order central differences approximations

$$(\Delta_h u)_{i,j} = \frac{u_{i+1,j} + u_{i-1,j} - 4u_{i,j} + u_{i,j-1} + u_{i,j+1}}{h^2}, \quad 1 \le i, j \le M, \tag{14}$$

with the boundary conditions approximated by central differences, using artificial nodes, and where $u_{i,j}$ stands for the component of u at the pixel (i, j), [29]. This is shown to satisfy conditions (R1), (R2). Other examples are given by the Collatz's nine-point scheme and generalizations, [7, 35], the use of finite element matrix methods, [24], and the application of spectral methods, [4, 15, 30].

4 Numerical Experiments

4.1 Some Implementation Details

Before illustrating the behaviour of the model (3) with numerical examples, some previous comments on the implementation are required. From the semi-discrete version (13) (where a certain degree of approximation of L_h to L is assumed), the practical implementation is carried out throughout a suitable time discretization of (13) and in this sense a large variety of numerical methods is available. (A detailed analysis is out of the scope of the paper, and we refer the reader to a future work.) In order to obtain stable numerical approximations, one of the key points is the choice of a suitable treatment of the convolution integral. The general formulation for the advance in time will then be of the form

$$\mathbf{u}_n = \mathbf{u}_0 + \sum_{j=0}^{n} \mathbf{Q}_{n-j}\mathbf{u}_j, \quad n \ge 1, \tag{15}$$

In (15), for a given time step $\tau > 0$, $\mathbf{u}_n$ stands for the approximation to the solution of (13) at time level $t_n = n\tau, n \ge 0$. Thus, for a given initial image $\mathbf{u}_0$, the system of difference equations is implemented up to the final time T. The weights $\mathbf{Q}_n$, $n \ge 1$, depend on the matrix of kernels $D(t)$, and the discrete operator L_h in (13), in a

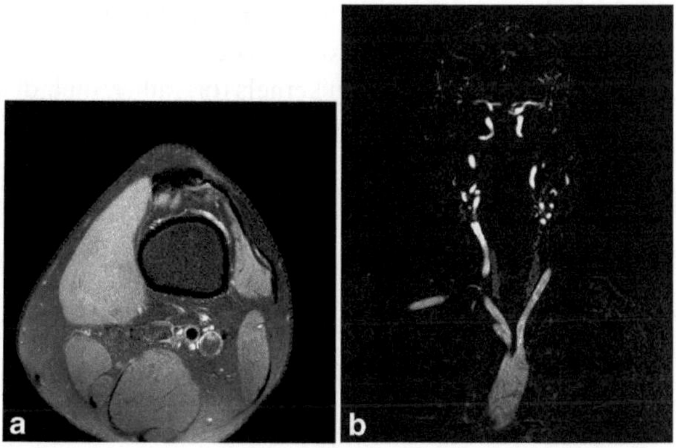

Fig. 1 **a** A TAC of a human leg of size 800 × 800 (*left*), and **b** of a human aneurysm of size 576 × 448 (*right*)

way given by the chosen formula to treat the convolution integral. For the numerical experiments below, the operator (14) is considered, and the time discretization makes use of convolution quadratures, which are based on the backward Euler method (see [6, 19, 20] for details).

A second point of relevance for the implementation is the treatment of the operator $L_h D(t)$ in (13). In this sense, we observe that the time discretization (15) only requires the values of $L_h D(t)$ at times $t_n = n\tau, n = 0, \ldots N$. Then, each diagonal component $k_n(t)$ can be computed via the stair function

$$\widetilde{k}_n(t) = k_n^0 + \sum_{j\geq 1} (k_n^j - k_n^{j-1}) U(t - t_j), \quad 1 \leq n \leq N, \tag{16}$$

where $U : [0, T] \to \mathbb{R}$ is the Heaviside function, and $k_n^j := k_n(t_j)$, $j \geq 0$. The introduction of (16) is justified by the requirement, presented in some discretizations (in particular, the one considered here) of making use of the Laplace transform, $\mathcal{L}(\tilde{k})$, which is not guaranteed for any choice of functions k_n. In fact,

$$\mathcal{L}\left(\widetilde{k}_n(t)\right)(z) = \frac{k_n^0}{z} + \sum_{j=1}^{N} \frac{k_n^j - k_n^{j-1}}{z} e^{-zt_j}.$$

The advantages of this implementation was mentioned in [10] for kernels of fractional type, and will be illustrated in the numerical experiments below with some other choices.

4.2 *Numerical Illustration*

Considered here are two types of experiments. The first one has an illustrative purpose: different choices of the kernel generate restored images $\mathbf{u}_n$ from simple, small, and synthetic initial images $\mathbf{u}_0$ by using (15), and several features, mainly related to denoising and edge detection, are observed. The second group of experiments consider zoomed parts of a human leg and aneurysm TACs (Fig. 1), with the aim of showing the previous effects, and calibrating the computational effort on more sophisticated and of larger size images.

Two kinds of convolution kernels (or, rather, their discrete versions) are used. The corresponding numerical experiments are explained below.

1. The first choice is an improved version of fractional-type kernels (5), analyzed and implemented in [8, 11]. Note that the kernel function in (5) can be selected to control the smoothing effect on the image via the parameter α, which is chosen, at each pixel, to this task. This idea can now be generalized by considering more adaptable kernels. Two natural choices can be the following, for each pixel $n = 1, \ldots, N$, (that is, each diagonal entry of D in (13)):

   (a)

$$k_n(t) := \frac{t^{\alpha_n(t)-1}}{\Gamma(\alpha_n(t))}, \qquad t \geq 0, \quad 1 \leq n \leq N, \tag{17}$$

   for some viscosity function $\alpha_n : [0, +\infty) \to \mathbb{R}$, with $1 \leq \alpha_n(t) \leq 2$, $t \geq 0$ (see [28]).

   (b) $k_n(t)$ as the inverse Laplace transform of

$$K_n(\alpha, z) = \frac{1}{z^{\mathcal{L}(\alpha_n)(z)\,z}}, \quad 1 \leq n \leq N, \tag{18}$$

   where $\mathcal{L}(\alpha_n)(z)$ stands for the Laplace transform of some $\alpha_n(t)$, [10, 26].

   Note that these kernels would correspond to fractional-type models, but where the order may vary with time; in this sense, they can be considered as an extension of those treated in [8, 11], since in the case of $\alpha_n(t) = \alpha_n$ is constant, the two kernels (17) and (18) coincide with (5). In computational terms, (a) is less suitable since the Laplace transform cannot be in general explicitly computed.

   The role of the kernels is illustrated by taking (18) with different choices of the viscosity parameters $\alpha_n(t)$. For instance, assume that the restoration requires some preservation of edges and vertices and, at the same time, removes isolated spots (noisy pixels), and let $\alpha_n^{(m)}$ be the value of the viscosity parameter at n-th pixel in the vector representation), and at time step t_m. Hence, *grosso modo*, automatic selection of the values $\alpha_n^{(m)}$ must satisfy the following criteria: pixels where the gradient is large (vertices, edges, isolated spots, etc) should be associated with values of the corresponding α_n close to two (low diffusion), and pixels with lower gradients (flat areas) should be associated with values of α_n close to one (hight diffusion). In this context, for example, spots (*isolated* noisy pixels, i.e. pixels with very high gradient variation), should be associated with values of α_n close to one, while very flat areas should correspond to values of α_n close to two.

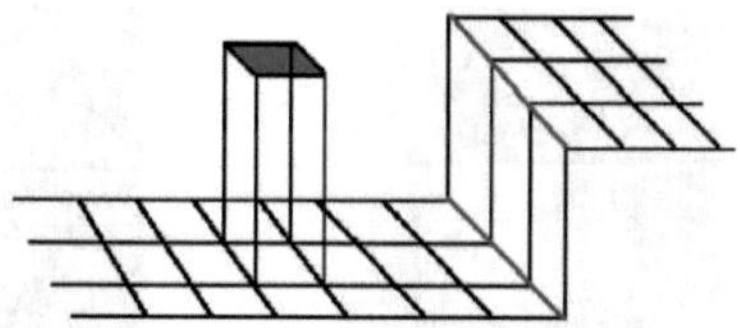

Fig. 2 Three dimensional representation of a spot for a gray-scale image

The influence of the parameters $\alpha_n^{(m)}$ is shown by the following, simple example. We try to remove the white spot in Fig. 2, by processing an initial 6×6 image with three kernels of the form (18): the first two are computed by using the profiles 1 and 2, for the viscosity parameter, given in Fig. 3 . The third method considers an initial selection which remains constant during the whole evolution. The evolution of the image with these three kernels is illustrated in Figs. 4, 5, and 6, respectively.

Their comparison suggests that Profile 2 gives better results: the edge has not been damaged, and the noisy pixel is well removed, that is, spurious perturbations in the neighboring pixels are not present, contrary to what is happening in the case of the two other kernels.

The nonlocal method (15) associated to Profile 2 has been applied to zoomed parts of Fig. 1a, b. The corresponding evolution is illustrated, at different times, in Figs. 7 and 8, respectively. Observe that the noise (meaningless information in this case) has been removed and, additionally, the main structures (including contours and edges) are well preserved. This is useful, for example, if a posterior contour detection, or a meaningful localization of structures, is required.

The effect of longer time integration on the image is illustrated in Fig. 9, where a zoomed subimage of Fig. 1b is taken as initial condition for (15) and evolved up to two different final times T. The results suggest a good behaviour for (always) moderately long times, since the smoothing effect (which removes the meaningless information) affects the preservation of the edges in a less expected way (having in mind that the model (3) is linear).

2. A second choice of the kernel makes use of (16), where the advantage given by the freedom to select the discrete values k_j, $j \geq 0$, has been taken into account. Thus, the following strategy has been adopted (this will generalize that considered in the

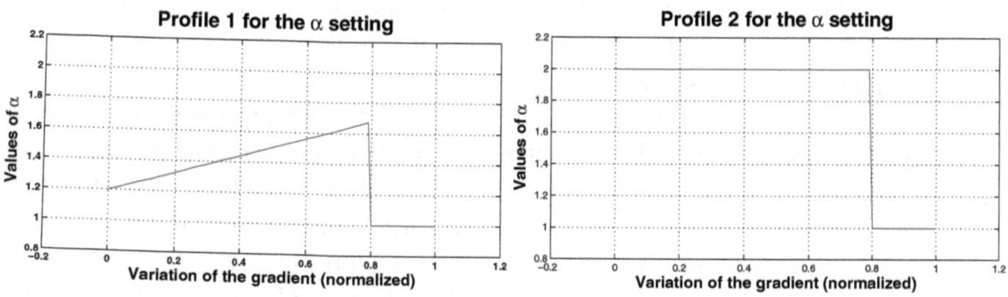

Fig. 3 Profiles 1 and 2 for the viscosity parameter α

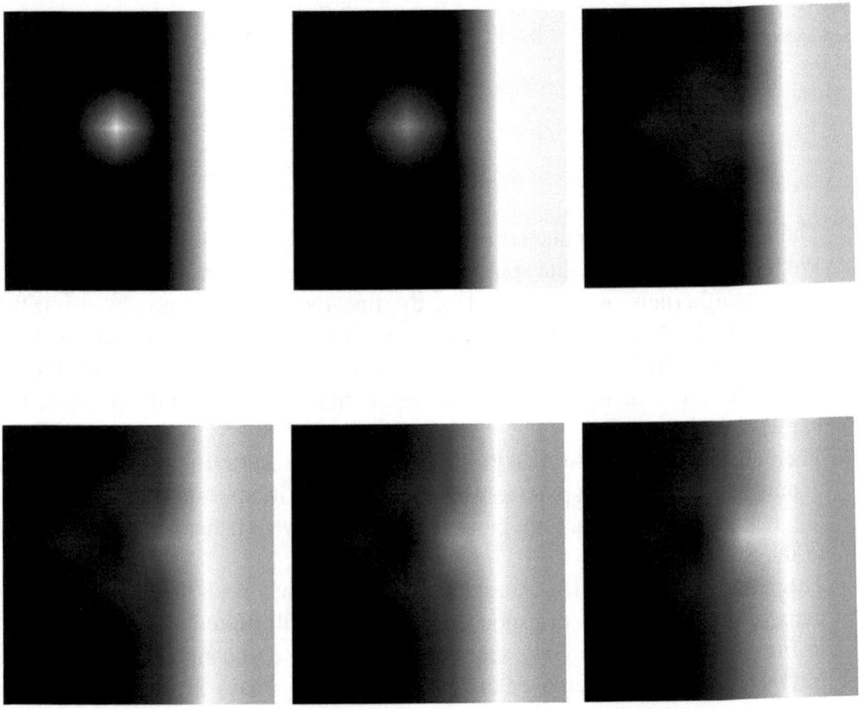

Fig. 4 Evolved spot at times $t_n = 0, 0.05, 0.5, 1, 1.5, 2$, with the profile of Fig. 3a

previous item): For those pixels that will remain unchanged, the corresponding kernel in the matrix $D(t)$ will approach zero from some time level value t_j (making the evolution almost stationary); for those pixels to be removed, the corresponding kernel will approach one from some time (in this case, the evolution behaves like that of the heat equation).

This strategy has been first applied to two synthetic, simple images, with inner structure. The evolution of the first one is represented in Fig. 10. In this case, no isolated pixels are present and the choice of the discrete values of the kernel helps to preserve the structure (edges, corners and the inner square). In a second image (Fig. 11), the inner square is replaced by an inner spot (representing an isolated pixel) and the same strategy for the choice of k in the model removes the spot without a relevant worsening of the rest of the structure.

The conclusions, derived from these simple examples, are arguments in favour of the application of the model (15) with this adaptative choice of the kernel to more complex images. *A priori*, the nonlocal character of (15) suggests the drawback of the computational cost of the implementation. In this sense, the selection of the kernel can also be managed to overcome this problem. An example of this is given in Fig. 12, where a subimage of Fig. 1b is evolved with (15), and the same kernel as in Figs. 10 and 11. Note that the previously described effects are

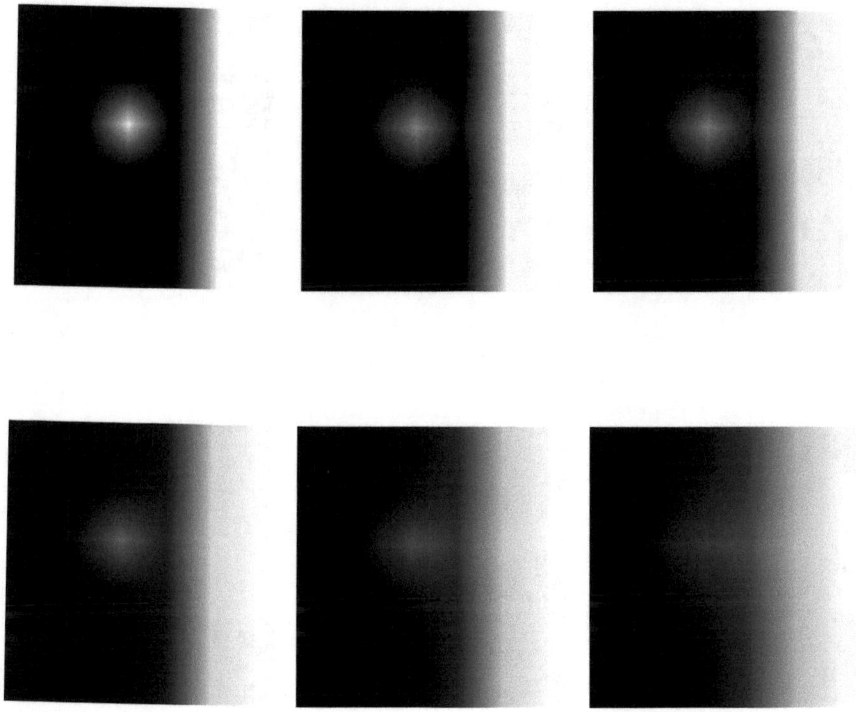

Fig. 5 Evolved spot at times $t_n = 0, 0.05, 0.5, 1, 1.5, 2$, with the profile of Fig. 3b

obtained in a short final time ($T = 1$), and with a small number of steps ($N = 10$ in this case; that is $\tau = 10^{-1}$).

In order to emphasize the freedom provided by the choice of the kernel via (16), a final example is displayed. In this case, the discrete values of the kernels are distributed by setting diffusion within a suitable range of values. More specifically, we modify the strategy as follows: two thresholds $0 < \varepsilon_1 < \varepsilon_2 < 1$ for the values of the gradient of the image (normalized to one) at the pixels are first fixed. Then, if the gradient at a pixel is below ε_1 or above ε_2 then the pixel will be removed, and the corresponding kernel will approach one (high diffusion is applied). Otherwise, the kernel will go to zero as in the previous strategy. The resulting system (15) is able to improve the detection of the contours. This is first observed in Fig. 13 where, from the same original image as in Fig. 11a, the method locates the border of a square (and still removes the isolated inner spot). This improved effect is also generated in a subimage of the aneurysm in Fig. 1b (displayed in Fig. 14) in a short time.

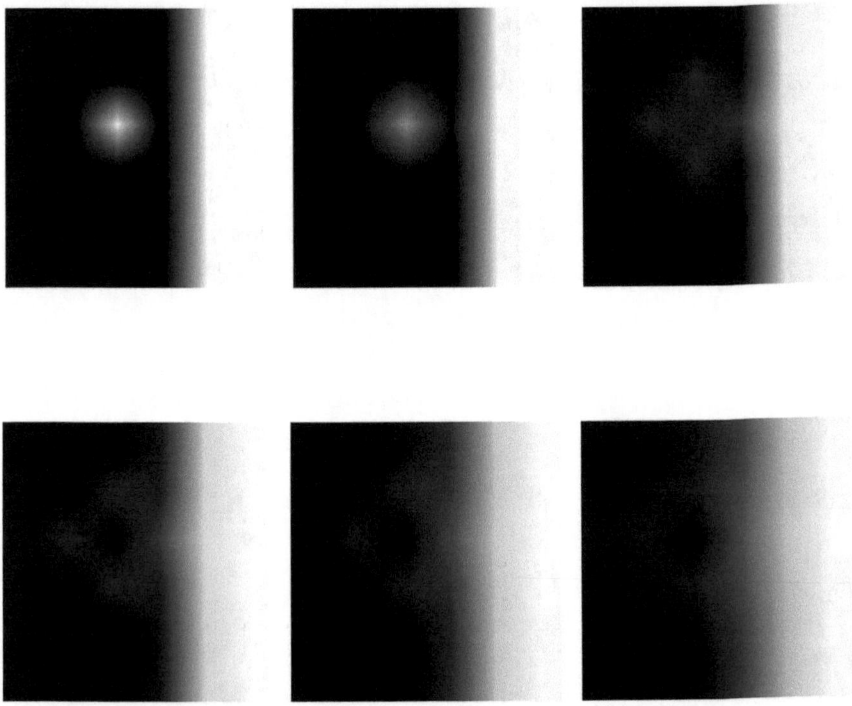

Fig. 6 Evolved spot at times $t_n = 0,\ 0.05,\ 0.5,\ 1,\ 1.5,\ 2$, with a constant profile α

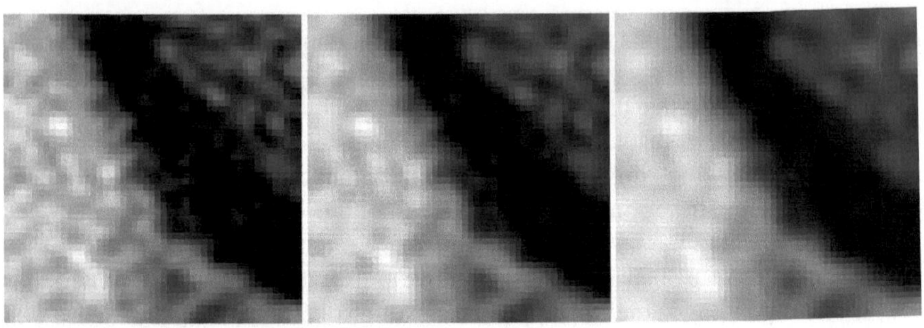

Fig. 7 Subimage $400-450 \times 320-370$ of the Fig. 1a (*left*), and processed with $T = 3$, $\tau = T/50$, at time levels t_{25} (*middle*), and t_{50} (*right*)

5 Conclusions and Future Works

In this paper, evolutionary integral models for image restoration, where the image evolves according to a linear, and nonlocal equation of Volterra type, are studied. It is shown that under non-restrictive hypotheses on the convolution kernel, the

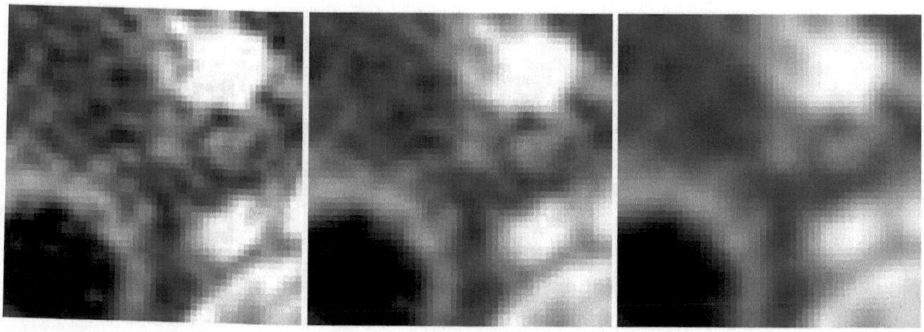

Fig. 8 Subimage $500-550 \times 450-500$ of the Fig. 1a (*left*), and processed with $T = 3$, $\tau = T/30$, at time levels t_{15} (*middle*), and t_{30} (*right*)

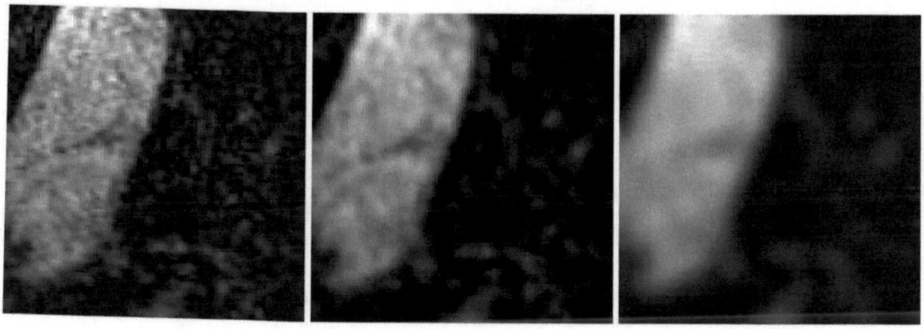

Fig. 9 Subimage $470 - 550 \times 200 - 300$ of the Fig. 1b (*left*), processed with $T = 3$, $\tau = T/40$, and at time level t_{40} (*middle*), and processed with $T = 5$, $\tau = T/30$, and at time level t_{30} (*right*)

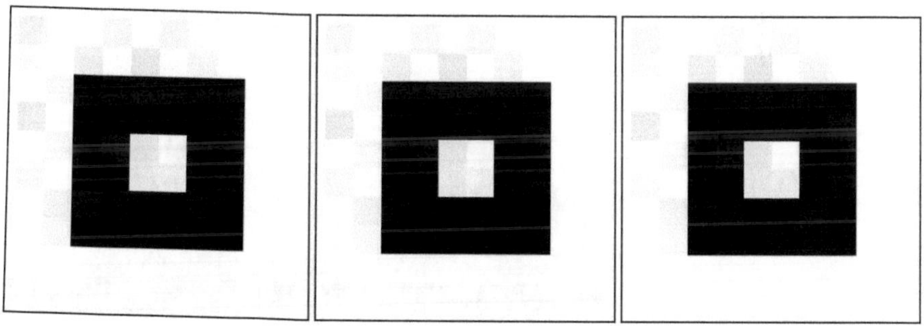

Fig. 10 Original Syntetic image 10×10 (*left*), processed with $T = 7$, $\tau = T/70$, at time level t_{40} (*middle*), and t_{70} (*right*)

continuous and semi-discrete (in space) models are well-posed, satisfy some scale-space properties and behave like a constant (the average value) for long times. One of the advantages of the models is the freedom when selecting the discrete values of the kernel for the implementation. This provides the method with a relevant adaptability to the image to be restored. Several examples of this property are shown in the

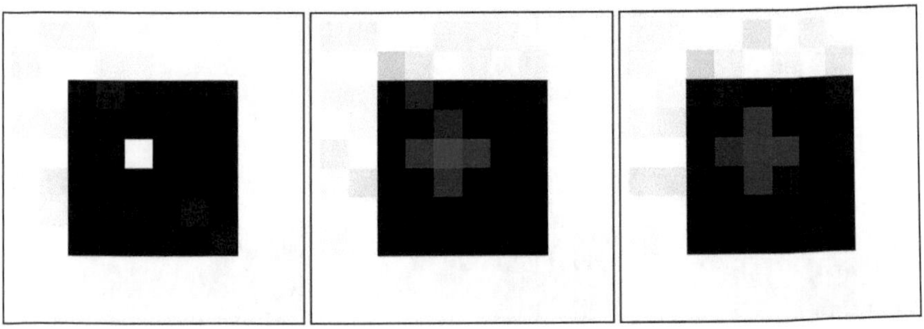

Fig. 11 Original Syntetic image 10 × 10 (*left*), processed with $T = 7$, $\tau = T/70$, at time level t_{40} (*middle*), and t_{70} (*right*)

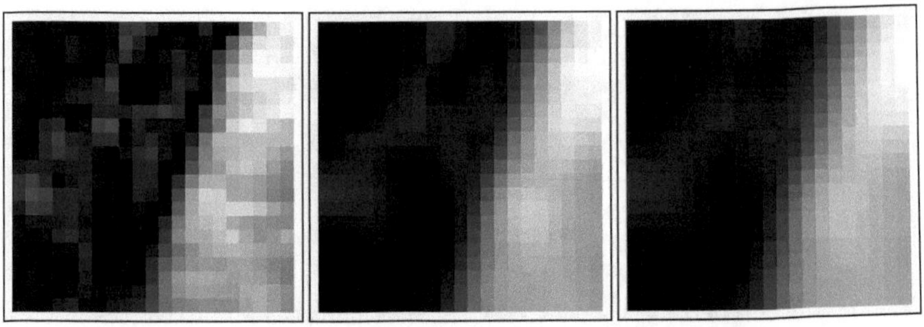

Fig. 12 Subimage 470 − 490 × 200 − 220 of the Fig. 1b (*left*), processed with $T = 1$, $\tau = T/10$, and at time level t_5 (*middle*), and l t_{10} (*right*)

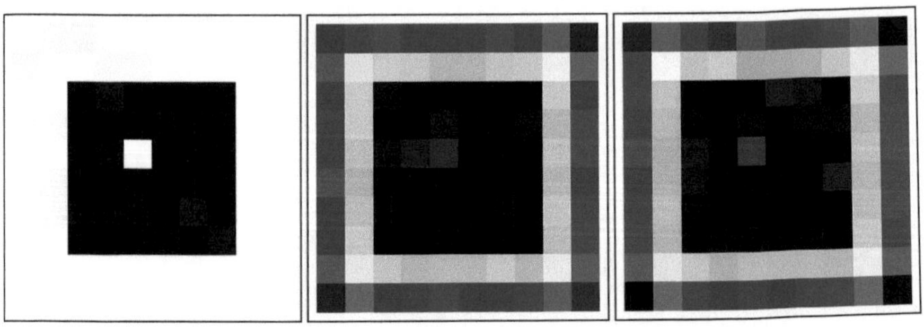

Fig. 13 Original Syntetic image 10 × 10 (*left*), processed with $T = 7$, $\tau = T/70$, at time level t_{20} (*middle*), and t_{40} (*right*)

numerical experiments presented in the paper. They are mainly focused on the ability of the method (according to the selection of the kernel) for denoising and contour detection for short time integration. The promising results encourage us to analyze the fully discrete model in more detail and to incorporate nonlinearities as subjects of a future work.

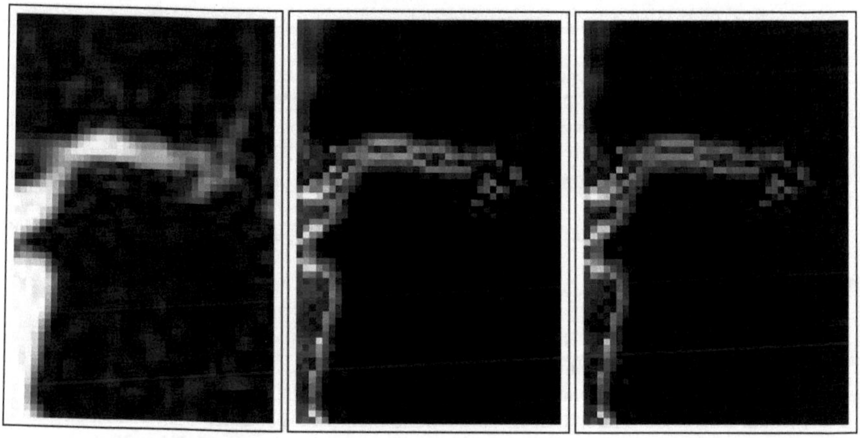

Fig. 14 Subimage $110 - 170 \times 240 - 280$ of the Fig. 1b (*left*), processed with $T = 3$, $\tau = T/30$, and at time level t_{15} (*middle*), and l t_{30} (*right*)

References

1. Álvarez L, Guichard F, Lions P-L, Morel J-M (1993) Axioms and fundamental equations for image processing. Arch Ration Mech Anal 123:199–257
2. Aubert J, Kornprobst P (2001) Mathematical problems in image processing. Springer-Verlag, Berlin
3. Bartels S, Prohl A (2007) Stable discretization of scalar and constrained vectorial Perona–Malik equation. Interfaces Free Bound 4:431–453
4. Boyd, JP (2001) Chebyshev and Fourier spectral methods, 2nd edn. Dover, New York
5. Brezis H (2011) Functional analysis, Sobolev spaces and partial differential equations. Springer, New York
6. Calvo MP, Cuesta E, Palencia C (2007) Runge–Kutta convolution quadrature methods for well-posed equations with memory. Numer Math 107:589–614
7. Collatz L (1960) The numerical treatment of differential equations. Springer-Verlag, New York
8. Cuesta E, Finat J (2003) Image processing by means of a linear integro–differential equation. IASTED1:438–442
9. Cuesta E, Palencia C (2003) A numerical method for an integro–differential equation with memory in Banach spaces. SIAM J Numer Anal 41:1232–1241
10. Cuesta E, Durán A, Kirane M, Malik SA (2012) Image filtering with generalized fractional integrals. In: Proceedings of the 12th international conference on computational and mathematical methods in science and engineering. CMMSE 2012:553–563
11. Cuesta E, Kirane M, Malik SA (2012) Image structure preserve denoising using generalized fractional time integrals. Signal Process 92:553–563
12. Deng T-B, Qin W (2013) Coefficient relation-based minimax design and low-complexity structure of variable fractional-delay digital filters. Signal Process 93:923–932
13. Didas S, Burgeth B, Imiya A, Weickert J (2005) Regularity and scale-space properties of fractional high order linear filtering. In: Kimmel R, Sochen N, Weickert J (eds) Scale-space and PDE methods in computer vision, LNCS, vol 3459. Springer-Verlag, Berlin, pp 13–25
14. Guidotti P, Lambers JV (2009) Two new nonlinear diffusion for noise reduction. J Math Imaging Vision 33:25–37
15. Kuo T-Y, Chen H-Ch, Horng T-L (2013) A fast Poisson solver by Chebyshev pseudospectral method using reflexive decomposition. Taiwan J Math 17:1167–1181

16. Lee JS (1983) Digital image smoothing and the sigma filter. Comput Vision Graph Image Process 24:253–269
17. López–Fernández M, Palencia C (2004) On the numerical inversion of the Laplace transform of certain holomorphic mappings. Appl Numer Math 51:289–303
18. López–Fernández M, Lubich Ch, Schadle A (2008) Adaptive, fast and oblivious convolution in evolution equations with memory. SIAM J Sci Comput 30:1015–1037
19. Lubich Ch (1988) Convolution quadrature and discretized operational calculus I. Numer Math 52:129–145
20. Lubich Ch (1988) Convolution quadrature and discretized operational calculus II. Numer Math 52:413–425
21. Magin R, Ortigueira MD, Podlubny I, Trujillo J (2011) On the fractional signals and systems. Signal Process 91:350–371
22. Perona P, Malik J (1990) Scale-space and edge detection using anisotropic diffusion. IEEE Trans Pattern Anal Mach Intell 12:629–639
23. Podlubny I (1999) Fractional differential equations. Academic, London
24. Proskurowsky W, Widlund O (1980) A finite element-capacitance matrix method for the Neumann problem for Laplace's equation. SIAM J Sci Stat Comput 1:410–425
25. Pruss J (1993) Evolutionary integral equations and applications. Birkhäuser, Basel
26. Ross B, Samko S (1995) Fractional integration operator of variable order in the holder spaces $h^{\lambda(x)}$. Int J Math Math Sci 18:777–788
27. Rudin L, Osher S, Fatemi E (1992) Nonlinear total variation based noise removal algorithm. Phys D 60:259–268
28. Scarpi G (1972) Sulla possibilita di un modello reologico di tipo evolutivo. Rend Sc Nat Fis Mat II 52:570–575
29. Strickwerda JC (1989) Difference schemes and partial differential equations. Wadsworth and Brooks, Pacific Grove
30. Trefethen Ll N (2000) Spectral methods in MATLAB. SIAM, Philadelphia
31. Tseng Ch-Ch, Lee S-L (2013) Designs of two-dimensional linear phase FIR filters using fractional derivative constrains. Signal Process 93:1141–1151
32. Weickert J (1997) A review of nonlinear diffusion filtering, Lecture notes in computer science—scale space theory in computer science. Springer, Berlin
33. Weickert J (1998) Anisotropic diffusion in image processing. B. G. Teubner, Stuttgart
34. Yaroslavsky LP (1985) Digital picture processing. An introduction. Springer-Verlag, New York
35. Zhuang Y, Sun XH (2001) A high-order fast direct solver for singular Poisson equations. J Comput Phys 171:79–94

Colour Image Quantisation using KM and KHM Clustering Techniques with Outlier-Based Initialisation

Henryk Palus and Mariusz Frackiewicz

Abstract This chapter deals with some problems of using clustering techniques K-means (KM) and K-harmonic means (KHM) in colour image quantisation. A lot of attention has been paid to initialisation procedures, because they strongly affect the results of the quantisation. Classical versions of KM and KHM start with randomly selected centres. Authors are more interested in using deterministic initialisations based on the distribution of image pixels in the colour space. In addition to two previously proposed initialisations (DC and SD), here is considered a new outlier-based initialisation. It is based on the modified Mirkin's algorithm (MM) and places the cluster centres in peripheral (outlier) colours of pixels cloud. New approach takes into account small clusters, sometimes representing colours important for proper perception of quantised image. Pixel clustering was created in the *RGB*, *YCbCr* and *CIELAB* colour spaces. Finally, resulting quantised images were evaluated by means of average colour differences in *RGB* (*PSNR*) and *CIELAB*(ΔE) colour spaces and additionally by the loss of colourfulness (ΔM).

1 Introduction

True colour images acquired by a camera contain only a small subset of all possible 16.7 million colours. Therefore, it makes sense to further reduce the number of colours in the image. Nowadays, the colour image quantisation (CIQ) is an important auxiliary operation in the field of colour image processing and is very useful in image compression, image pre-segmentation, image watermarking and content-based image retrieval (CBIR). These algorithms are also still used to present the true colour images on devices with limited number of colours. CIQ reduces significantly the

H. Palus (✉) · M. Frackiewicz
Silesian University of Technology, ul. Akademicka 16,
44-100 Gliwice, Poland
e-mail: Henryk.Palus@polsl.pl

M. Frackiewicz
e-mail: Mariusz.Frackiewicz@polsl.pl

J. M. R. S. Tavares, R. Natal Jorge (eds.), *Developments in Medical Image Processing and Computational Vision*, Lecture Notes in Computational Vision and Biomechanics 19,
DOI 10.1007/978-3-319-13407-9_16

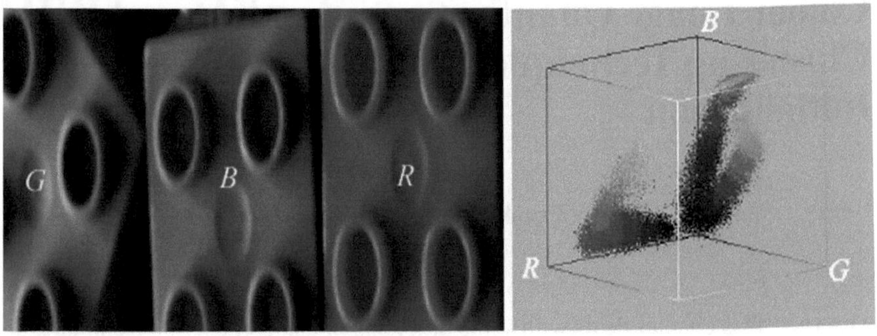

a b

Fig. 1 Simple colour image and its clusters in *RGB* colour space

number of colours in the image to the specially selected set of representative colours (colour palette). Colour palette generation is the most important step in any CIQ method. Proper choice of the colour palette helps minimize the colour difference between the original image and the quantised image.

There exist two main classes of CIQ techniques: splitting techniques and clustering techniques [1]. The splitting techniques divide the colour space into smaller disjoined subspaces and then a colour palette is built by choosing representative colours from these subspaces. Good examples of such techniques are the Median Cut [8], Octree [5] and Wu's [16] algorithms. For example, the Median Cut method first locates a tightest box in *RGB* colour space, that encloses all image colours. Then, the box is cut on the longest side and two subboxes are formed. As a result of a such cut both subboxes should contain the same number of colours and from here comes the name of the method. Next, a subbox with longest side is cut. This process continues until the total number of subboxes is smaller than the number of colours in the palette chosen for the quantised image. All colours in one subbox are represented by their mean value.

On the other hand, the clustering techniques are the optimization tasks that minimize the quantisation errors by minimization the sums of distances between the cluster centres and cluster points. One of the most popular clustering techniques is the K-means (KM) technique [10] and its existing modifications e.g. K-harmonic means (KHM) technique [19]. The clustering has a long tradition of use to quantize colour images [18]. It can be easily to see that each of the dominant colours in natural image corresponds to a separate fragment of pixels cloud in the colour space, which can be called a cluster (Fig. 1). As a generally statement, it may be found that the splitting techniques are faster than the clustering techniques but they have larger quantisation errors.

The results of many clustering techniques depend on method of determination of initial cluster centres, used colour space, applied colour metric etc. Such sensitivity to initialisation is an important disadvantage of these clustering techniques. A random selection of the initial centres, used in classical KM version, is not able to achieve repeatable results in colour image quantisation. Therefore, in our previous paper [3] we attempted to use two new heuristic methods of initialisation. The first method, which is an arbitrary one, is based on uniform partitioning of diagonal of *RGB* cube (DC) into k segments. Gray levels in the middle of segments are used as initial centres. If an image is clustered into k clusters, k initial cluster centres are located on the gray level axis. The second method, which is an adaptive one, uses a size of pixel cloud of a colour image and the method has been marked as SD. First, the mean value and standard deviation (SD) for each *RGB* component of all image pixels are calculated. Then, around the point of mean colour (a pixel cloud centre) a rectangular cuboid with sides equal $2\sigma_R$, $2\sigma_G$ and $2\sigma_B$ is constructed. We assume that it lies within the *RGB* cube. Next, the main diagonal of the cuboid is divided into k equal segments. The centres of these segments are used as initial cluster centres. Initial cluster centres in KM can also come directly from splitting algorithms e.g. from MC or Wu's algorithms and such combined approach (MC+KM, Wu+KM) was proposed few years ago [14]. Experiments have shown that Wu+KM technique offers a slightly better performance than MC+KM and KM initialised by SD approach.

Appropriate initialisation provides the high quality clustering achieved by running small number of iterations and avoids the formation of empty clusters, which sometimes occurs in the case of DC initialisation. The result of empty clusters is a reduction in the number of colours in quantised image. Removing empty clusters needs changing the cluster centres or splitting a newly created cluster. Good initialisation for the KM technique, used in colour quantisation, is still looked for by many researchers [2].

The KHM is based on harmonic means, instead of arithmetic means and additionally uses fuzzy membership of pixels to clusters and dynamic weight functions, what means different influence an individual pixel on calculating new values of centres in each iteration. KHM is robust to initialisation and creates non-empty clusters. A disadvantage of KHM in relation to KM is greater computational complexity, resulting in a longer computation time.

The clustering process can be conducted not only in the *RGB* colour space, but also in other colour spaces. Here a special role is played by recommended in 1976 the *CIELAB* colour space [17]. It is a perceptually uniform colour space which approximately expresses a way of human colour perception. The Euclidean distance in this space is approximately equal to the perceptual colour difference. This should be of great importance in the process of clustering. Unfortunately, the transform from *RGB* to *CIELAB* is complicated and nonlinear.

The *YCbCr* colour space is applied in CIQ task among other used colour spaces. Its advantage, in comparison to *CIELAB* colour space, is a linearity of transformation from *RGB* space, which results in faster calculation of the *YCbCr* components. Although the colour difference in the *YCbCr* space less corresponds to the human colour perception than the colour difference calculated in *CIELAB*, however makes it better than the Euclidean distance calculated in *RGB* space. The *YCbCr* components can be received from the following transformation [9]:

$$Y = 0.257R + 0.504G + 0.098B + 16 \tag{1}$$

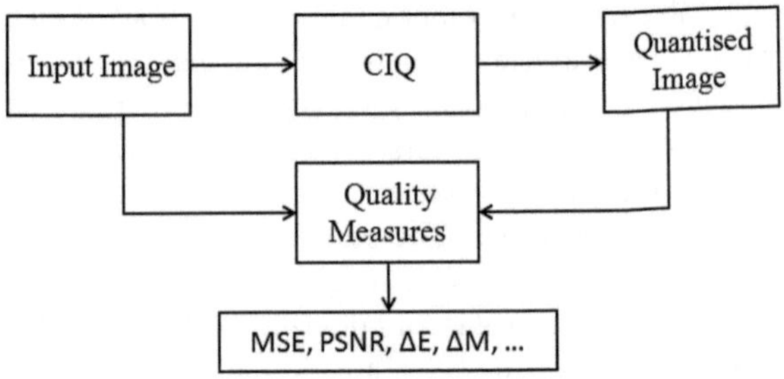

Fig. 2 The general idea of CIQ quality measure

$$Cb = -0.148R - 0.291G + 0.439B + 128 \tag{2}$$

$$Cr = 0.439R - 0.368G - 0.071B + 128 \tag{3}$$

Therefore, later in this chapter, are tested the CIQ methods in the following colour spaces: basic *RGB*, *YCbCr* and perceptually uniform *CIELAB*.

This chapter is organized as follows. In Sect. 2, we present two typical and one untypical quality measures used for CIQ quality evaluation. The results of experimental tests for determination of factors influencing the quantisation errors are described in Sect. 3. The idea of the new proposed initialisation method (modified Mirkin's algorithm) is illustrated on several images in Sect. 4. Section 5 shows on a larger set of images a usefulness of a new MM initialisation in quantisation process, which is oriented toward image segmentation. Finally we conclude the chapter in Sect. 6.

2 CIQ Quality Measures

The colour quantisation error depends on the number of colours in palette (e.g. 256, 64, 16, 8, 4 colours): the smaller number of colours in palette, then larger is the quantisation error. Objective CIQ quality measures (Fig. 2) are very important in the evaluation process of different colour quantizers.

Commonly used most popular measure is the Mean Squared Error (*MSE*) defined by:

$$MSE = \frac{1}{3MN}\sum_{i=1}^{M}\sum_{j=1}^{N}\left[(R_{ij} - R^*_{ij})^2 + (G_{ij} - G^*_{ij})^2 + (B_{ij} - B^*_{ij})^2\right] \tag{4}$$

where M and N are the image dimensions in pixels, R_{ij}, G_{ij}, B_{ij} are the colour components of the pixel at location (i, j) in the original image and R^*_{ij}, G^*_{ij}, B^*_{ij} are the colour components of the pixel in quantised image. The smaller the *MSE* value, the better is the quantised image. Other error measure applied to evaluation of quantisation is Peak Signal-to-Noise Ratio (*PSNR*), good correlated with *MSE* value and expressed in decibel scale:

$$PSNR = 20\log_{10}\frac{255}{\sqrt{MSE}} \tag{5}$$

Unfortunately, these both measures that come from the signal processing field are poorly correlated with subjective visual quality of an image. The quantisation error can be treated as a colour error that should be determined in a perceptually uniform colour space. Therefore, an average colour difference in *CIELAB* colour space (ΔE) is sometimes applied as a quantisation error:

$$\Delta E = \frac{1}{MN}\sum_{i=1}^{M}\sum_{j=1}^{N}\sqrt{(L_{ij}-L^*_{ij})^2+(a_{ij}-a^*_{ij})^2+(b_{ij}-b^*_{ij})^2} \tag{6}$$

where: L_{ij}, a_{ij}, b_{ij} are the colour components of the pixel at location (i, j) in the original image and L^*_{ij}, a^*_{ij}, b^*_{ij} are the *CIELAB* colour components of the pixel in the quantised image. Also the loss of image colourfulness due to colour quantisation can be used as an additional tool for evaluation of quantisation error [13].

$$\Delta M = \left| M_{orig} - M_{quant} \right| \tag{7}$$

where: M_{orig} - colourfulness of the original image, M_{quant} - colourfulness of the quantised image. Formulas for computing of image colourfulness are simple and good correlate with the perceptual colourfulness of the image [6]:

$$M = \sqrt{\sigma_{rg}^2 + \sigma_{yb}^2} + 0.3 \times \sqrt{\mu_{rg}^2 + \mu_{yb}^2} \tag{8}$$

where σ_{rg}, σ_{yb} are the standard deviations and μ_{rg}, μ_{yb} are the mean values of opponent colour components of the image pixels. The opponent components are approximated by following simplified equations:

$$rg = R - G \tag{9}$$

$$yb = 0.5(R + G) - B \tag{10}$$

where *rg* - red-green opponency and *yb* - yellow-blue opponency.

It should be noted here that a common drawback of all these quality measures based on colour similarity is that they compare the images by using pixel to pixel comparison, without taking into account an impact of neighbouring pixels on the perception of colour of considered pixel. The additional factors, defining the quality of quantised image can include the edge similarity and structural similarity [7]. In this paper a new quality measure as a combination of all three similarities was proposed. However, in many cases the human visual system is the best final judge of quality of quantised image (subjective quality measures).

3 Preliminary Experimental Tests

A set of five natural images has been randomly chosen from Berkeley's image database [11] and presented in Fig. 3 in order of their number of unique colours.

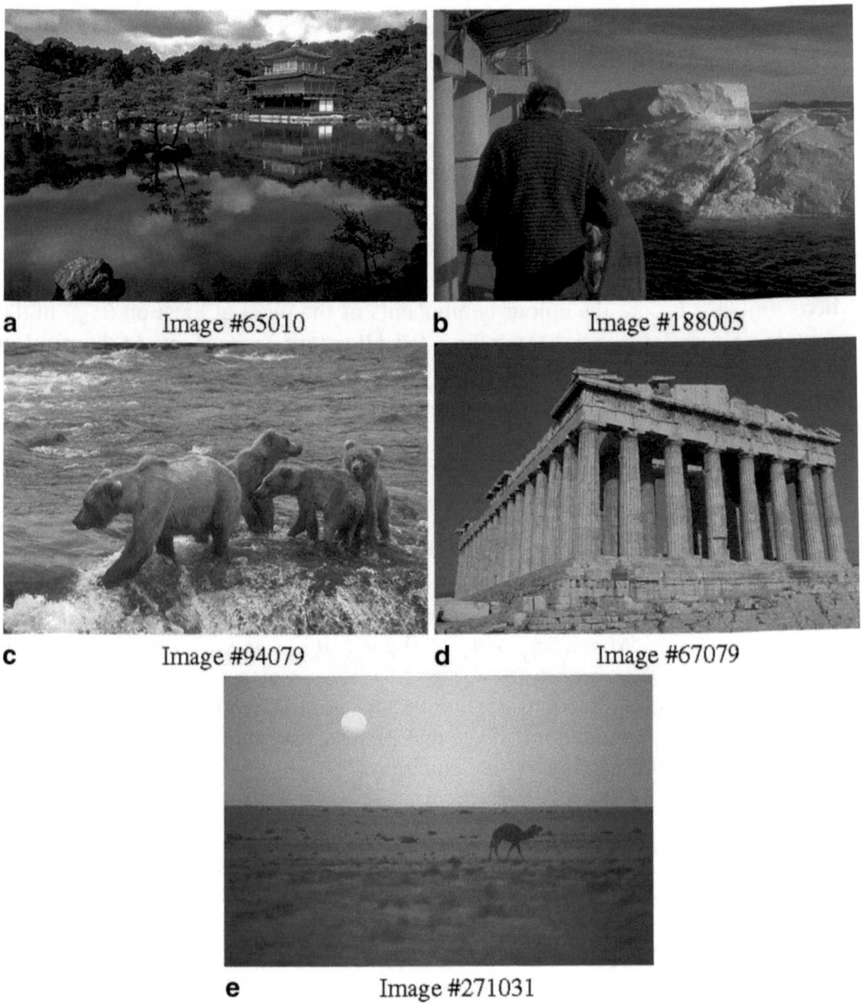

Fig. 3 A set of five test images from Berkeley image database

All these images were acquired at the same spatial resolution, i.e. 481×321 pixels. First tests were conducted to show that the larger unique number of colours in the original image, the larger also quantisation errors for a given size of the palette (here eight colours). The number of iterations in used clustering techniques was equal to 15 and the quantisation was realised by KM and KHM techniques in the *RGB* colour space. The data in Table 1 shows the error values for KM technique with two different initialisations: DC and SD. Similarly, Table 2 contains error values calculated for more efficient KHM technique. It should be noted that in both cases with the decreasing numbers of unique colours in images in Fig. 3 generally decreases the values of

Table 1 Quantisation results of the KM technique ($k = 8$)

Image	Colours	$PSNR$ (dB)		ΔE		ΔM	
		DC	SD	DC	SD	DC	SD
#65010	49404	24.8	25.0	11.3	9.8	9.9	7.0
#188005	31797	26.4	26.4	8.6	8.5	9.3	8.2
#94079	31225	27.1	27.6	6.1	5.3	9.1	4.6
#67079	22217	27.9	29.4	5.0	4.3	1.8	1.0
#271031	7652	30.1	32.1	3.7	3.2	1.2	1.5

Table 2 Quantisation results of the KHM technique ($k = 8$)

Image	Colours	$PSNR$ (dB)		ΔE		ΔM	
		DC	SD	DC	SD	DC	SD
#65010	49404	24.9	24.9	11.1	10.8	11.1	10.8
#188005	31797	26.8	26.5	8.1	9.0	8.1	9.0
#94079	31225	27.2	27.2	6.0	5.8	6.0	5.8
#67079	22217	28.2	29.0	4.9	4.4	4.9	4.4
#271031	7652	32.1	32.1	3.2	3.2	3.2	3.2

Table 3 Quantisation results of the splitting techniques ($k = 8$)

Image	Colours	$PSNR$ (dB)		ΔE		ΔM	
		MC	Wu's	MC	Wu's	MC	Wu's
#65010	49404	22.3	24.7	11.2	10.0	4.1	9.4
#188005	31797	25.7	26.1	8.6	8.9	6.9	10.4
#94079	31225	26.4	27.1	6.2	5.7	7.4	7.5
#67079	22217	28.1	28.6	5.2	4.7	1.1	1.6
#271031	7652	30.3	32.0	3.4	3.2	1.3	1.2

quantisation errors, i.e. increases $PSNR$ and decrease ΔE and ΔM. A similar effect also occurs for two tested splitting algorithms: MC and Wu's (see Table 3).

In this way we confirmed a quite obvious hypothesis about the impact of the number of unique colours in the image on the quantisation error.

4 Idea of Outlier-Based Initialisation

Both DC and SD initialisations generate the starting centres of clusters located close to gray line. In the case of KM these locations of centres largely determine the final colours of the quantised image. There exist colour images for which the KM technique with earlier presented initialisations (DC, SD) does not give good results, particularly when the size of colour palette is small (e.g. four or eight colours).

Good example of such image is shown in Fig. 4a. This image is not very colourful, but it contains 138 877 unique colours! Colour pixels, as in other images, are generally grouped along diagonal of the *RGB* cube. Small red part of pixel cloud represents a red letter lying in the middle of the image (see Fig. 4b). The formation of the separate red cluster can be very important for CIQ application in image segmentation.

Unfortunately, the colour quantisation into 4 colours by KM and KHM techniques with initialisations DC and SD does not permit to obtain the red letter in quantised image (see Fig. 4c, d). Therefore we looked for a better method of initialisation for our clustering techniques and we have found an intelligent initialisation of KM proposed by Mirkin [12]. In this method the initialisation of KM is based on so-called Anomalous Pattern (AP) clusters, which are the most distant from the centre of cloud of points. Such outliers (peripheral points of the cloud) are the most important in this initialisation. This algorithm is general in nature and can be used in many different pattern recognition tasks.

Mirkin's algorithm consists of the following steps:

1. Find the centre of cloud of points in *RGB* colour space and mark it as C.
2. Find a furthest point away from centre C and mark it as $Cout$.
3. Perform the KM clustering into two clusters based on appointed previously centres: C and $Cout$ and just the centre $Cout$ is repositioned after each iteration.
4. Add the *RGB* components of $Cout$ to the list of stored centres.
5. Remove all points belonging to the cluster with centre $Cout$.
6. Check that there are still points in the cloud. If so, go back to the pt.2.
7. Sort obtained clusters by size (the number of elements) and select k largest clusters. Their centres are final starting centres for KM clustering.

Modification of Mirkin's (MM) algorithm proposed below is based on two important changes in relation to the original Mirkin's algorithm. First, the initial centres $Cout$ are used as starting centres instead of the final centres, which, in original algorithm, are found after clustering into two clusters. Second, clusters are not sorted according to size in the final step of the algorithm. In this way, the MM initialisation locates the starting cluster centres in outlier points (colours) i.e. points, which are furthest from the centre of pixels cloud. This allows to take into account the small clusters, which represent the colours of small, but perceptually essential regions [4, 15].

Modified Mirkin's algorithm looks as follows:

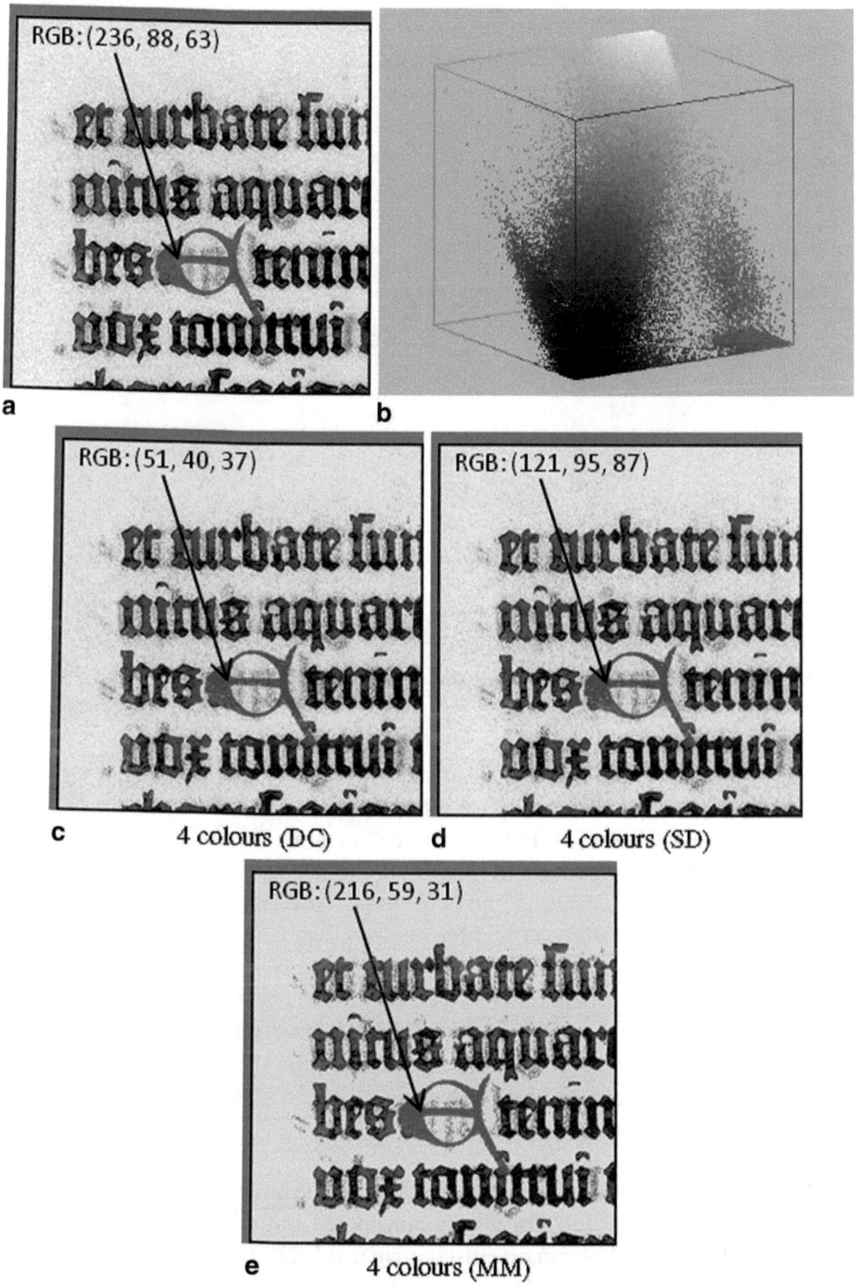

Fig. 4 Results of colour quantisation: **a** original image, **b** colour gamut, **c** KM with DC (4 colours), **d** KM with SD (4 colours), **e** KM with MM (4 colours)

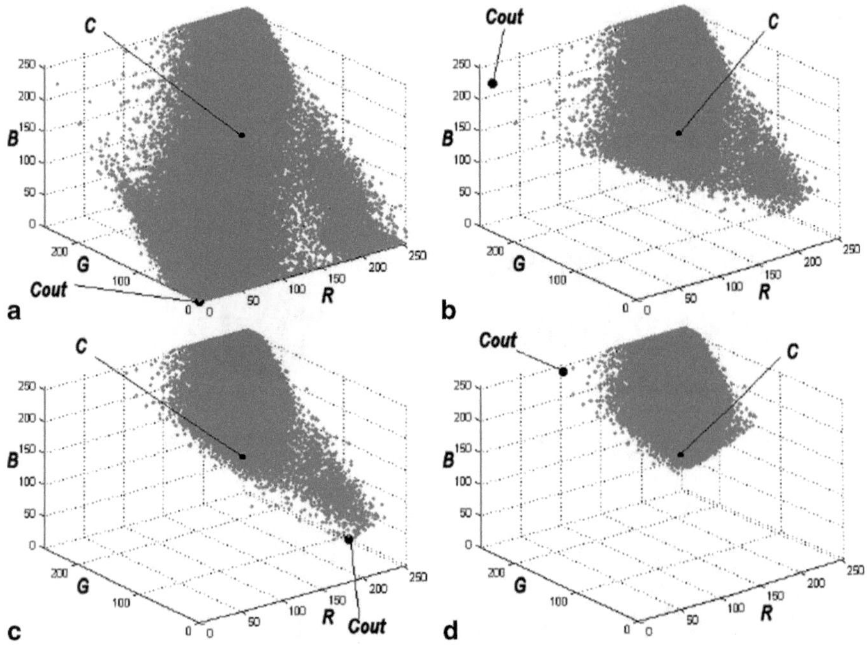

Fig. 5 Outlier cluster centres found during MM initialisation

1. Find the centre of cloud of points in *RGB* colour space and mark it as C.
2. Find a furthest point away from centre C and mark it as $Cout$.
3. Add the *RGB* components of $Cout$ to the list of stored centres.
4. Perform the KM clustering into two clusters based on appointed previously centres: C and $Cout$ and just the centre $Cout$ is repositioned after each iteration.
5. Remove all points belonging to the cluster with centre $Cout$.
6. Check that there are still points in the cloud. If so, go back to the pt.2.
7. Select the first k clusters determined by this algorithm. Their centres are final starting centres for KM clustering.

The MM initialisation permits to get the red letter in the image during the quantisation into 4 colours (see Fig. 4e). For all the considered initialisations we calculated a colour error for the red letter in quantised image: $\Delta E(\text{DC}) = 77$, $\Delta E(\text{SD}) = 60$ and $\Delta E(\text{MM}) = 11$. These results demonstrate the superiority of MM initialisation over other tested initialisations.

Figure 5 illustrates subsequent eliminations of outlier clusters from the cloud of points presented as 3D scatter plot and helps to understand the algorithm. Here, the

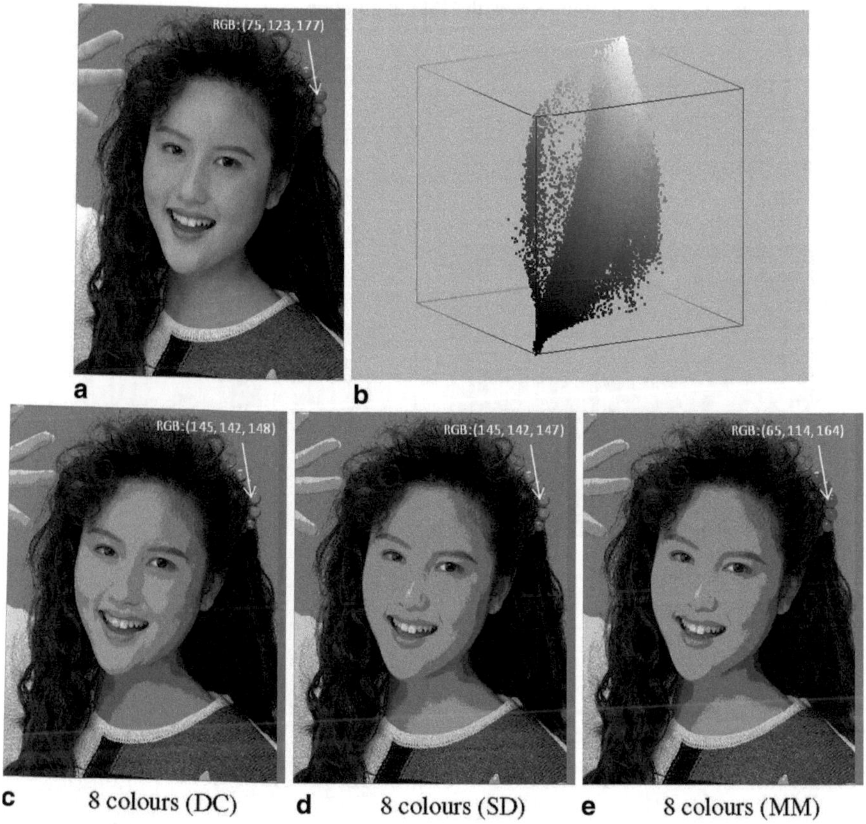

Fig. 6 Results of colour quantisation **a** original image, **b** colour gamut for original image, **c** KM with DC initialisation, **d** KM with SD initialisation, **e** KM with MM initialisation

third step of MM (see Fig. 5c) has particular importance, because a centre of red cluster is detected.

Another example of usefulness of MM initialisation is the quantisation of the image shown in Fig. 6. Particular attention should be paid to the blue beads, which are perceptually important region in the original image. The image is quantised into 8 colours. The colour quantisation by KM technique with initialisations DC and SD generates the images without blue pixels in quantised image; the beads are gray (see *RGB* values in Fig. 6c, d). This problem is solved by using the MM initialisation, as shown in Fig. 6e. We calculated appropriate colour errors for the blue beads: $\Delta E(\text{DC}) = 32$, $\Delta E(\text{SD}) = 33$ and $\Delta E(\text{MM}) = 4$. Definitely the smallest error again achieved the MM initialisation.

Similar experiments were also carried out with other images. Their visual evaluation confirmed the advantages of the MM initialisation. Despite the limited palette, each quantised image contained the perceptually significant colours. On the other hand, generally accepted image quality measures for quantised images do not give clear results (see Table 4). Only ΔM, the loss of image colourfulness, that is strongly related to colour perception, shows the advantage of MM initialisation.

Table 4 Quantisation results of the KM with MM initialisation

Image	*PSNR* (dB)			ΔE			ΔM		
	DC	SD	MM	DC	SD	MM	DC	SD	MM
Fig. 4	20.7	20.7	20.4	13.4	13.4	12.9	32.0	31.4	14.2
Fig. 6	26.5	26.2	25.9	6.0	5.7	6.1	4.7	3.9	3.6

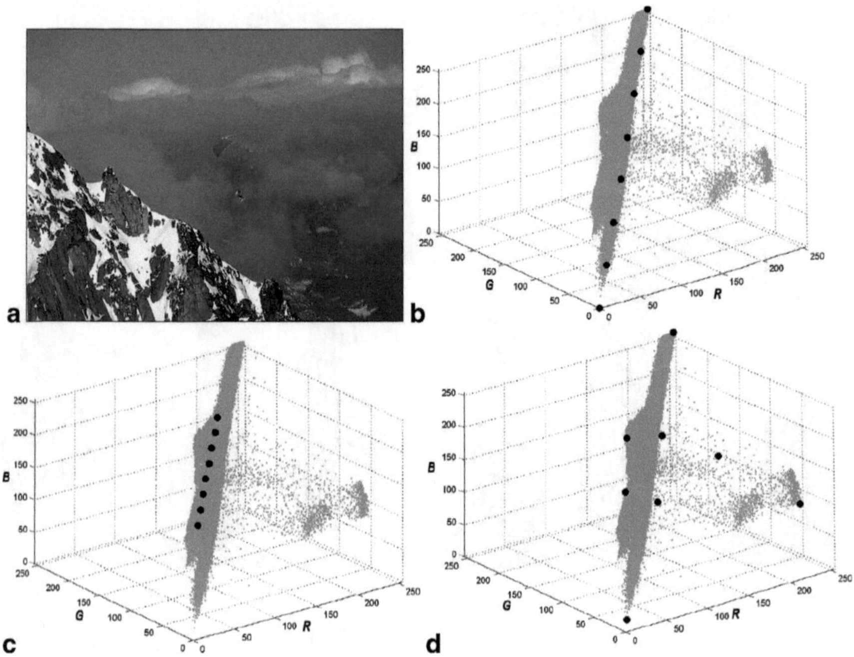

Fig. 7 An original image, **b** Centres found in DC initialisation, **c** Centres found in SD initialisation, **d** Centres found in MM initialisation. All clusterings for 8 clusters

5 Further Tests of New Initialisation

In the first group of tests were determined the positions of starting centres of clusters for three compared initialisations: DC, SD and MM. The colour pixels in pixels cloud of natural images are generally grouped along diagonal of the *RGB* cube. Black dots plotted on a pixels cloud present the location of these centres. All clusterings presented in this section were achieved after 30 iterations of KM technique.

5.1 Distributions of Clustering Starting Centres

The first test image (Fig. 7a) contains perceptually important red area lying in the middle of the image and showing a paraglider, which can be seen in Fig. 7b, c, d as a small part of pixels cloud directed to the red colour. In the case of DC and SD

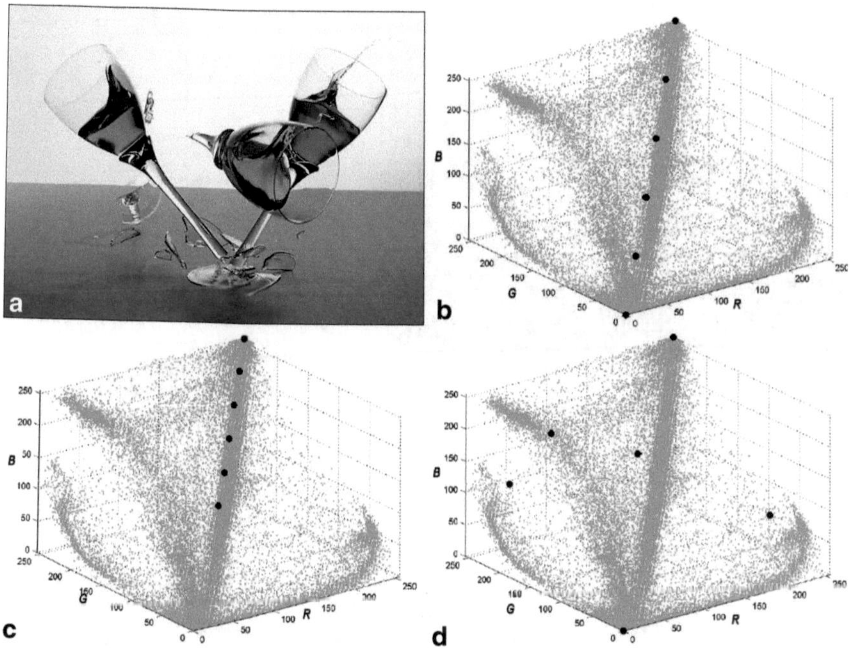

Fig. 8 An original image, b Centres found in DC initialisation, c Centres found in SD initialisation, d Centres found in MM initialisation. All clusterings for 8 clusters

initialisation all eight initial centres are located on the diagonal of the *RGB* cube, only the MM initialisation (Fig. 7d) generates two peripherally located centres, one of which is contained in a cluster of red pixels. This gives a chance to get a good CIQ result using the KM technique with MM initialisation.

The second test image (Fig. 8a), quantised into 6 colours, creates a specific pixels cloud (Fig. 8 b, c, d) in the *RGB* space with three branches for three colours *R*, *G* and *B*. Only the MM initialisation puts the initial centres in these sectors, which are important for further clustering (Fig. 8d).

The third considered test image (Fig. 9a) presents a book cover and contains six colour characters with distinct chromatic colours and it is characterized by more complex pixels cloud (Fig. 9b, c, d). Again, only the MM initialisation (Fig. 9d) settles a part of centres outside of the main pixels cloud, which gives a opportunity to obtain a good CIQ result.

5.2 *CIQ for Salient Region Detection*

The second part of tests serves to compare the quality of images quantised with different initialisations. These tests were performed in the *RGB* colour space and two

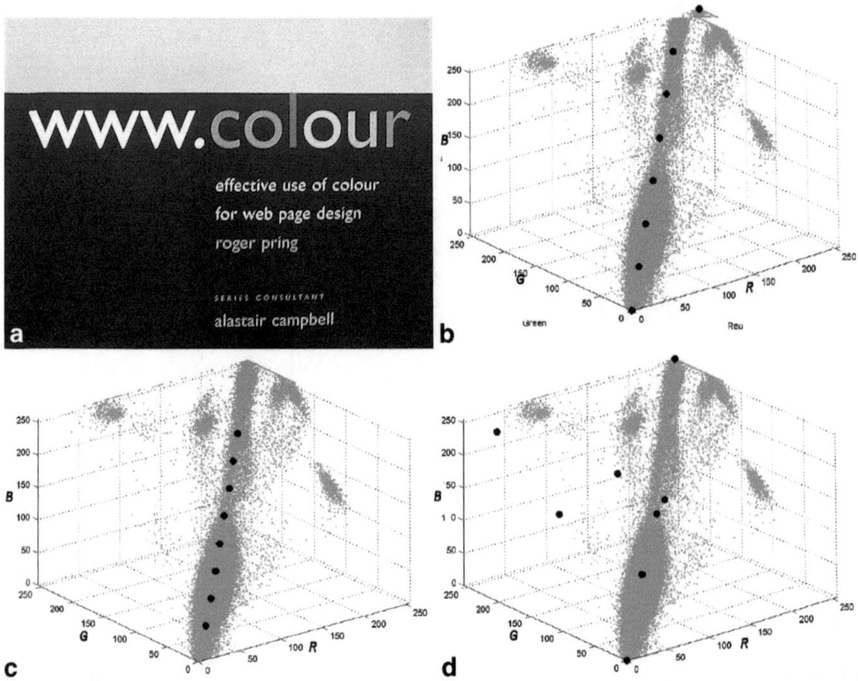

Fig. 9 An original image, **b** Centres found in DC initialisation, **c** Centres found in SD initialisation, **d** Centres found in MM initialisation. All clusterings for 8 clusters

additional colour spaces: *YCbCr* (linear transformation of *RGB* space) and perceptually uniform *CIELAB* colour space (non-linear transformation of *RGB* space). In addition to the subjective visual assessment a loss of image colourfulness ΔM was used, and the other typical quality measures described in Sect. 2 were rejected. Their nature makes that the colours of the perceptually significant regions with small areas do not play a noticeable role.

Figure 10 shows quantised versions of the original image presented in Fig. 7a. The visual assessment indicates a dominance of the MM initialisation since regardless of the type of colour space a reddish paraglider remains in quantised image. Particular attention is paid the quantisation in the *CIELAB* colour space, where the loss of image colourfulness ΔM regardless of initialisation is smallest.

Figure 11 shows quantised versions of the original image presented in Fig. 8a. Original image contains the three chromatic colours only, so it is easy to visually assess the results of quantisation. These three chromatic colours remained in the quantised images in four of nine cases only. There are three images quantised after MM initialisation and one image quantised in *CIELAB* space after SD initialisation. The original image is not a natural image. Perhaps that is why the relation between the results is here not so clear.

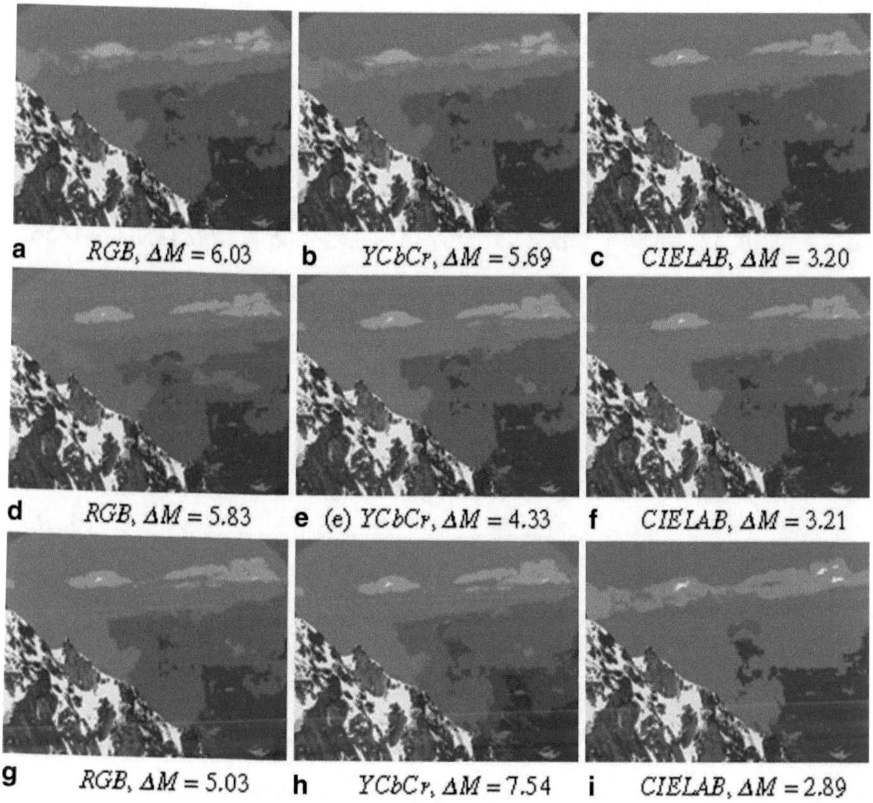

Fig. 10 KM results for the image from Fig. 7a, **a**, **b**, **c**, results with DC initialisation, **d**, **e**, **f** results with SD initialisation, **g**, **h**, **i** results with MM initialisation ($k = 8$)

Figure 12 shows quantised versions of the original image in Fig. 9a. The original image contains six characters with distinct chromatic colours, making easy a visually assessment of the quantised images. The caption below Fig. 12 includes a number of chromatic colours recognized by the observer. You can notice that the maximal number of chromatic colours obtained after CIQ is 4 and it has been achieved only in case of MM initialisation in the *YCbCr* and *CIELAB* spaces. These results occur simultaneously with the least loss of image colourfulness ΔM.

6 Conclusions

In this chapter we showed for two different CIQ techniques that the number of unique colours in the natural image significantly influences on the value of quantisation error. But the main contribution of the work is a new alternative way for initialisation of KM, which provides better CIQ results. This approach based on detection and elimination

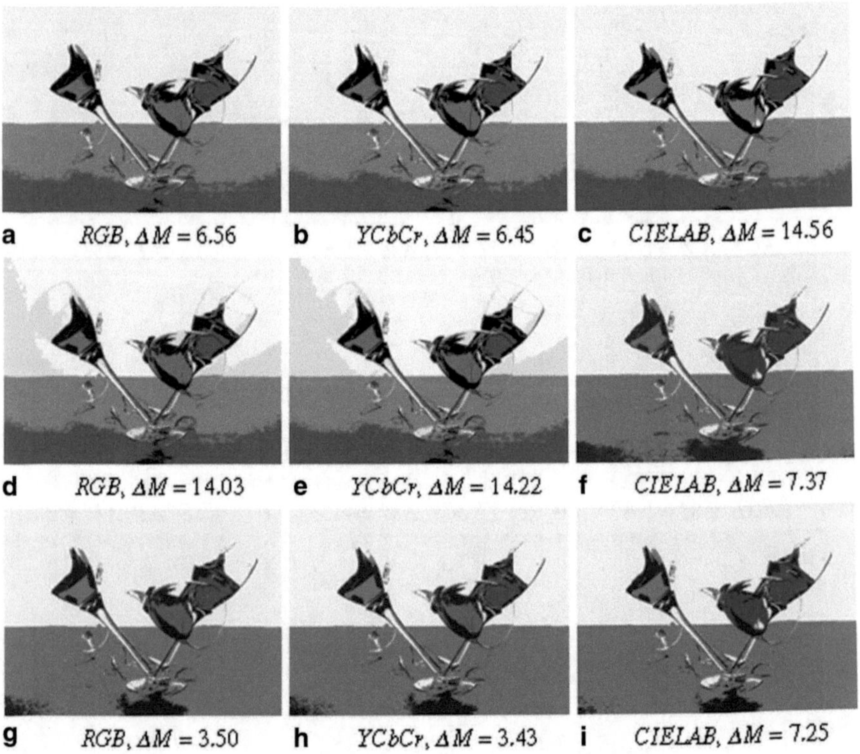

Fig. 11 KM results for the image from Fig. 8a, **a**, **b**, **c** results with DC initialisation, **d**, **e**, **f** results with SD initialisation, **g**, **h**, **i** results with MM initialisation ($k = 6$)

outlier clusters, named here MM, does not lose the perceptually important colour regions of the original image. Additionally, the usefulness of quality measure called the loss of colourfulness to CIQ assessment has been confirmed.

Acknowledgements This work was supported by Polish Ministry for Science and Higher Education under internal grant BK-/RAu1/2014 for Institute of Automatic Control, Silesian University of Technology, Gliwice, Poland.

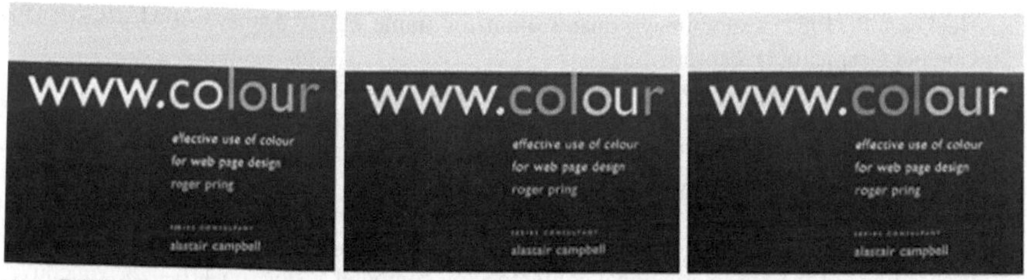

a RGB, 2 col., $\Delta M = 7.79$ **b** $YCbCr$, 3 col., $\Delta M = 5.43$ **c** $CIELAB$, 3 col., $\Delta M = 6.24$

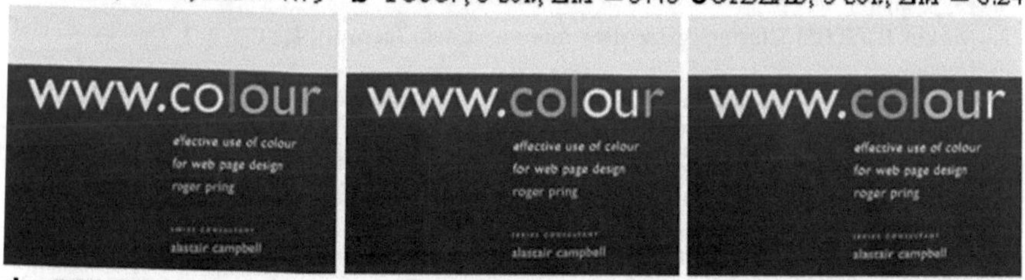

d RGB, 2 col., $\Delta M = 11.43$ **e** $YCbCr$, 2 col., $\Delta M = 11.04$ **f** $CIELAB$, 2 col., $\Delta M = 6.72$

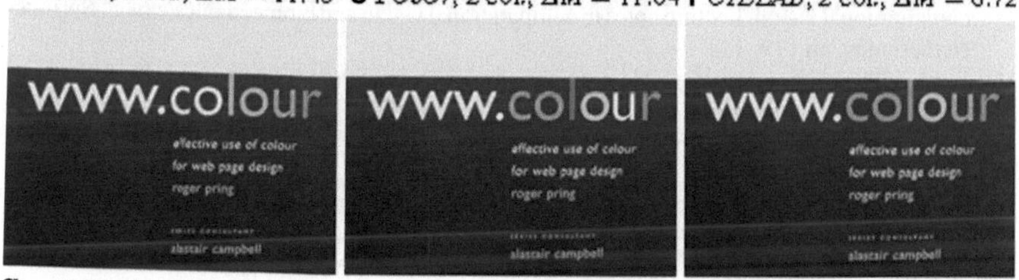

g RGB, 2 col., $\Delta M = 5.98$ **h** $YCbCr$, 4 col., $\Delta M = 4.35$ **i** $CIELAB$, 4 col., $\Delta M = 3.72$

Fig. 12 KM results for the image from Fig. 9a, **a**, **b**, **c** results with DC initialisation, **d**, **e**, **f** results with SD initialisation, **g**, **h**, **i** results with MM initialisation ($k = 8$)

References

1. Brun L, Tremeau A (2003) Color quantization. In: Sharma G (ed) Digital color imaging handbook. CRC, Boca Raton, pp 589–637
2. Celebi ME (2011) Improving the performance of k-means for color quantization. Image Vision Comput 29(4):260–271
3. Frackiewicz M, Palus H (2011) KM and KHM clustering techniques for colour image quantisation. In: Tavares JMR, Jorge RN (eds) Computational vision and medical image processing, vol. 19. Springer, Netherlands, pp 161–174
4. Frackiewicz M, Palus H (2013) Outlier-based initialisation of k-means in colour image quantisation. In: Informatics and Applications (ICIA), Lodz, Poland, Second International Conference on Informatics and Applications, pp 36–41
5. Gervautz M, Purgathofer W (1990) A simple method for color quantization: octree quantization. In: Glassner AS (ed) Graphics gems. Academic, San Diego pp 287–293
6. Hasler D, Suesstrunk S (2003) Measuring colourfulness for natural images. In: Electronic imaging 2003: human vision and electronic imaging VIII, Proceedings of SPIE, vol. 5007, pp 87–95
7. Hassan M, Bhagvati C (2012) Color image quantization quality assessment. In: Venugopal K, Patnaik L (eds) Wireless networks and computational intelligence, vol. 292. Springer, Berlin, pp 139–148

8. Heckbert P (1982) Color image quantization for frame buffer display. ACM SIGGRAPH Comput Graph 16(3):297–307
9. Koschan A, Abidi M (2008) Digital color image processing. Wiley, New York
10. Mac Queen J (1967) Some methods for classification and analysis of multivariate observations. In: Proceedings of the 5th Berkeley symposium on mathematics, statistics, and probabilities, vol. I, pp 281–297. Berkeley and Los Angeles, CA, USA
11. Martin D, Fowlkes C, Tal D, Malik J (2001) A database of human segmented natural images and its application to evaluating segmentation algorithms and measuring ecological statistics. In: Proceedings of the 8th international conference on computer vision, pp 416–423. Vancouver, BC, Canada
12. Mirkin B (2005) Clustering for data mining: a data recovery approach. Chapman & Hall, London
13. Palus H (2004) On color image quantization by the k-means algorithm. In: Droege D, Paulus D (eds) Proceedings of 10. Workshop Farbbildverarbeitung, pp 58–65
14. Palus H, Frackiewicz M (2010) New approach for initialization of k-means technique applied to color quantization. In: Information Technology (ICIT), Gdansk, Poland, 2nd international conference on information technology, pp 205–209
15. Palus H, Frackiewicz M (2013) Colour quantisation as a preprocessing step for image segmentation. In: Tavares JMR, Natal Jorge RM (eds) Topics in medical image processing and computational vision, Lecture notes in computational vision and biomechanics, vol. 8. Springer, Netherlands, pp 119–138
16. Wu X (1991) Efficient statistical computations for optimal color quantization. In: Arvo J (ed) Graphic gems II. Academic Press, New York, pp 126–133
17. Wyszecki G, Stiles W (1982) Color science: concepts and methods, quantitative data and formulae. Wiley, New York
18. Xiang Z, Joy G (1994) Color image quantization by agglomerative clustering. IEEE Comput Graph Appl 14(3):44–48
19. Zhang B, Hsu M, Dayal U (1999) K-harmonic means-data clustering algorithm. Tech. Rep. TR HPL-1999-124, Hewlett Packard Labs, Palo Alto, CA, USA

A Study of a Firefly Meta-Heuristics for Multithreshold Image Segmentation

H. Erdmann, G. Wachs-Lopes, C. Gallão, M. P. Ribeiro and P. S. Rodrigues

Abstract Thresholding-based image segmentation algorithms are usually developed for a specific set of images because the objective of these algorithms is strongly related to their applications. The binarization of the image is generally preferred over multi-segmentation, mainly because it's simple and easy to implement. However, in this paper we demonstrate that a scene separation with three threshold levels can be more effective and closer to a manually performed segmentation. Also, we show that similar results can be achieved through a firefly-based meta-heuristic. Finally, we suggest a similarity measure that can be used for the comparison between the distances of the automatic and manual segmentation.

1 Introduction

Image segmentation is a task with applications in several areas related to digital image processing. It can be done by estimating the number of thresholds used to partition an image into regions of interest. The most simple thresholding technique is to divide the image in two regions, binarizing the search space.

Among the known techniques to define a threshold that splits an image in two clusters, there are those based on the probabilistic-distribution entropy for the color intensities. In [1], T. Pun wrote the first algorithm for image binarization based on the traditional Shannon entropy, assuming that the optimal threshold is the one that

H. Erdmann (✉) · G. W. -Lopes · C. Gallão · P. S. Rodrigues
Inaciana Educational Foundation, Sao Bernardo do Campo, Sao Paulo, Brazil
e-mail: horste@fei.edu.br

G. W. -Lopes
e-mail: gwachs@fei.edu.br

C. Gallão
e-mail: celsogallao@hotmail.com

M. P. Ribeiro
Federal University of Viçosa, Viçosa, Minas Gerais, Brazil
e-mail: monael@gmail.com

P. S. Rodrigues
e-mail: psergio@fei.edu.br

J. M. R. S. Tavares, R. Natal Jorge (eds.), *Developments in Medical Image Processing and Computational Vision*, Lecture Notes in Computational Vision and Biomechanics 19,
DOI 10.1007/978-3-319-13407-9_17

maximizes the additivity property for its entropy. Such property states that the total entropy for a whole physical system (represented by its probability distribution) can be calculated from the sum of entropies of its constituent subsystems (represented by their individual probability distributions).

Kapur et al. [2] maximized the upper threshold of the maximum entropy to obtain the optimal threshold, and Abutaleb [3] improved the method using bidimensional entropies. Furthermore, Li and Lee [4] and Pal [5] used the direct Kullback-Leibler divergence to define the optimal threshold. And some years before, Sahoo et al. [6] used the *Reiny*-entropy seeking the same objective. More details about these approaches can be found in [7], which presents a review of entropy-based methods for image segmentation.

Considering the restrictions of Shannon entropy, Albuquerque et al. [8] proposed an image segmentation method based on Tsallis non-extensive entropy [9], a new kind of entropy that is considered as a generalization of Shannon entropy through the inclusion of a real parameter q, called "non-extensive parameter". The work of Albuquerque [8] showed promising results and a vast literature demonstrating the performance of this method against the Optimal Threshold Problem. Although it is a new contribution to the field, this paper will not address the Tsallis entropy.

A logical extension of binarization is called multi-thresholding [10, 11], which consider multiple thresholds on the search space, leading to a larger number of regions in the process of segmentation.

However, since the optimal threshold calculation is a direct function of the thresholds quantity, the time required to search for the best combination between the thresholds tends to grow exponentially. Furthermore, the optimum quantity of thresholds is still a topic for discussion. Thus, the literature has proposed the use of meta-heuristics that may be efficient for the calculation of thresholds, one of them being the Firefly.

Recently, M. Horng [11] proposed an approach based on Minimum Cross-Entropy thresholding (MCET) for multilevel thresholding with the same objective function criterion as proposed by P. Yin [10]. The main conclusion of the work was that the Cross-Entropy based method, a linear time algorithm, obtained thresholds values very close to those found by equivalent exhaustive search (brute-force) algorithms. However, the results were inconclusive since their methodology to evaluate the experiment was subjective.

This article proposes an analysis of the Firefly meta-heuristics for multi-threshold-based image segmentation. We also present the use of a Golden Standard Image Base that allows us to compare the segmentation results of different algorithms in an objective manner.

2 The Proposed Methodology

The strategy used in this study is the comparison of the obtained results with exhaustive methods results, both manual and automatic. Although these methods have polynomial complexity in $O(n^{d+1})$ order, where d and n are the number of thresholds and histogram bins respectively. It is computationally expensive to calculate the results for $d \geq 3$.

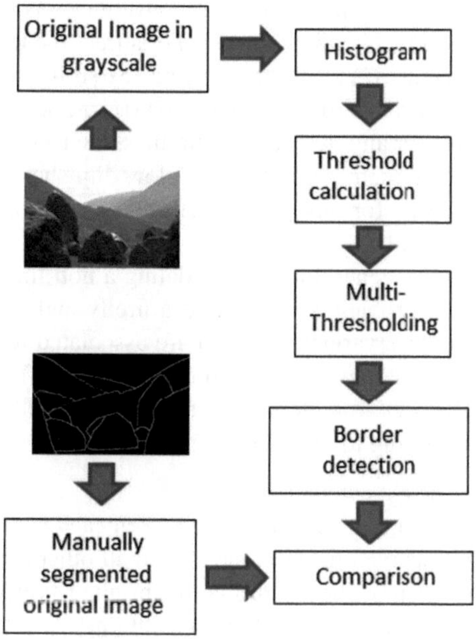

Fig. 1 Proposed comparison methodology scheme. The first row shows an example of original image and its manual segmentation taken as a basis of comparison

One important issue is to define the number of thresholds required to obtain a segmentation result as close as possible to that obtained manually. The answer seems subjective and dependent on cognitive factors that are outside the scope of this paper. Thus, the database used for comparison of the results consists of several images that were manually segmented during psychophysical experiments that were defined and performed in [12]. Moreover, the results will be compared in two directions. First, we compare the results of the exhaustive segmentation with the respective manual one. Then, we compare the results of the manual segmentation with the ones obtained with the Firefly meta-heuristics, allowing us to draw a comparison between both methods used.

Although answering cognitive questions is not the purpose of this paper, the exhaustive search of the entire result space, allows us to observe the minimum amount of thresholds required to obtain the closest result to the manual segmentation. This lower limit can be used for any segmentation algorithms besides those cited in this paper. The method used to compute the threshold-based multi segmentation with the Firefly meta-heuristics is shown in Fig. 1.

3 Firefly Meta-Heuristics

The Firefly (FF) algorithm was proposed by Xin-She Yang [13] and is a meta-heuristics inspired on the fireflies behavior, which are attracted among themselves according to their natural luminescence.

After their interactions, convergence is achieved through the creation of fireflies clusters, on which the brighter attract the less bright ones under certain restrictions, such as: (i) all fireflies are unisex so that one firefly will be attracted to any other fireflies regardless of their sex; (ii) attractiveness is proportional to their brightness, thus for any two flashing fireflies, the less bright one will move towards the brighter one, remembering that the glow dimishes as the distance between them increases; (iii) if, for any given firefly, there isn't any other brighter firefly, than it moves randomly.

The general idea is modeling a non-linear optimization problem by associating each problem's variable to a firefly and make the objective evaluation depending on these variables, which are associated to the fireflies brighten. Then, iteratively, the variables are updated (their brightens) under preestablished rules until the convergence to a global minimum. Generically, it is accomplished at each generation, according to the following main steps:

- bright evaluation;
- compute all distances between each par of fireflies;
- move all fireflies one toward all others, according to their brightens;
- keep the best solution (the brighter firefly);
- generate randomly new solutions;

The kernel of the algorithm is its Z-function evaluation, which depends on the current problem. Specifically for multi-level thresholding problem, as proposed in [13, 11] and [14], each firefly is considered a d-dimensional variable, where each dimension is a distinct threshold, partitioning the histogram space. In the specific case of the reference [14], the goal is to minimize an objective function under the non-extensive Tsallis entropy criterium of intensity histogram associated to each image to be segmented. The Algorithm 1, reproduced from [14], shows this idea in a more formal perspective, where the set of n initial firefly solutions is given in line 4. Each firefly f_i is a d-dimensional vector and x_k^i is the k-th threshold of the i-th firefly solution f_i.

In this implementation, for any firefly f_i, the strength of attractiveness for other brighter firefly f_j can be given by the update rule from lines 12 to 23. This equation states that at each iteration t, the solution f_i depends mainly on the f_j solution and the bright differences $r_{i,j}$ of all fireflies j, and the new random solution μ_t, which is drawn from a Gaussian or other distribution. The bright of a firefly i is only updated when i is less brighter than any other firefly j. Such update is proportional to the attractiveness factor β, the absorption coefficient γ and the step motion α.

The objective Z-function very much influences the final result and is application dependent. In this paper, we consider multi-level image thresholding problems in the step two of the proposed methodology and we investigate how the traditional Shannon entropy [1] and its generalization Tsallis entropy [8] influences in the final results of the proposed CAD system.

The algorithm is designed to model a non-linear optimizer associating the thresholds to fireflies. The kernel depends on these variables, which are associated with the fireflies glow and can be modified according to be more appropriate to the data

Algorithm 1 Firefly Algorithm to MLTP (adapted from [11])

Input: n : number of fireflies;
d: dimension;
γ: absorbing coefficient;
α: motion;
β: attracting factor;
MG: maximum number of generations;
Output: acceptable threshold set $f_i^* = \{x_1^i, x_2^i, \dots, x_d^i\}$
Define initial values: $t = 0$, $\alpha_0 = 1.0$
Randomly define the initial population $\{f_1, f_2, \dots, f_n\}$ where $f_i = \{x_1^i, x_2^i, \dots, x_d^i\}$ is the i-th d-dimensional solution of the firefly
while $t \leq MG$ **do**
  for $i = 1 \rightarrow n$ **do**
    for $j = 1 \rightarrow n$ **do**
      Calculate the $r_{i,j}$ distance between the glows $Z(f_i)$ and $Z(f_j)$
    end for
  end for
  for $i = 1 \rightarrow n$ **do**
    Glow evaluation $Z(f_i)$ using Tsallis entropy
    for $j = 1 \rightarrow n$ **do**
      if $Z(f_i)$ is less bright than $Z(f_j)$ **then**
        Move the f_i firefly towards the f_j firefly, according to the following update rule:
        Randomly generate a new solution $\mu_t = \{x_1, x_2, \dots, x_d\}$
        $\alpha_t = \alpha\alpha_t$
        $\beta_0 = \beta \exp(-\gamma r_{i,j}^2)$
        for $k = 1 \rightarrow d$ **do**
          $x_k^i = (1 - \beta_0)x_k^i + \beta_0 x_k^j + \alpha_t \mu_t$
        end for
      end if
    end for
  end for
  Sort the fireflies according to their glow $Z(.)$
  Define the brightest firefly f_i^* as the current result
  $t = t + 1$
end while

that is being manipulated. Then, the fireflies luminescences are updated iteratively under pre-established rules until the algorithm convergence to a global minimum.

The papers of Lukasik and Zak [15] and Yang [13] suggest that the FF overcome other meta-heuristics, such as the Ant Farm [16], Tabu search [17], PSO [18] and Genetic Algorithms [19]. Thus, the FF was presented as a computing-time efficient method to the Multilevel Thresholding Problem (MLTP). Recently, the work of [20] showed a computational time comparison of the FF against the other method, demonstrating that the FF is more efficient when the evaluation function is modeled with the maximum inter-cluster variance. Other works, such as [11] and [10] also showed similar results when applied to the MLTP.

Specifically for the MLTP modeling, each firefly is a d-dimensional vector, where each dimension is a single threshold that partitions the histogram space. In the specific work of M. H. Horng and R. J. Liou [11], the goal was to minimize the objective function using the Cross-Entropy of the intensities histogram associated with each segmented image criteria.

The Algorithm 1 describes the FF, where a solution set of n initial fireflies is given on line 3. Each firefly f_i is a d-dimensional vector and x_k^i is the k-th threshold of i-th solution. More details about the FF can be found in [11] and [13].

4 The Entropy Criteria for Evaluation Functions

In this paper we show the results obtained using a novel approach for the firefly algorithm. Our contribution is the use of Tsallis non-extensive entropy as a kernel evaluation function for the firefly algorithm. This type of entropy is described in the following sections.

4.1 The Shannon Entropy

The very celebrated Shannon entropy has been achieved several applications since C. Shannon proposed it for information theory [21]. Considering a probability distribution $P(H) = \{h(1), h(2), \ldots, h(n)\}$., the Shannon entropy, denoted by $S(H)$, is defined as:

$$S(H) = -\sum_{i=1}^{L} h_i \log(h_i) \tag{1}$$

As stated before, T. Pun [1] applied this concept for 1LTP through the following idea. Let two probability distributions from $P(H)$, one for the foreground, $P(H_1)$, and another for the background, $P(H_2)$, given by:

$$P(H_1) : \frac{h_1}{p_A}, \frac{h_2}{p_A}, \ldots, \frac{h_t}{p_A} \tag{2}$$

$$P(H_2) : \frac{h_{t+1}}{p_B}, \frac{h_{t+2}}{p_B}, \ldots, \frac{h_L}{p_B} \tag{3}$$

where $p_A = \sum_{i=1}^{t} p_i$ and $p_B = \sum_{i=t+1}^{L} p_i$.

If we assume that H_1 and H_2 are independent random variables, then the entropy of the composed distribution[1] verify the so called additivity rule:

$$S(H_1 * H_2) = S(H_1) + S(H_2). \tag{4}$$

[1] we define the composed distribution, also called direct product of $P = (p_1, \ldots, p_n)$ and $Q = (q_1, \ldots, q_m)$, as $P * Q = \{p_i q_j\}_{i,j}$, with $1 \leq i \leq n$ and $1 \leq j \leq m$

In the case of 1LTP, the optimal threshold t^* is that one which maximizes the Eq. (4), which can be computed in $O(L^2)$ time.

As before, by assuming independent distributions and under the same normalization restrictions, it is easy to extend the Eq. (4) for the case of $d > 1$ partitions, to obtain the following generalization of the additive rule:

$$S(H_1 * H_2 * \cdots * H_{d+1}) = S(H_1) + S(H_2) + \cdots + S(H_{d+1}) \tag{5}$$

which, as in the case of cross-entropy, requires $O(L^{d+1})$ in order to achieve the set of d optimal thresholds that maximizes the entropy in Expression (5).

4.2 The Non-Extensive Tsallis Entropy

As mentioned before, the Tsallis entropy is a generalization of the Shannon one (see [22] and references therein). The non-extensive Tsallis entropy of the distribution $P(H)$, denoted by $S_q(H)$, is given by:

$$S_q(H) = \frac{1 - \sum_{i=1}^{L} h_i^q}{1 - q} \tag{6}$$

The main feature observed in Eq. (6) is the introduction of a real parameter q, called non-extensive parameter. In [9] it is shown that, in the limit $q \to 1$, Eq. (6) meets the Eq. (1).

For Tsallis entropy we can find an analogous of the additivity property (Expression (4)), called pseudo-additivity due to the appearance of an extra term. For 1LTP ($d = 1$), given two independent probability distributions $P(H_1)$ and $P(H_2)$ from $P(H)$, the pseudo-additivity formalism of Tsallis entropy is given by the following expression:

$$S_q(H_1 * H_2) = S_q(H_1) + S_q(H_2) + (1 - q)S_q(H_1)S_q(H_2) \tag{7}$$

where $S_q(H_1)$ and $S_q(H_2)$ are calculated by applying Eq. (6) for the probability distributions $P(H_1)$ and $P(H_2)$.

For this 1LTP, the optimal threshold t^* is the one that maximizes the pseudo-additivity property (7), and is computed in $O(L^2)$. As in the case of Shannon entropy, we can easily derive a generalized version of Eq. (7) given by:

$$\begin{aligned} S_q(H_1 * \cdots * H_{d+1}) = S_q(H_1) + \cdots + S_q(H_{d+1}) + \\ (1 - q)S_q(H_1)S_q(H_2)\ldots S_q(H_{d+1}) \end{aligned} \tag{8}$$

which is useful for MLTP. However, for the same reasons of cross-entropy and Shannon entropy, the computational time for solving the corresponding MLTP (without a recursive technique) is $O(L^{d+1})$.

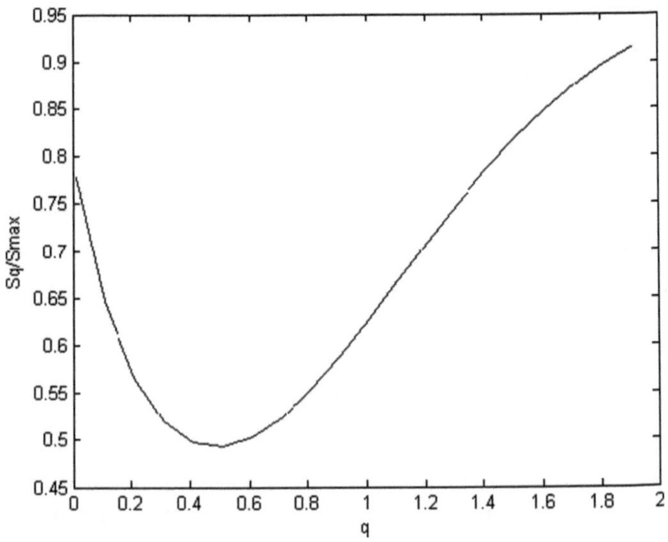

Fig. 2 Adapted from [24]. Automatic q value calculation. In this figure it is possible to see that the optimum value of q is 0.5

As Shannon Entropy (SE), Tsallis Entropy (TE) also tries to balance mutual information between partitions of a distribution, since it depends on the individual probabilities instead of their positions. Note that the parameter q powers the probability values, given a fine tuning in the pseudo-additivity maximization.

4.3 *Automatic q Calculation*

The main downside of the Tsallis entropy used by researchers such as Albuquerque et al. [8], and Rodrigues et al. [23], is the definition of the q parameter that usually is done manually. Thus, Rodrigues and Giraldi proposed a novel method for the automatic calculation of q value [24]. Since the maximal entropy of a probabilistic distribution X occur when all states of X, $(x_1, x_2, \ldots, x_n)$ have the same probability. So the maximum entropy of the X distribution, S_{MAX}, is given by Eq. (9).

$$S_{MAX} = \frac{1}{q-1}\left[1 - n(p^q(x))\right] \tag{9}$$

where: q is the entropic parameter and n is the amount of elements of the X distribution.

From the point of view of information theory , the lesser the relation between the entropy S_q produced by a q value and the maximal entropy S_{MAX} of a system, the greater is the information contained in that system. This is a well-known concept of the information theory and gives us the idea that an optimum q value can be calculated by minimizing the S_q/S_{MAX} function [24].

Thus for each distribution, we calculate the values of the relations between the S_q entropy and the maximal entropy S_{MAX} for each value of q varying in the range of $[0.01, 0.02, \ldots, 2.0]$ in order to find the q value that minimizes the relation. In Fig. 4, one can observe the behavior of the relation between S_q and S_{MAX} throughout the q variation.

5 The Image Database

In this work, we made use of 300 images from the Berkeley University database [12]. Such images are composed of various natural scenes, wherein each was manually segmented. The task to segment an image into different cognitive regions is still an open problem. It is possible to highlight two main reasons for it to be considered a difficult task: (i) a good segmentation depends on the context of the scene, as well as from the point of view of the person who is analyzing it; and (ii) it is rare to find a database for formal comparison of the results. Generally, researchers present their results comparing just a few images, pointing out what they believe is correct. In these cases, probably the same technique will work only with other images that belong to the same class. Still, the question that remains unresolved is: "What is a correct segmentation?".

In the absence of an answer to the question, a reference is necessary that allows the comparison of several techniques under the same database or parametrization. Regarding this, the image database used here can be considered as an attempt to establish such reference.

The Fig. 3 shows many examples of the pictures that belong to the database and the overlapping of 5 edge-maps derived from the manual segmentation, which denotes the high level of consistency between segmentations done by different persons. Additional details about this image database can be read on [12].

When overlapping the five edge-maps of the same image as in Fig. 3, some edges do not match, thus the final intensity of each edge of the overlapped image is going to be higher if it overlaps more edges and less intense otherwise. In this article, we made use of 300 images as comparison base (gold standard) for our experiments.

Furthermore, the divergence of information in the absolute value between the automatically-obtained segmentations and the golden standard (manually-obtained segmentations) were also not considered as a segmentation-quality measure. So, the image database is used as a tool for comparison between the results of the two evaluated methods.

6 Similarity Measure

We defined a function to measure the similarity between the manual and the automatic segmentation. However, this is a difficult task and the problem is still unsolved. Sezgin and Sankur [25] proposed 5 quantitative criteria for measuring the luminance

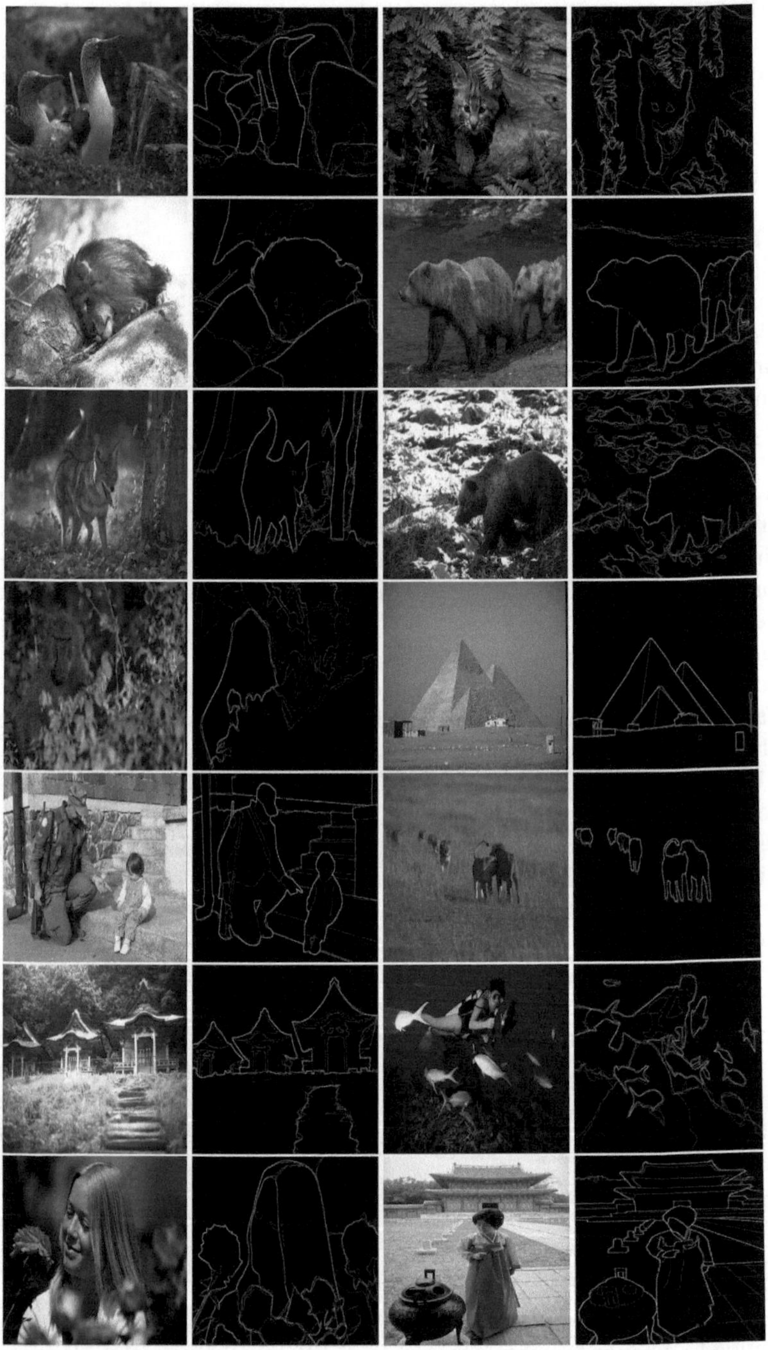

Fig. 3 Sample images from the Berkley University database [12] composed of 300 manually segmented images used on the experiments as ground truth

region and shaped 20 classical methods to measure the similarity between them. But the criterion they proposed was not based on a golden standard defined set of images, thus the method of comparison proposed in [25] can be used only as an intrinsic quality evaluation of the segmented areas: i.e, one output image segmented into uniformly molded regions cannot be considered as close as expected to the manual segmentation.

On the other side, golden standard based measuring techniques are also difficult to propose when the system needs to detect several regions of the image at the same time, a common task in computer vision. Besides that, to compare corresponding edges brings difficulty to detect entire regions, as well as their location in space. Also, in the area of computer vision, is an important demand to be able to deduct regions that are interrelated.

Although it is possible to design an algorithm which tolerates localization errors, it is likely that detecting only the matching pixels and assuming all others are flaws or false positive and may provide a poor performance.

One can speculate from Fig. 3 that the comparison between the edge-maps derived from the automatic and manual segmentations must tolerate localization errors as long as there are also divergences on the edges of the golden standard. Thus, the consideration of some differences can be useful in the final result as shown in [12].

On the other hand, from 2D edge-maps, such as the one we used, one can obtain two types of information: geometrical dispersion and intensity dispersion. The geometric dispersion measures the size and the location of the edges; the intensity dispersion measures how common is that edge among all manual segmentations that were overlapped. Thus, the geometric dispersion between two edge-maps has its information measured in a quantitative manner, in the x and y dimensions, while the luminance dispersion can be represented by the z dimension.

The divergence of information between the two edge-maps of an $M \times N$ image in the x dimension is calculated by the Euclidean distance between the two maps, where the H_x as vertical projection at the edge map for automatic segmentation and the M_x is the corresponding vertical projection for the manual one.

So, in this article, we propose a similarity function between the two edge-vertical-projection M_x and H_x of the x dimension presented in Eq. (10) to measure how different the automatically-obtained segmentation (AS_x) is from the manual one (golden standard, GS_x), in this specific direction:

$$Sim_x(GS_x|AS_x) = \sqrt{\sum_{i=1}^{M}(M_x(i) - H_x(i))^2}, \tag{10}$$

where M is the size of x distribution, M_x and H_x are the image edges projections in the x direction, manual and automatic respectively. M_x and H_x are obtained by sum of values greater than 0 in each column.

Similarly, the corresponding function to y direction is given for

$$Sim_y(GS_y|AS_y) = \sqrt{\sum_{i=1}^{N}(M_y(i) - H_y(i))^2}, \tag{11}$$

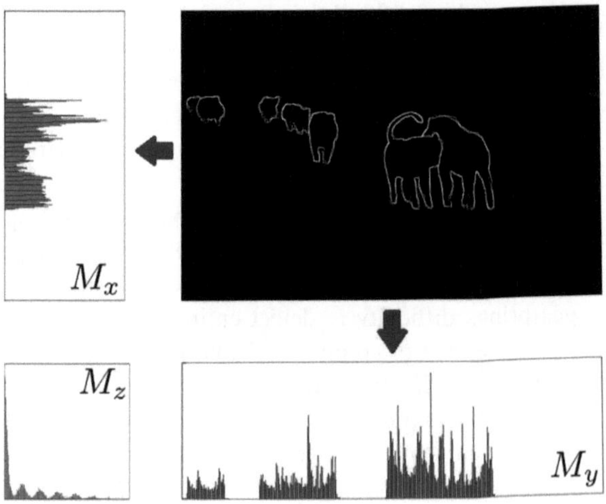

Fig. 4 Method used to obtain the vertical (M_x) and horizontal (M_y) projections of the edge map. The M_z distribution is the grayscale histogram

where N is the size of y distribution and M_y and H_y are obtained by sum of values greater than 0 in each line. The corresponding function to z direction is given for

$$Sim_z(GS_z|AS_z) = \sqrt{\sum_{i=0}^{L} (M_z(i) - H_z(i))^2}, \tag{12}$$

where $L = [0, 1, ..., 255]$ is the total of image gray levels. AS_z and GS_z represent the grayscale histogram.

Thus, in this study, we propose the following evaluation function to measure the similarity between two edge-maps:

$$Sim(GS|AS) = Sim_x + Sim_y + Sim_z \tag{13}$$

7 Experiments and Discussion

The methodology shown in Fig. 1 describes both scenarios used in this paper: (i) the segmentation with 1, 2 and 3 thresholds found by an exhaustive search; and (ii) the segmentation with 1, 2 and 3 thresholds obtained with the use of the FF meta-heuristic.

The main reason for using the exhaustive search was to guarantee that the whole solution space is explored in order to find the thresholds that provide the closest results to the golden standard for each image.

The authors of [13] and [11] presented multi-thresholding approaches based on the FF algorithm and made a comparison with the exhaustive strategy, where the FF's kernel was chosen as being the Cross-Entropy approach. This type of comparison is limited, since it is only a relative matching between the FF result and the one obtained with the entropic method (achieved in an exhaustive manner). So there is no way of knowing if there are other better solutions (threshold levels), since the search space was not entirely explored. Another limitation of the method presented in [13] and [11] is the similarity measure used, since they used the noise difference of each segmentation as a metric.

In this article the two limitations listed above were addressed in the following manner: we explored the entire solution space, for 1, 2 and 3 thresholds, ensuring that there was no better solution from the similarity measure point of view. And we also used the manually segmented image set presented previously as the basis for comparing the results of our experiments.

7.1 Exhaustive Segmentation

As in Fig. 1, we applied a threshold (1 level) for each image. Then, for each possible threshold, the image was segmented. Then we applied a gradient-based edge detector which returns the boundaries of the regions that were found. Next, the comparison between the newly obtained edge-map and the golden standard is given by Eq. (13). If $T = \{t_1, t_2, \ldots, t_L\}$, where $L = 256$, then the optimal threshold $t_{opt} \in T$ is the one that minimizes Eq. (13). These procedure was then repeated for 2 and 3 levels, remembering that the solutions space grows exponentially, since we need $|T|^2$ and $|T|^3$ tests for segmentating with 2 and 3 levels respectively.

Despite being an exhaustive strategy, the algorithm surely returns the optimal results. This means that no other thresholding-based segmentation algorithm can outmatch this algorithm's results because it searches through all possible threshold combinations in the solution's space. Thus, the distance between the exhaustive search and the Golden Standard are the lowest possible and can be used as a lower boundary for minimizing the Eq. (13). This strategy is more appropriate than the noise minimization that was proposed in [13] and [11].

If $I = \{i_1, i_2, \ldots, i_{300}\}$ is the 300 image set, for each $i_j \in I$, we can associate an array $S_i = [s_{i1}, s_{i2}, s_{i3}]$, where s_{i1} is the value given by Eq. (13) for the binarization of i_j with the optimal t_{opt}; s_{i2} is the following value for the multi-thresholding of i_j with the optimal thresholds $\{t_{opt1}, t_{opt2}\} \in T$; and finally, s_{i3} is the corresponding array with 3 thresholds $\{t_{opt1}, t_{opt2}, t_{opt3}\} \in T$.

For better visualization of the results, we created an $M_{300\times3}$ matrix, where each M_{ij} ($1 \le i \le 300$ and $1 \le j \le 3$) element is the value of $s_{ij} \in S_i$ associated with the i image. Each i line of M was normalized into 3 intensity values $L \in \{0, 128, 255\}$, so that $M_{ij} = 0$ if $s_{ij} = max S_i$; $M_{ij} = 255$, if $s_{ij} = min S_i$; and $M_{i,j} = 128$, if s_{ij} is the median of S_i. The Fig. 5 shows M as one single image with dimensions 300×3 resized to 300×300 for better visualization.

Thus, for cell (i, j) of M on Fig. 5, the brighter the pixel, the more the image segmented with the j-th threshold resembles the manually segmented image. The darker the pixel, greater the difference between them.

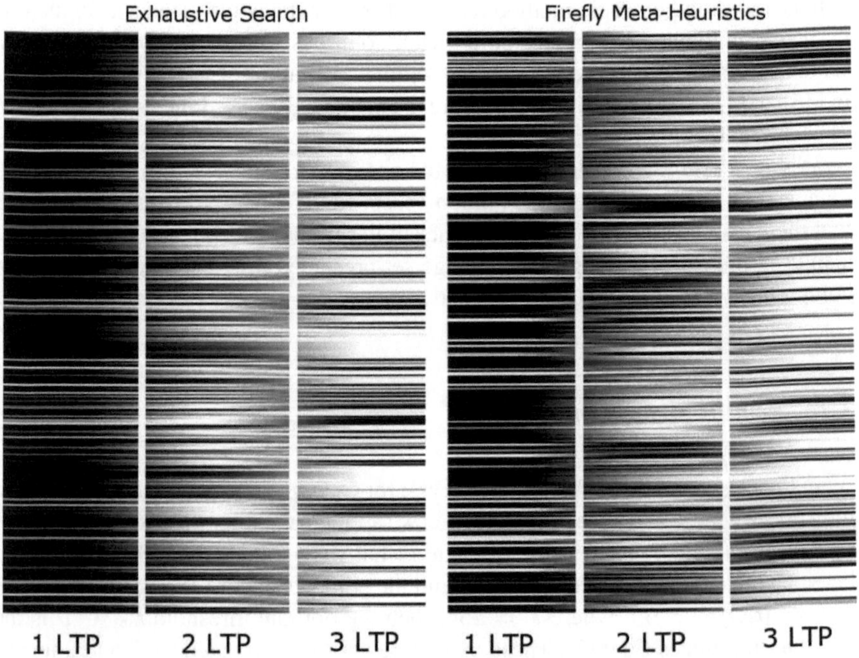

Fig. 5 Exhaustive segmentation results (*left*) and FF Meta-Heuristics segmentation results (*right*). Each row represents one of the 300 images from the database. The columns are the results of the segmentation with 1, 2 and 3 thresholds. For each row, the brighter the column, the more the image segmented with the corresponding threshold resembles the manually segmented image

7.2 Segmentation with the Firefly Meta-Heuristics

The experiments were repeated using the FF segmentation, except for the threshold calculation, that is done with the Algorithm 1. Just like the experiments with the exhaustive search method, we also created a $M_{300\times3}$ matrix with the same properties as the previous one. Comparing the Fig. 5, it is possible to notice a similarity between them, indicating that the FF results are close to the exhaustive method.

7.3 Discussion

Looking closer to the Fig. 5, one can perceive a gradient from dark to bright in both methods used, so that, for most rows (images), the columns that correspond to the segmentation with 3 thresholds are brighter (more similar) than the others. This means that, in our experiments, segmentating an image into 4 levels (3 thresholds), generally, gives us better results than with lesser threshold levels. The opposite applies to the first column, which is darker than the other 2, meaning that although

Table 1 Comparison between the exhaustive search (BF) and the FF results

Avg. Dist. with GS	Exhaustive search	Firefly algorithm	Difference (%)
FF = BF	21.41	24.15	11.33
FF ≠ BF	21.36	23.69	9.85
Total	21.39	23.93	10.61

Table 2 Quantitative comparison between the exhaustive search (BF) and the FF results

Threshold results	Exhaustive search	Firefly algorithm
1 Threshold	5	53
2 Thresholds	114	73
3 Thresholds	181	174
1 Threshold (when FF=BF)	1	1
2 Thresholds (when FF=BF)	36	36
3 Thresholds (when FF=BF)	116	116

it's the fastest and easiest way to segmentate an image, binarizing generally produces the worst segmentation results when compared with the results obtained with more thresholds.

In a more detailed analysis, we listed on Table 1 a general comparison between the results of the FF Meta-Heuristics and the exhaustive search (or brute-force, BF). The columns 2 and 3 represent the average distance between the golden standard (GS) and the BF and FF methods respectively. The last column represents the percent difference between the FF and BF. The first line describes the average distances when the BF and the FF thresholds are equal. The second line lists the distances when the results are not equal. And the final line summarizes all the results.

The main observation that can be made from the results listed on Table 1 is that the FF algorithm's results are very close to the exhaustive search. The average difference between them is 10.61 %. This shows that even when the FF does not find the optimum threshold, the distance between the segmentation obtained from its result is only 10.61 % different from the desired. As the threshold quantity grows, the levels combination tends to a combinatory explosion that causes the exhaustive search method to be impossible to calculate. The FF methods responds well in these cases, finding a result that is only 10.61 % different from the optimum but with linear processing time.

The Table 2 describes a quantitative comparison between the exhaustive search and the FF Meta-Heuristics. On the first line, it shows how many images where best segmented with 1 threshold with the BF and the FF methods (columns 2 and 3 respectively). The second and third lines describe how many images were best segmented with 2 and 3 thresholds respectively. The other three lines describe how many images where best segmented with 1,2 and 3 thresholds respectively with the FF and BF methods resulting in the same thresholds amount.

From Table 2, it is possible to reaffirm the observations made from Fig. 5, that generally, 3 thresholds produce a better segmentation than 2 which, in turn, is still better than 1 threshold (binarization). This can be explained due to the matrix normalization. The brighter the $M_{i,j}$ cell, the closer the j-th threshold segmentation is to the manual segmentation. So, it is possible to conclude that this approximation gets higher as the j value increases. That is, if the goal of the threshold segmentation is to find the threshold set that results in a segmentation that is close to the manual one, then, to use 3 thresholds is more efficient than 2 which in turn is better than 1. However, one can speculate that beyond 3 thresholds, the results tend to get worse since this leads to the over-segmentation of the image. But this is a further investigation out of the current scope.

8 Conclusions

This paper presented the application of a meta-heuristic inspired by the fireflies behavior for multi-thresholding image segmentation. The proposed method's results were compared with the results of exhaustive search for 1, 2 and 3 thresholds through a manually segmented database. By searching all the solution's up to 3 thresholds space, we were able to establish a lower limit for the comparison with the manual segmentation results. This limit is useful for other algorithms or thresholds-based segmentation strategies.

The experiments indicate that the FF results are close to the exhaustive search. Moreover, these results suggest that, for threshold-based segmentation, separating the image into four groups with three thresholds, provides better chances to reach the edges obtained with the manual segmentation as a final result than dividing into three groups. Furthermore, this last separation is still closer to the manual results than the separation in two groups, the so-called binarization.

Another important point is that, as the thresholds quantity raises, the exhaustive search method's computing time tend to grow exponentially. Since the results of the FF Meta-Heuristics are very close to the brute-force method, its linear computing time is an attractive alternative to find a solution that is approximately 10 % different from the optimum result.

References

1. Pun T (1981) Entropic thresholding: a new approach. Comput Graphics Image Process 16:210–239
2. Kapur JN, Sahoo PK, Wong AKC (1985) A new method for gray-level picture thresholding using the entropy of the histogram. Comput. Graphics Image Process 29:273–285
3. Abutaleb AS (1989) A new method for gray-level picture thresholding using the entropy of the histogram. Comput Graphics Image Process 47:22–32
4. Li CH, Lee CK (1993) Minimum cross entropy thresholding. Pattern Recognit 26:617–625
5. Pal NR (1996) On minimum cross entropy thresholding. Pattern Recognit 26:575–580

6. Sahoo P, Soltani S, Wong A, Chen Y (1988) A survay of thresholding techniques. Comput Vis Gr Image Process 41(1):233–260
7. Chang C-I, Du Y, Wang J, Guo S-M, Thouin P (2006, Dec.) Survey and comparative analysis of entropy and relative entropy thresholding techniques. IEEE Proc, Vis, Image Signal Process 153(6):837–850
8. Albuquerque M, Esquef I, Mello A (2004) Image thresholding using tsallis entropy. J Stat Phys 25:1059–1065
9. Tsallis C (1999, March) Nonextensive statistics: theoretical, experimental and computational evidences and connections. Braz J Phys 29(1):1–35
10. Yin PY (2007) Multilevel minimum cross entropy threshold selection based on particle swarm optimization. Appl Math Comput 184:503–513
11. Horng MH, Liou RJ (2011) Multilevel minimum cross entropy threshold selection based on firefly algorithm. Expert Syst Appl 38:14805–14811
12. Martin D, Fowlkes C, Tal D, Malik J (2001, July) A database of human segmented natural images and its application to evaluating segmentation algorithms and measuring ecological statistics. In: Proc. 8th Int'l Conf. Computer Vision, vol 2, pp 416–423
13. Yang XS (2009) Firefly algorithms for multimodal optimization. Stochastic algorithms: fundation and applications, SAGA 2009. Lecture Notes Computer Science 5792:169–178
14. Erdmann H, Lopes LA, Wachs-Lopes G, Ribeiro MP, Rodrigues PS (2013) A study of firefly meta-heuristic for multithresholding image segmentation. In: VIpImage: Thematic Conference on Computational Vision and Medical Image Processing, Ilha da Madeira, Portugal, October, 14 to 16 2013, pp 211–217
15. Lukasik S, Zak S (2009) Firefly algorithm for continuous constrained optimization tasks. In: 1st International Conference on Computational Collective Intelligence, Semantic Web, 5-7 October 2009.
16. Dorigo M (1992) Optimization, learning, and natural algorithms. Ph. D. Thesis, Dipartimento di Elettronica e Informazione, Politecnico di Milano, Italy
17. Glover F (1989) Tabu search. PART I, ORSA J Comput 1:190–206
18. Kennedy J, Goldberg RC (1997) Particle swarm optimization. In: Proceedings of IEEE International Conference on Neural Networks, vol IV, pp 1942–1948
19. Goldberg DE (1997) Genetic algorithms in search, optimization, and machine learning. Addison Wesley, Reading
20. Hassanzadeh T, Vojodi H, Eftekhari AM (2011) An image segmentation approach based on maximum variance intra-cluster method and firefly algorithm. In: Seventh International Conference on Natural Computation, IEEE, Ed., Shanghai, China, pp 1844–1848
21. Shannon C, Weaver W (1948) The mathematical theory of communication. University of Illinois Press, Urbana
22. Tavares AHMP (2003) Aspectos matemáticos da entropia. Master Thesis, Universidade de Aveiro
23. Giraldi G, Rodrigues P (2009) Improving the non-extensive tsallis non-extensive medical image segmentation based on tsallis entropy. Pattern Analysis and Application, vol. Submitted
24. Rodrigues P, Giraldi G (2009) Computing the q-index for tsallis non-extensive image segmentation. In XXII Brazilian Symposium on Computer Graphics and Image Processing (Sibgrapi 2009), SBC, Ed., vol. To Appear
25. Sezgin M, Sankur B (2004, Jan) Survay ove image thresholding techniques and quantitative performance evaluation. J Eletr Imaging 13(1):146–165

Visual-Inertial 2D Feature Tracking based on an Affine Photometric Model

Dominik Aufderheide, Gerard Edwards and Werner Krybus

Abstract The robust tracking of point features throughout an image sequence is one fundamental stage in many different computer vision algorithms (e.g. visual modelling, object tracking, etc.). In most cases, this tracking is realised by means of a feature detection step and then a subsequent re-identification of the same feature point, based on some variant of a template matching algorithm. Without any auxiliary knowledge about the movement of the camera, actual tracking techniques are only robust for relatively moderate frame-to-frame feature displacements. This paper presents a framework for a visual-inertial feature tracking scheme, where images and measurements of an inertial measurement unit (IMU) are fused in order to allow a wider range of camera movements. The inertial measurements are used to estimate the visual appearance of a feature's local neighbourhood based on a affine photometric warping model.

1 Introduction

Many different applications in the field of computer vision (CV) require the robust identification and tracking of distinctive feature points in monocular image sequences acquired by a moving camera. Prominent examples of such applications are 3D scene modelling following the structure-from-motion (SfM) principle or the simultaneous localisation and mapping (SLAM) for mobile robot applications. The general procedure of feature point tracking can be subdivided in two distinctive phases:

D. Aufderheide (✉) · W. Krybus
Division Soest, Institute for Computer Science, Vision and Computational Intelligence,
South Westphalia University of Applied Sciences, Luebecker Ring 2, 59494 Soest, Germany
e-mail: aufderheide@fh-swf.de

W. Krybus
e-mail: krybus@fh-swf.de

G. Edwards
Department of Electronic & Electrical Engineering,
Faculty of Science and Engineering, The University of Chester,
Thornton Science Park, Pool Lane, Ince, Chester CH2 4NU, UK
e-mail: gerard.edwards@chester.ac.uk

J. M. R. S. Tavares, R. Natal Jorge (eds.), *Developments in Medical Image Processing and Computational Vision*, Lecture Notes in Computational Vision and Biomechanics 19,
DOI 10.1007/978-3-319-13407-9_18

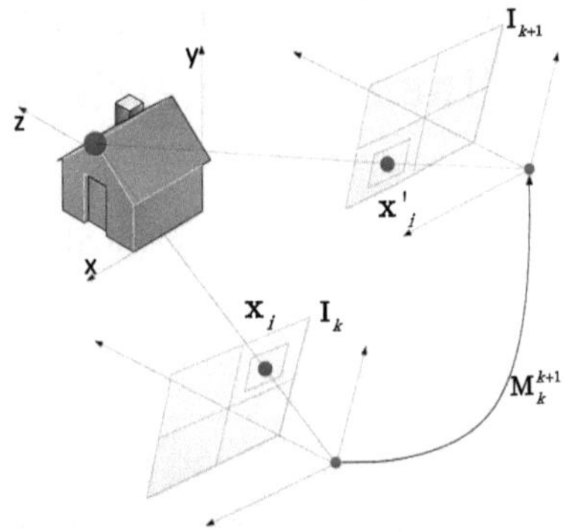

Fig. 1 Re-identification of single feature point in two subsequent frames of an image sequence

- *Detection*—The first stage is the identification of a set of distinctive point features ${}^kX = \{\mathbf{x}_1, \cdots, \mathbf{x}_n\}$ with $\mathbf{x}_i = (x, y)^T$ in image $\mathbf{I}_k$, e.g. based on computing the *cornerness* of each pixel (see [5]). At this stage each feature point is typically assigned with some kind of a descriptor $\theta\left(\mathbf{I}_{k(\mathbf{x}_i)}\right)$, which is used in the second stage for the re-identification of the feature. This descriptor could be a simple local neighbourhood of pixels around $\mathbf{x}_i$ or a more abstract descriptor such as the SIFT/SURF descriptors described by [9].
- *Re-identification*—The general task of feature tracking is the successful re-identification of the initial set of features ${}^kX$ from image $\mathbf{I}_k$ in the subsequent frame $\mathbf{I}_{k+1}$. Generally this can be described as an optimisation problem where the distance between a descriptor for pixel $\mathbf{x}'$ from $\mathbf{I}_{k+1}$ and the given descriptor $\theta\left(\mathbf{I}_{k(\mathbf{x}_i)}\right)$ should be minimised by varying $\mathbf{x}'$ within the image boundaries. In most cases the optimisation problem is not just driven by varying the image coordinates, but also by using some kind of a motion model $\Omega\left[\theta\left(\mathbf{I}_{k(\mathbf{x}_i)}\right)\right]_{\mathbf{M}_k^{k+1}}$ which tries to compensate the change in the descriptors appearance based on an estimation of the cameras movement $\mathbf{M}_k^{k+1}$ between $\mathbf{I}_k$ and $\mathbf{I}_{k+1}$. In order to reduce the computational complexity of the minimisation the range for varying both the pixel coordinates and the motion model parameters are limited to certain *search regions*. The general procedure of feature tracking is visualised in Fig. 1.

As it was shown by Aufderheide et al. [2], there are many ways for a feature tracking method to fail completely or produce a non-negligible number of incorrect matches. This can be clearly seen from a mathematical point of view by the fact that either the optimisation problem converges within a local minimum or not at all.

In Aufderheide et al. [1], we described a general approach for the combination of visual and inertial measurements within a parallel multi-sensory data fusion network for 3D scene reconstruction called *VISrec!*. Closely related to this work is the adaptation of ideas presented by Hwangbo et al. [6] for using the inertial measurements not only as an aiding modality during the estimation of the cameras egomotion, but also during the feature tracking itself.

The first stage for realising this was the development of an inertial smart sensor system (S^3) based on a bank of inertial measurement units in MEMS[1] technology. The S^3 is able to compute the actual absolute camera pose (position and orientation) for each frame. The hardware employed and the corresponding navigation algorithm are described in Sect. 2. As a second step a visual feature tracking algorithm, as described in Sect. 3, needs to be implemented. This algorithm considers prior motion estimates from the inertial S^3 in order to guarantee a greater convergence region of the optimisation problem and deliver an improved overall tracking performance. The results are briefly discussed in Sect. 4. Finally Sect. 5 concludes the whole work and describes potential future work.

2 Inertial Smart Sensor System S^3

For the implementation of an Inertial Fusion Cell (IFC) a smart sensor system (S^3) is suggested here, which is composed as a bank of different micro-electromechanical systems (MEMS). The proposed system contains accelerometers, gyroscopes and magnetometers. All of them are sensory units with three degrees of freedom (DoF). The S^3 contains the sensors itself, signal conditioning (filtering) and a multi-sensor data fusion (MSDF) scheme for pose (position and orientation) estimation.

2.1 General S^3 Architecture

The general architecture of the S^3 is shown in the following Fig. 2, where the overall architecture contains the main 'organ' consisting of the sensory units as described in Sect. 2.2. A single micro controller is used for analogue-digital-conversion (ADC), signal conditioning (SC) and the transfer of sensor data to a PC. The actual sensor fusion scheme is realised on the PC.

2.2 Hardware

The hardware setup of the S^3 is inspired by the standard configuration of a multi-sensor orientation system (MODS) as defined in [13]. The used system consists of a LY530AL single-axis gyro and a LPR530AL dual-axis gyro both from STMicroelectronics, which are measure the rotational velocities around the three main axis of the inertial coordinate system ICS (see Fig. 3). The accelerations of translational movements are measured by a triple-axis accelerometer ADXL345 from Analog Devices. Finally a 3-DoF magnetometer from Honeywell (HMC5843) is used to measure

[1] MEMS—micro-electromechanical systems.

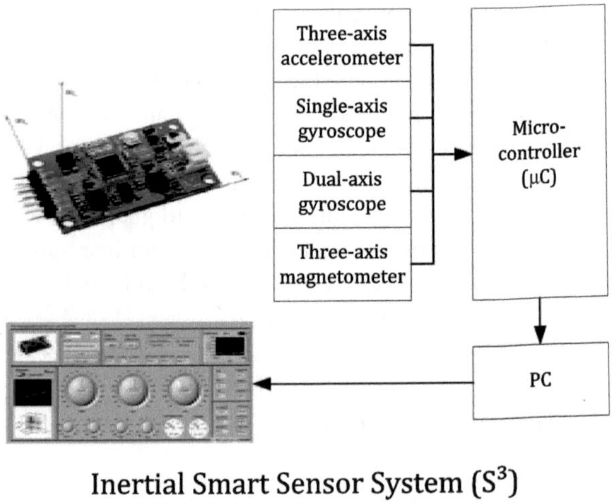

Fig. 2 General architecture of the inertial S^3

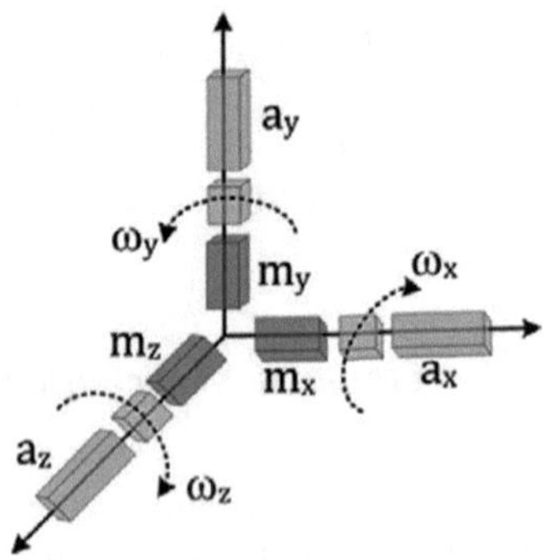

Fig. 3 General architecture of the inertial measurement units and measured entities

the earth's magnetic field. All IMU sensors are connected to a micro controller (ATMega328) which is responsible for initialisation, signal conditioning and communication. The interface between sensor and micro controller is based on I^2C-Bus for the accelerometer and magnetometer, while the gyroscope is directly connected to ADC channels of the AVR. So the used sensor setup consists of three orthogonal arranged accelerometers measuring a three dimensional acceleration $\mathbf{a}^b = \left[a_x \, a_y \, a_z\right]^T$ normalised with the gravitational acceleration constant g. Here b indicates the actual body coordinate system in which the entities are measured. The triple-axis gyroscope measures the corresponding angular velocities $\boldsymbol{\omega}^b = \left[\omega_x \, \omega_y \, \omega_z\right]^T$ around the sensitivity axes of the accelerometers. The magnetometer is used to sense the earth's magnetic field $\mathbf{m}^b = \left[m_x \, m_y \, m_z\right]^T$. Figure 3 shows the general configuration of all sensory units and the corresponding measured entities.

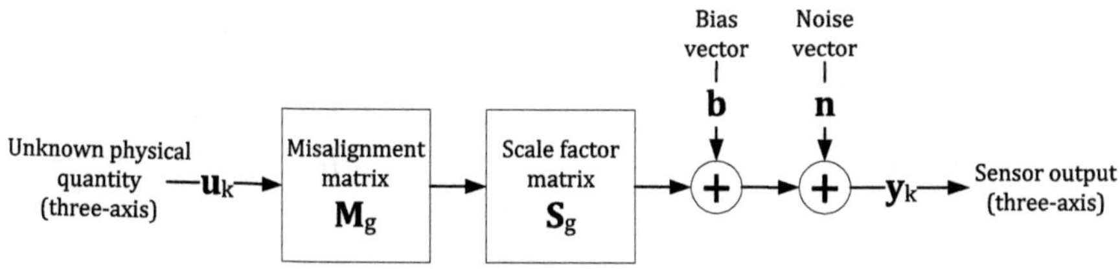

Fig. 4 General sensor model

2.3 *Sensor Modelling and Signal Conditioning*

Measurements from MEMS devices in general and inertial MEMS sensors in particular suffer from different error sources. Due to this it is necessary to implement both: an adequate calibration framework and a signal conditioning routine. The calibration of the sensory units is only possible if a reasonable sensor model is available in advance. The sensor model should address all possible error sources. Here the proposed model from [14] was utilised and adapted for the given context. It contains:

- Misalignment of sensitivity axes—Ideally the three independent sensitivity axes of each inertial sensor should be orthogonal. Due to imprecise construction of MEMS-based IMUs this is not the case for the vast majority of sensory packages. The misalignment can be compensated by finding a matrix **M** which transforms the non-orthogonal axis to a orthogonal setup.
- Biases—The output of the gyroscopes and accelerometers should be exactly zero if the S^3 is not moved at all. However there is typically a time-varying offset for real sensors. It is possible to differentiate *g-independent* biases (e.g. for gyroscopes) and *g-dependent* biases. For the latter there is a relation between the applied acceleration and the bias. The bias is modelled by incorporation of a bias vector **b**.
- Measurement noise—The general measurement noise has to be taken into account. The standard sensor model contains a white noise term **n**.
- Scaling factors—In most cases there is an unknown scaling factor between the measured physical quantity and the real signal. The scaling can be compensated for by introducing a scale matrix $\mathbf{S} = diag\left(s_x, s_y, s_z\right)$.

A block-diagram of the general sensor model is shown in the following figure (Fig. 4).

Based on this it is possible to define three separate sensor models for all three sensor types[2], as shown in the following equations:

$$\boldsymbol{\omega}_b = \mathbf{M}_g \cdot \mathbf{S}_g \cdot \boldsymbol{\omega}_b' + \mathbf{b}_g + \mathbf{n}_g \tag{1}$$

$$\mathbf{a}_b = \mathbf{M}_a \cdot \mathbf{S}_a \cdot \mathbf{a}_b' + \mathbf{b}_a + \mathbf{n}_a \tag{2}$$

[2] The different sensor types are indicated by the subscript indices at the entities in the different equations.

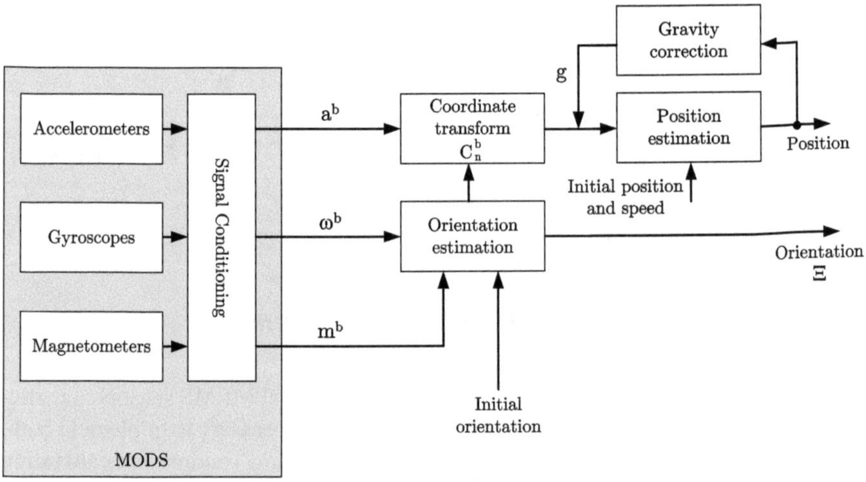

Fig. 5 Computational elements of an INS

$$\mathbf{m}_b = \mathbf{M}_m \cdot \mathbf{S}_m \cdot \mathbf{m}'_b + \mathbf{b}_m + \mathbf{n}_m \tag{3}$$

It was shown that **M** and **S** can be determined by sensor calibration procedure in which the sensor array is moved to different known locations to determine the calibration parameters. Due to their time-varying character, the noise and bias terms cannot be determined a-priori. The signal conditioning step on the μC takes care of the measurement noise by integrating an FIR digital filter structure. The implementation realises a low-pass FIR filter based on the assumption that the frequencies of the measurement noise are much higher than the frequencies of the signal itself. The complete filter was realised in software on the μC, where the cut-off-frequencies for the different sensory units were determined by an experimental evaluation.

2.4 *Basic Principles of Inertial Navigation*

Classical approaches for inertial navigation are stable-platform systems which are isolated from any external rotational motion by specialised mechanical platforms. In comparison to those classical stable platform systems, the MEMS sensors are mounted rigidly to the device (here: the camera). In such a strapdown system, it is necessary to transform the measured quantities of the accelerometers, into a global coordinate system by using known orientations computed from gyroscope measurements. In general the mechanis system level operation of a strapdown inertial navigation systems (INS) can be described by the computational elements indicated in Fig. 5. The main problem with this classical framework is that location is determined by integrating measurements from gyros (orientation) and accelerometers (position). Due to superimposed sensor drift and noise, which is especially significant for MEMS devices, the errors for the egomotion estimation tend to grow unbounded.

The necessary computation of the orientation ξ of the S^3 based on the gyroscope measurements ω_b and a start orientation $\xi_{(t_0)}$ can be described as follows:

$$\xi = \xi_{(t_0)} + \int \omega_b dt \tag{4}$$

The integration of the measured rotational velocities would lead to an unbounded drifting error in the absolute orientation estimates. Figure 6 shows two examples for this typical drifting behaviour for all three Euler angles. For the two experiments shown in Fig. 6, the S^3 was not moved, but even after a short period of time (here: $6000 \cdot 0.01s = 60s$) there is an absolute orientation error of up to 4° clearly recognisable. For the estimation of the absolute position these problems are even more severe, because the position ϕ can be computed from acceleration measurements, in the inertial reference frame $\mathbf{a}_i$, only by double integration:

$$\phi = \phi_{(t_0)} + \int\int \mathbf{a}_i dt \tag{5}$$

Possible errors in the orientation estimation stage would lead also to a wrong position, due to the necessity to transform the accelerations in the body coordinate frame $\mathbf{a}_b$ to the inertial reference frame (here indicated by the subscript i).

The following figure (Fig. 7) demonstrates the typical drifting error for the absolute position (one axis) computed by using the classical strapdown methodology.

By using only gyroscopes, there is actually no way to control the drifting error for the orientation in a reasonable way. It is necessary to use other information channels. So the final framework for pose estimation considers two steps: an orientation estimation and a position estimation as shown in Fig. 8. In comparison to the classical strapdown method, the suggested approach here incorporates also the accelerometers for orientation estimation. The suggested fusion network is given in the following figure, and the different sub-fusion processes are described in Sects. 2.5 and 2.6.

2.5 *Fusion for orientation*

The general idea for compensating the drift error of the gyroscopes is based on using the accelerometers as an additional attitude sensor. Due to the fact that the 3-DoF accelerometer measures not only (external) translational motion, but also the influence of the gravity, it is possible to calculate the attitude based on the single components of the measured acceleration. At this point it should be noted that measurements from the accelerometers can only provide roll and pitch angle Thus, the heading angle of the unit has to be derived by using the magnetometer instead.

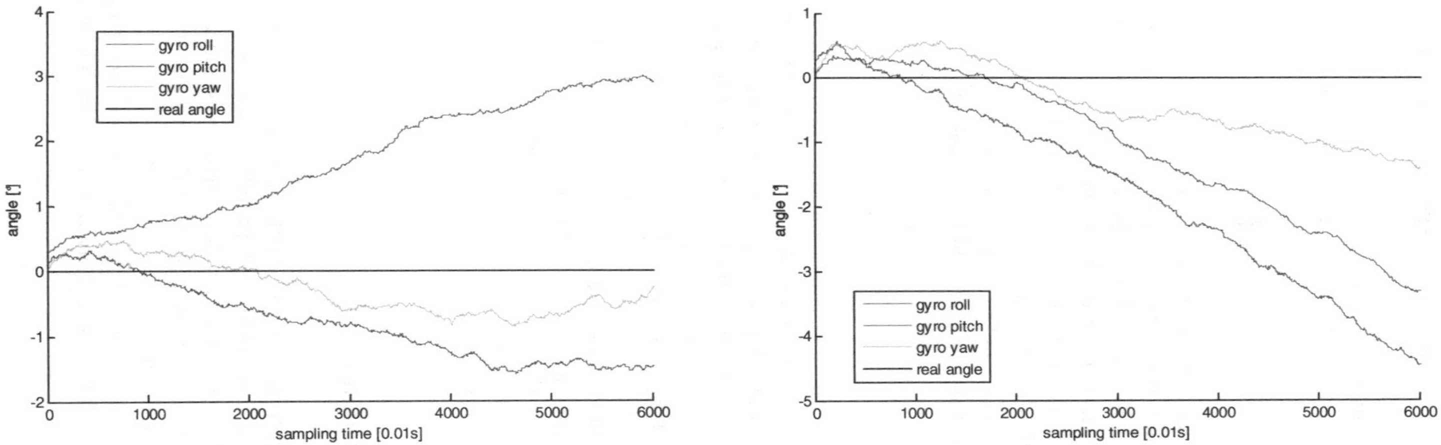

Fig. 6 Drifting error for orientation estimates based on gyroscope measurements, for two separate experiments

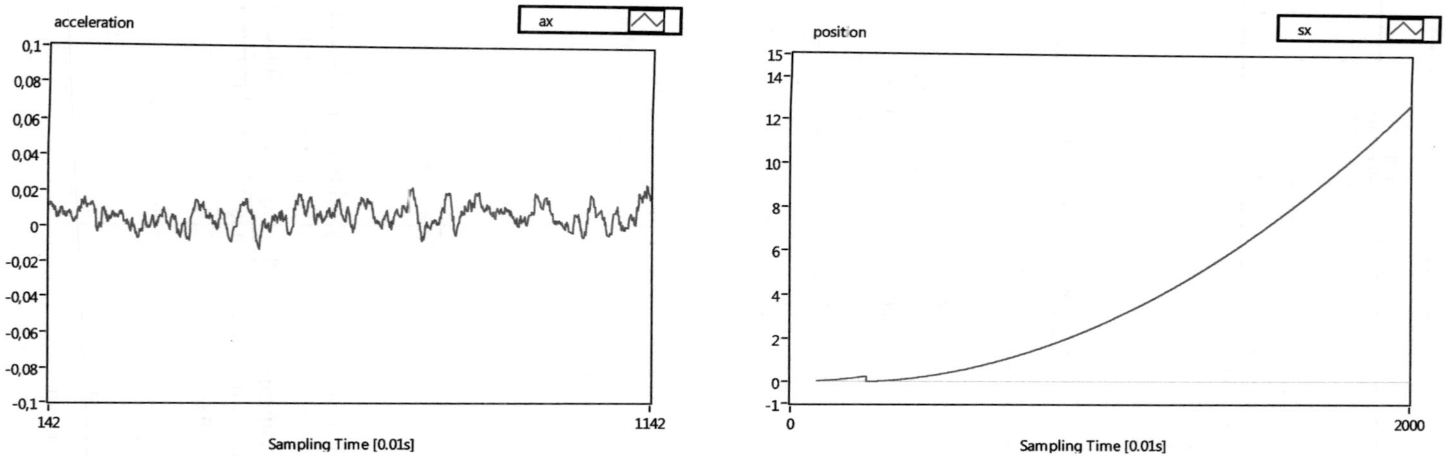

Fig. 7 Drifting error for absolute position estimates based on classical strapdown mechanisation of an inertial navigation system (*left*: acceleration measurements; *right*: absolute position estimate)

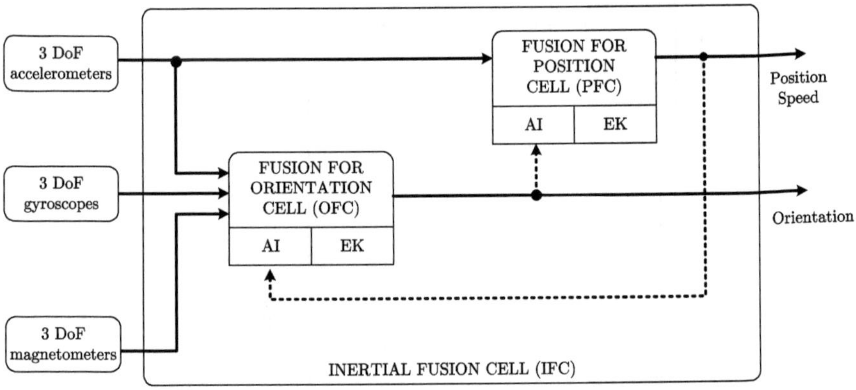

Fig. 8 System design of the inertial fusion cell (IFC)

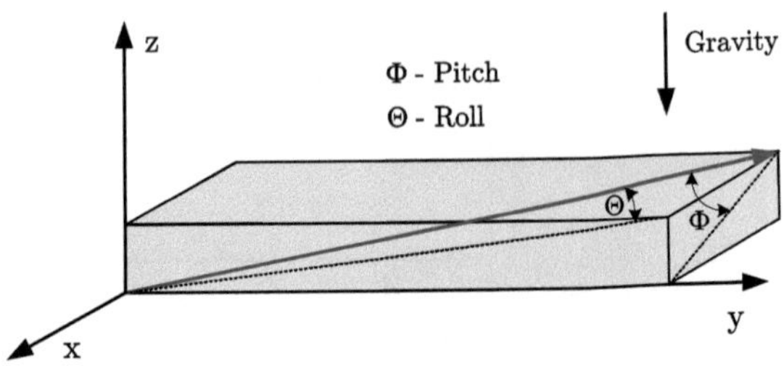

Fig. 9 Geometrical relations between measured accelerations due to gravity and the roll and pitch angle of the attitude

Figure 9 gives an illustration showing the geometrical relations between measured accelerations due to gravity and the roll and pitch angle of the attitude. The angles can be determined by following relations:

$$\theta = arctan2\left(a_x^2, \sqrt{(a_y + a_z)^2}\right) \tag{6}$$

$$\phi = arctan2\left(a_y^2, \sqrt{(a_x + a_z)^2}\right) \tag{7}$$

The missing heading angle can be obtained by using the readings from the magnetometer and the already determined roll and pitch angles. Here it is important to be aware that the measured elements of the earth magnetic field have to be transformed to the local horizontal plane (tilt compensation is illustrated in Fig. 10) as indicating in the corresponding relations

$$\begin{aligned} X_h &= m_x \cdot c\varphi + m_y \cdot s\theta \cdot s\varphi - m_z \cdot s\theta \cdot s\varphi \\ Y_h &= m_y \cdot c\theta + m_z \cdot s\theta \\ \psi &= \arctan 2\,(Y_h, X_h) \end{aligned} \tag{8}$$

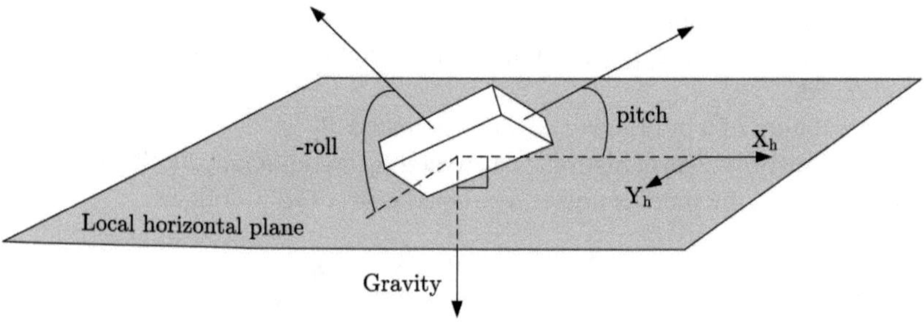

Fig. 10 Local horizontal plane as a reference

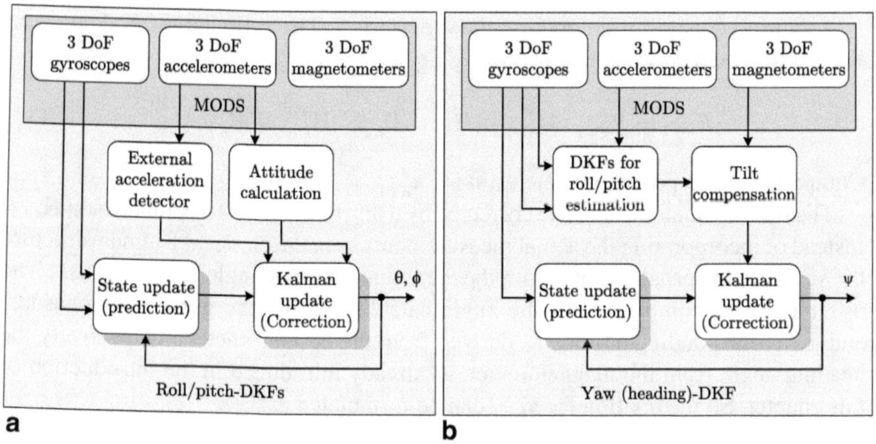

Fig. 11 **a** Discrete Kalman filter (DKF) for estimation of roll and pitch angles based on gyroscope and accelerometer measurements. **b** DKF for estimation of yaw (heading) angle from gyroscope and magnetometer measurements

Based on this approach a discrete Kalman filter bank (DKF-bank) is implemented which is responsible for the estimation of all three angles of the camera's orientation. For the pitch and the roll angle the same DKF-architecture is used, as indicated in Fig. 11a. In comparison the heading angle is estimated by an alternative architecture as shown in Fig. 11b.

The Kalman filtering process is composed from the following classical steps, where the following descriptions are simplified by referrring to just a single angle ξ.

Computation of an a priori state estimate $\mathbf{x}_{\mathbf{k+1}}^{-}$

As mentioned earlier the hidden states of the system are $\mathbf{x} = [\xi, \mathbf{b_{gyro}}]^{\mathbf{T}}$. The a priori estimates are computed by following the following relations:

$$\begin{aligned} \widehat{\omega}_{k+1} &= \omega_{k+1} - b_{gyro_k} \\ \xi_{k+1} &= \xi_k + \int \widehat{\omega}_{k+1} dt \\ b_{gyro_{k+1}} &= b_{gyro_k} \end{aligned} \tag{9}$$

Here the actual measurements from the gyroscopes ω_{k+1} are corrected for by the actually estimated bias b_{gyro_k} from the former iteration, before the actual angle ξ_{k+1} is computed.

Computation of a priori error covariance matrix $\mathbf{P^-_{k+1}}$

The a priori covariance matrix is calculated by incorporating the Jacobi matrix **A** of the states and the process noise covariance matrix $\mathbf{Q_K}$ as follows:

$$\mathbf{P^-_{k+1}} = \mathbf{A} \cdot \mathbf{P_k} \cdot \mathbf{A^T} + \mathbf{Q_K} \tag{10}$$

The two steps (1) and (2) are the elements of the prediction step as indicated in Fig. 11.

Computation of Kalman gain $\mathbf{K}_{k+1}$

As a prerequisite for computing the a posteriori state estimate the Kalman gain $\mathbf{K}_{k+1}$ has to be determined by following Eq. 11.

$$K_{k+1} = \mathbf{P^-_{k+1}} \cdot \mathbf{H}^T_{k+1} \cdot \left(\mathbf{H}_{k+1} \cdot \mathbf{P^-_{k+1}} \cdot \mathbf{H}^T_{k+1} + \mathbf{R}_{k+1}\right)^{-1} \tag{11}$$

Computation of a posteriori state estimate $\mathbf{x^+_{k+1}}$

The state estimate can now be corrected by using the calculated Kalman gain $\mathbf{K}_{k+1}$. Instead of incorporating the actual measurements as in the classical Kalman structure the suggested approach is based on the computation of an angle difference $\Delta\xi$. The difference is a comparison of the angle calculated from the gyroscope measures and the corresponding attitude as derived from the accelerometers, respectively the heading angle from the magnetometer, as already introduced in the introduction of this chapter. So the relation for $\mathbf{x^+_{k+1}}$ can be formulated as:

$$\mathbf{x^+_{k+1}} = \mathbf{x^-_{k+1}} - \mathbf{K}_{k+1} \cdot \Delta\xi \tag{12}$$

At this point it is important to consider the fact that the attitude measurements from the accelerometers are only reliable if there is no external translational motion. Thus an external acceleration detection is also needs to be part of the fusion procedure. For this reason the following condition (see Rehbinder et al. [12]) is evaluated continuously:

$$\|\mathbf{a}\| = \sqrt{(a_x^2 + a_y^2 + a_z^2)} \overset{!}{=} 1 \tag{13}$$

If the relation is fulfilled there is no external acceleration and the estimation of the attitude from accelerometers is more reliable than the one computed from rotational velocities as provided by the gyroscopes. For real sensors, a threshold $\varepsilon_\mathbf{g}$ is introduced to define an allowed variation from this ideal case. If the camera is not at rest the observation variance for the gyroscope data σ_g^2 is set to zero. By representing the magnitude of the acceleration measurements as $\|\mathbf{a}\|$ and the earth gravitational field $\mathbf{g} = [0, 0, -g]^T$ the observation variance can be defined by following Eq. 14.

$$\sigma_g^2 = \begin{cases} \sigma_g^2, & \|\mathbf{a}\| - \|\mathbf{g}\| < \varepsilon_\mathbf{g} \\ 0, & otherwise \end{cases} \tag{14}$$

A similar approach is chosen to overcome problems with the magnetometer measurements, in magnetically distorted environments for the DKF for the heading angle. The magnitude of the earth magnetic field $\mathbf{m}$ is evaluated as shown in the following Eq. 15[3], in an analogous way to Eq. 14 for describing variation due to gravity:

$$\sigma_g^2 = \begin{cases} \sigma_g^2, & \|\mathbf{m}\| - m_{des} < \varepsilon_{\mathbf{m}} \\ 0, & otherwise \end{cases} \tag{15}$$

Computation of posteriori error covariance matrix $\mathbf{P}^+_{\mathbf{k+1}}$

Finally the error covariance matrix is updated in the following way:

$$\mathbf{P}^+_{k+1} = \mathbf{P}^-_{k+1} - \mathbf{K}_{k+1} \cdot \mathbf{H}_{k+1} \cdot \mathbf{P}^-_{k+1} \tag{16}$$

It was shown in Aufderheide et al. [3], that the proposed strategy is able to outperform other classical algorithms for inertial sensor fusion, such as complementarity filtering or heuristic methods, in terms of accuracy and long-time stability.

If there is a robust estimate of the camera orientation available, it is possible to compute a 2D homography $\mathcal{H}$ which describes the optical flow (motion of all image pixels) between two successive image frames. According to Hwangbo et al. [7], it is possible to compute $\mathcal{H}$ for a pure rotational camera movement by using the following relation.

$$\mathcal{H}_k^{k+1} = \mathbf{K}\mathbf{R}_{CI}\mathbf{R}_k^{k+1}\mathbf{K}^{-1} \tag{17}$$

Here $\mathbf{K}$ represents the intrinsic camera parameters (such as focal length f, pixel size k, etc.), $\mathbf{R}_{CI}$ describes relative orientation between inertial and visual reference coordinate system and $\mathbf{R}_k^{k+1}$ describes the rotation of the camera between frame k and $k+1$, within the general frame-to-frame relative pose $\widetilde{\mathbf{M}}_k^{k+1}$.

2.6 *Fusion for Position*

At this point the orientation of the camera is known by following the classical strapdown approach. Hence, the position $\mathbf{p}$ can only be obtained by double integration of the body accelerations $\mathbf{a}$, when a known orientation $\Xi = [\phi\,\theta\,\psi]^T$ is available that allows a rotation from body frame B to reference (or navigation) frame N by using the direct cosine matrix (DCM) $\mathbf{C}_n^b$, defined as follows[4]:

$$\mathbf{C}_n^b = \begin{bmatrix} c\theta c\psi & s\varphi s\theta c\psi - c\varphi s\psi & c\varphi s\theta c\psi + s\varphi s\psi \\ c\theta s\psi & s\varphi s\theta s\psi + c\varphi c\psi & c\varphi s\theta s\psi - s\varphi c\psi \\ -s\theta & s\varphi c\theta & c\varphi c\theta \end{bmatrix} \tag{18}$$

[3] m_{des} describes the magnitude of the earth's magnetic field (e.g. 48 μT in Western Europe).
[4] For simplification: $s\alpha = sin(\alpha)$ and $c\beta = cos(\beta)$.

$$\mathbf{C}_n^b(\mathbf{q}) = \frac{1}{\sqrt{q_4^2 + \|\mathbf{e}\|^2}} \cdot \begin{bmatrix} q_1^2 - q_2^2 - q_3^2 + q_4^2 & 2(q_1q_2 + q_3q_4) & 2(q_1q_3 - q_2q_4) \\ 2(q_1q_2 - q_3q_4) & -q_1^2 + q_2^2 - q_3^2 + q_4^2 & 2(q_2q_3 + q_1q_4) \\ 2(q_1q_3 + q_2q_4) & 2(q_2q_3 - q_1q_4) & -q_1^2 - q_2^2 + q_3^2 + q_4^2 \end{bmatrix} \tag{19}$$

The DCM can also be expressed in terms of an orientation quaternion $\mathbf{q} = [\mathbf{e}^T, q_4]^T$, where $\mathbf{e} = [q_1, q_2, q_3]^T$ describes the vector part and q_4 is the scalar part of $\mathbf{q}$. Equation 19 shows the relation between $\mathbf{C}_n^b$ and a computed $\mathbf{q}$. The actual position is computed by double integration of accelerometer measurements.

It should be noted here, that the absolute position estimate is affected by a much higher rate of uncertainty, because the double integration leads to an enormous drift which can not be bounded. The proposed approach for the visual-inertial feature tracking uses mainly frame-to-frame motion estimates, so that the drift within the absolute camera pose can be neglected.

3 Visual-Inertial Feature Tracking

Once there is a reliable motion estimate available it is very important to synchronise the inertial and the visual measurements. For this a basic clock signal is used to trigger both inertial sampling and acquiring images. The inertial measurements are available with a much higher frequency than the 30 frames per seconds (FPS) delivered by a standard camera module. Thus it is necessary to accumulate motion estimates from the S^3 to compute the frame-to-frame relative pose $\widetilde{\mathbf{M}}_k^{k+1}$.

Figure 12 shows the general architecture of the visual-inertial feature tracking system (VIFtrack!) for two subsequent frames of an image sequence.

The two camera positions for the frames $\mathbf{I_k}$ and $\mathbf{I_{k+1}}$ are related by a relative motion $\mathbf{M}_k^{k+1}$. The inertial smart sensor system is able to generate an estimate of that motion (translation and orientation) $\widetilde{\mathbf{M}}_k^{k+1}$ which can be used to update a set of parameters of the affine photometric motion model $\widehat{\mathbf{p}}_k^{k+1}$.

The chosen motion model should be able to compensate typical changes of the visual appearance of a descriptor over time. Here both photometric (illumination changes, etc.) and geometric changes of an image patch need to be considered. For this Jin et al. [8] propose a model which extended the classical affine geometric distortion proposed by Tomasi and Shi [15] by adding an photometric term.

The following equation shows the implementation of the model by using a parameter vector $\mathbf{p} = \left(\mathbf{A}_{[1,1]}, \mathbf{A}_{[1,2]}, \mathbf{A}_{[2,1]}, \mathbf{A}_{[2,2]}, \mathbf{d}_{[1]}, \mathbf{d}_{[2]}, \sigma, o\right)$ which contains the different elements of the affine warp ($\mathbf{A}$ and $\mathbf{d}$) and two photometric parameters (σ, o).

$$\Omega\left[\theta\left(\mathbf{I}_{k(\mathbf{x}_i)}\right)\right]_{\mathbf{p}} = (\sigma + 1)\,\theta\,(\mathbf{I}_k(\mathbf{A}\mathbf{x}_i + \mathbf{d})) + o \tag{20}$$

The photometric model is illustrated by Fig. 13, where a light source Λ illuminates a scene and the emitted light is reflected by the main surface S to the image plane Π, which is modelled by parameter σ.

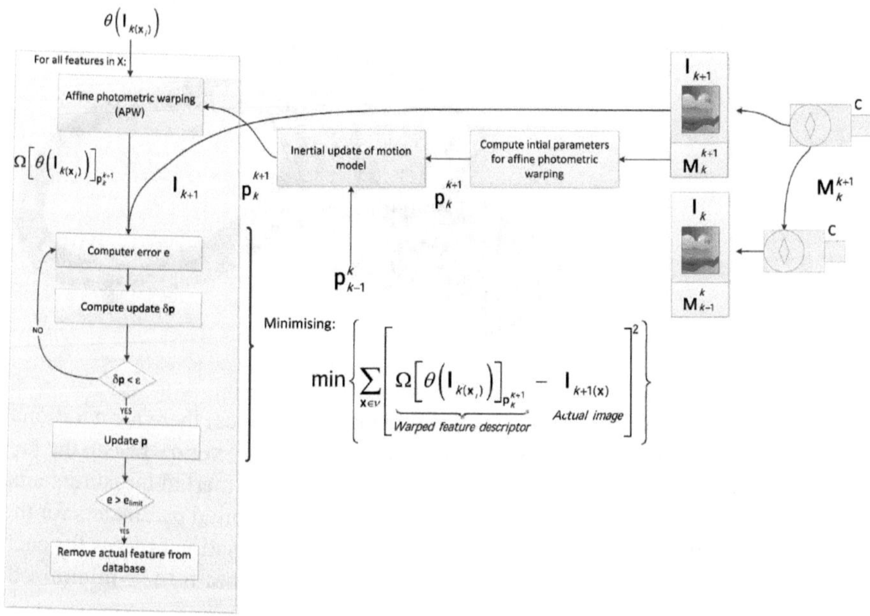

Fig. 12 General scheme of the VIFtrack! approach

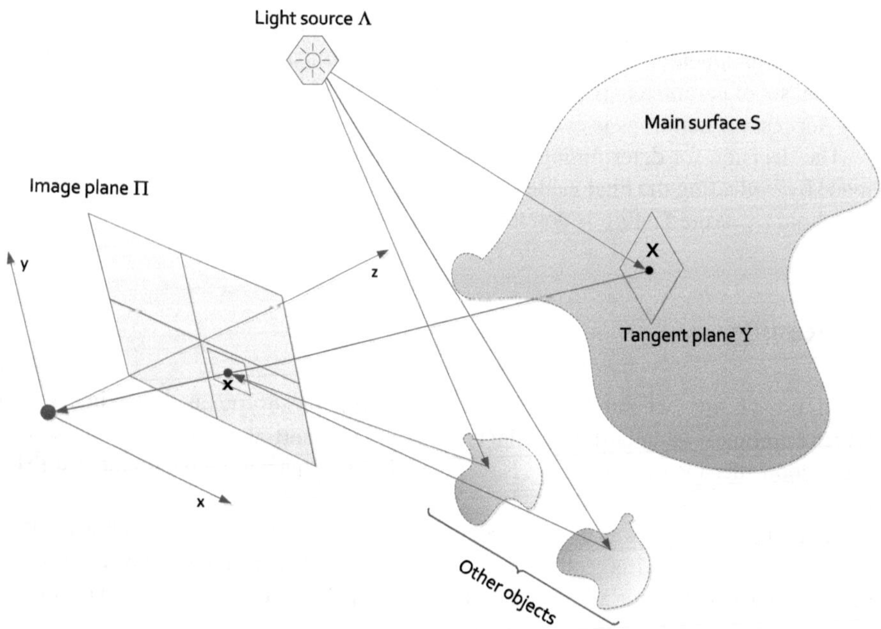

Fig. 13 Illustration of the photometric model with light rays reflected by the surface of the main object and reflectance from other objects

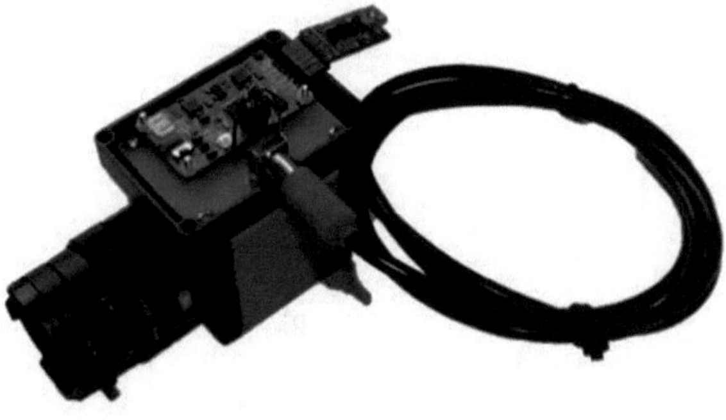

Fig. 14 Prototype of a visual-inertial sensor for VIFtrack!

Due to reflectance from other objects (ambient light sources) there are additional rays, which also change the intensity of an image pixel (parameter o). Due to the fact that the photometric motion cannot be estimated by using the inertial measurements, the corresponding values from the former frame are used as initial parameters for the optimisation. After the warping of the descriptors the optimisation process for each feature in X starts. For this optimisation, the following term needs to be minimized:

$$e = \min \left\{ \sum_{\mathbf{x} \in \nu} \left[\Omega \left[\theta \left(\mathbf{I}_{k(\mathbf{x}_i)} \right) \right]_{\mathbf{p}_{k}k+1} - \mathbf{I}_{k+1(\mathbf{x})} \right]^2 \right\} \quad (21)$$

The minimisation problem can be approximated by a linearisation[5] around the actual set of parameters. Classical Gauss–Newton optimisation is used for finding the optimal set of parameters $\mathbf{p}$. As an abort criterion the actual change rate of $\mathbf{p}$ between two successive iterations is evaluated ($\delta\mathbf{p} < \varepsilon$).

The decision for determining whether a feature was successfully tracked can be made by evaluating the final value for e after the last iteration. If e lies above a certain threshold e_{limit} the feature is deleted from the feature database.

4 Results

The approach was evaluated by using a visual-inertial prototype (as shown in Fig. 14) which combines a standard industrial camera and the inertial smart sensor system. A microcontroller located on the S^3 is responsible for synchronising camera and IMU data.

An industrial robot was used in order to generate measurements with known motion, which can be used as ground truth sequences. Due to the fact that the background of the project is the area of 3D modelling, the used sequences contain only single

[5] For this a simple first-order Taylor expansion of the minimisation term is used.

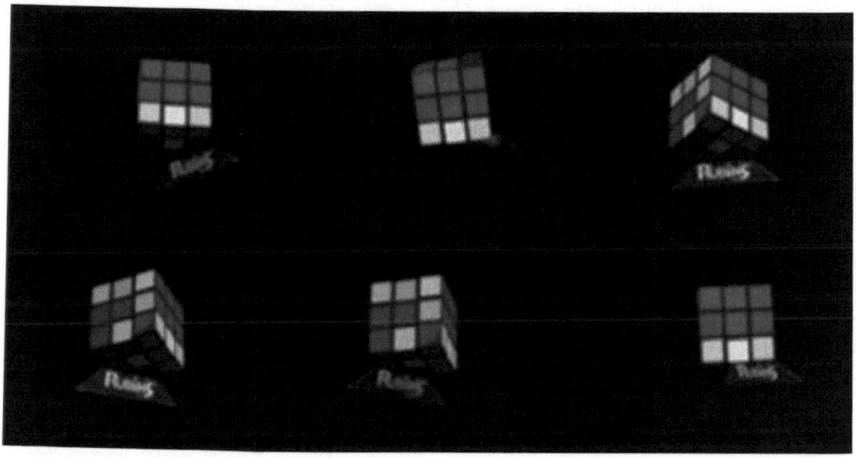

Fig. 15 Different frames of a test sequence "Object"

objects and a uniform background. The following figure illustrates exemplary frames of a typical sequence (Fig. 15).

We tested different motion patterns and optimised the corresponding parameters of the algorithm in order to produce best results. It was found that especially for high rotational velocities of the camera the VIFtrack! approach is able to outperform other feature tracking methods. Due to the fact that classical methods, such as the KLT-tracker from [11], utilise a purely translational model it is quite clear that especially a rolling camera leads to non-converging behaviour for many feature points. Figure 16 shows a typical motion pattern (slow camera speed) which we used for the evaluation. The suggested scheme can increase the number of successfully tracked features[6] up to 60 % in comparison to classical KLT for sequences with a rolling camera.

Figure 17 shows a comparison of the tracking performance for the VIFtrack!-method and the same principle (affine-photometric warping) only based on visual information for a given sequence. The mean number of successfully tracked features increases from 74 for visual-alone feature tracking up to 91 for the VIFtrack! scheme respectively. Especially for applications where a specific number of corresponding features is necessary (e.g. visual odometry) the VIFtrack!-method is useful, because while the visual-alone feature tracker loses up to 54 % of its feature points, VIFtrack! loses only up to 21 %.

The algorithm was also tested for a hand-held camera which was moved through an indoor environment. Figure 18 shows two typical examples for the tracking of features between two subsequent frames of the sequence. This sequence is more complex because the camera is freely moving within an indoor environment and no

[6] Here a successfully tracked feature is a feature which is not neglected based on the error threshold e_{limit}.

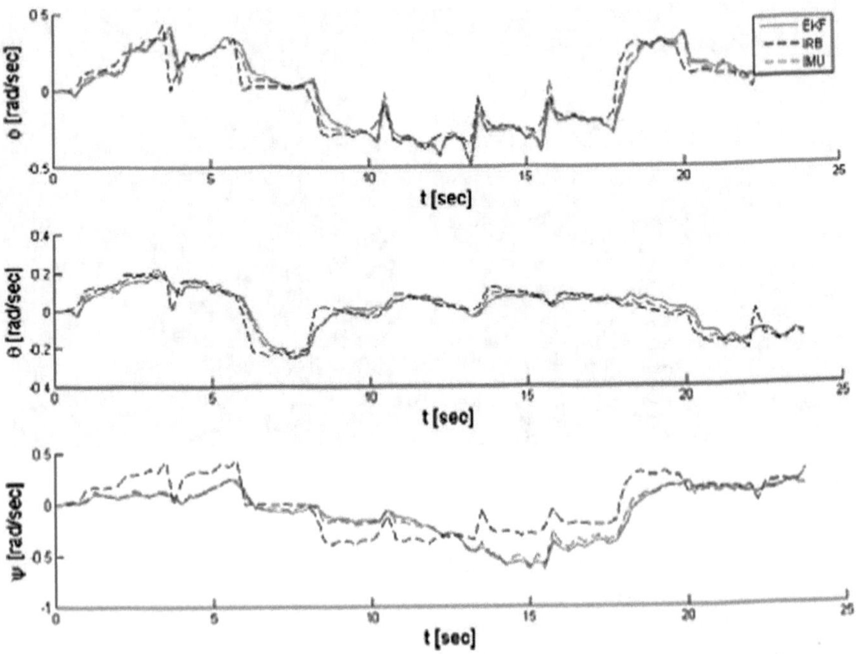

Fig. 16 Typical motion pattern for the evaluation describing rotation around the three Euler angles: *Black*: ground truth motion from industrial robot (IRB), *red*: measured angles from inertial measurements (IMU), *green*: estimated angles by fusion inertial and visual motion estimates (EKF))

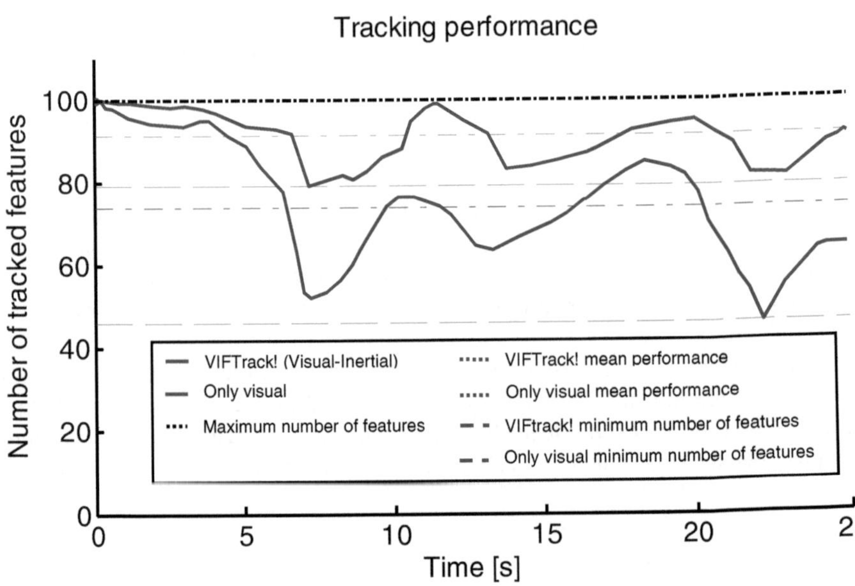

Fig. 17 Performance comparison between VIFtrack! and affine-photometric warping only based on visual information for the "object" sequence

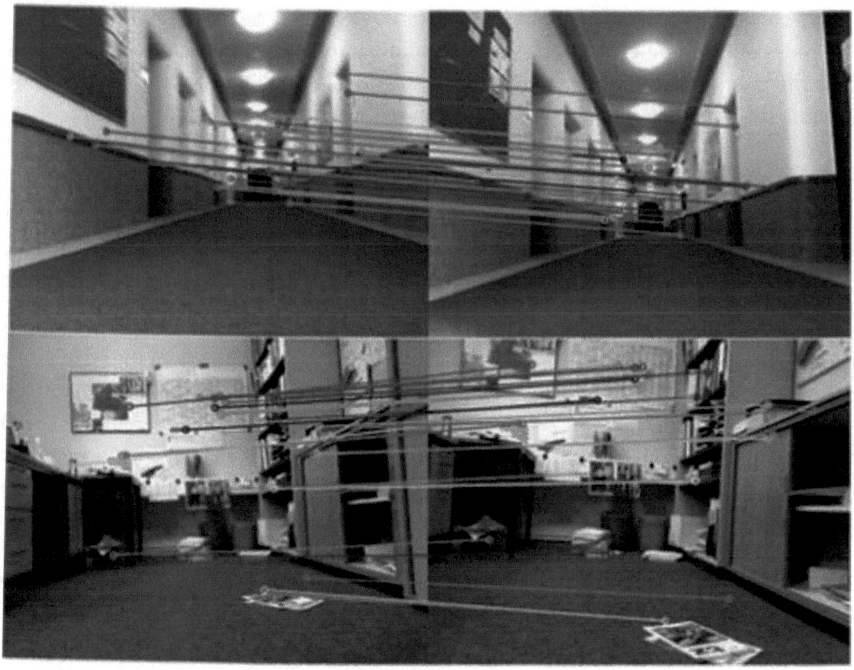

Fig. 18 Two examples for subsequent feature tracking results for the sequence gathered from a hand-held camera moved within an indoor environment

feature detected initially, within the first frame, remains visible for the entire sequence. For evaluating the VIFtrack! procedure a simple routine was introduced, which generates a set of feature candidates ${}^{1}X$ from the first frame. During the motion of the camera the number of successfully tracked features n decreases over time. Once n reaches a certain threshold ϖ, the algorithms generates a new set of feature candidates ${}^{k}X$ from the actual frame k of the sequence. This simple procedure should avoid that the tracking algorithm looses its track completely. The following table (Table 1) shows how often the algorithm generates a new set of feature candidates for the visual-inertial approach r_{VI} and classical KLT r_{KLT}.

Table 1 Comparison of the number of reinitialisation of feature candidates for VIFtrack! and classical KLT

n	r_{VI}	r_{KLT}	$\frac{r_{KLT}-r_{VI}}{r_{VI}}$ (%)
100	13	18	38
80	16	23	44
60	21	31	48
40	35	53	51
20	44	75	70

It can be seen from Table 1, that the usage of the VIFtrack! scheme is able to reduce the number of necessary re-initialisations of feature candidates due to the more robust feature tracking. Especially for a small number of initial feature candidates the visual-inertial feature tracking outperforms classical KLT.

5 Conclusion

The general problem of tracking a point feature throughout an image sequence acquired by a moving camera requires the implementation of an algorithm which is able to model the change of the visual appearance of each feature over time. The state of the art motion model used for feature tracking is an affine-photometric warping model, which models both changes in geometry and photometric conditions. For camera movements which involve high rotational velocities the 2D displacement of a point feature between two successive frames will increase dramatically. This leads to a non-converging behaviour of the minimisation problem, which adjusts a set of parameters in order to find the optimal match of the corresponding feature.

The usage of motion estimates, generated by an inertial smart sensor system as initial estimates for the motion model, leads to an increasing number of feature points, which can be successfully tracked throughout the whole sequence.

Future work will look into the possibility of fusing different motion estimates from visual and inertial cues, which would hopefully lead to a higher robustness against incorrect inertial measurements. For this visual-based relative pose estimators need to be evaluated to get a handle on the accuracy (see Aufderheide et al. [4]).

References

1. Aufderheide D, Krybus W (2010) Towards real-time camera egomotion estimation and three-dimensional scene acquisition from monocular image streams. In: Proceedings of the 2010 international conference on Indoor Positioning and Indoor Navigation (IPIN 2010). Zurich, Switzerland, September, 15–17 2010, pp 1–10. IEEE – ISBN 978-1-4244-5862-2
2. Aufderheide D, Steffens M, Kieneke S, Krybus W, Kohring C, Morton D (2009) Detection of salient regions for stereo matching by a probabilistic scene analysis. In: Proceedings of the 9th conference on optical 3-D measurement techniques. Vienna, Austria, July, 1–3 2009, pp 328–331. ISBN 978-3-9501492-5-8
3. Aufderheide D, Krybus W, Dodds D (2011) A MEMS-based smart sensor system for estimation of camera pose for computer vision applications. In: Proceedings of the University of Bolton Research and Innovation Conference 2011, Bolton, U.K., June, 28–29 2011, The University of Bolton Institutional Repository
4. Aufderheide D, Krybus W, Witkowski U, Edwards G (2012) Solving the PnP problem for visual odometry—an evaluation of methodologies for mobile robots. In: Advances in autonomous robotics—joint proceedings of the 13th annual TAROS conference and the 15th annual FIRA RoboWorld Congress Bristol, UK, August 20–23, pp 461–462
5. Harris C, Stephens M (1988) A combined corner and edge detector. In: Proceedings of the 4th Alvey vision conference, pp 147–151

6. Hwangbo M, Kim JS, Kanade T (2009) Inertial-aided KLT feature tracking for a moving camera. In: 2009 IEEE/RJS international conference on intelligent robots and systems. St. Louis, USA, pp 1909–1916
7. Hwangbo M, Kim JS, Kanade T (2011) Gyro-aided feature tracking for a moving camera: fusion, auto-calibration and GPU implementation. Int J Robot Res 30(14):1755–1774
8. Jin H, Favaro P, Soatto S (2001) Real-time feature tracking and outlier rejection with changes in illumination. In: Proceedings of the International Conference on Computer Vision (ICCV), July 2001
9. Juan L, Gwun O (2009) A comparison of SIFT, PCA-SIFT and SURF. Int J Image Process (IJIP) 3(4):143–152. CSC Journals
10. Kim J, Hwangbo M, Kanade T (2009) Realtime affine-photometric KLT feature tracker on GPU in CUDA framework. The fifth IEEE workshop on embedded computer vision in ICCV 2009, Sept 2009, pp 1306–1311
11. Lucas B, Kanade T (1981) An iterative image registration technique with an application to Stereo vision. In: International joint conference on artificial intelligence, pp 674–679
12. Rehbinder H, Hu X (2004) Drift-free attitude estimation for accelerated rigid bodies. Automatica 40(4):653–659
13. Sabatini A (2006) Quaternion-based extended Kalman filter for determining orientations by inertial and magnetic sensing. IEEE Trans Biomed Eng 53(7):1346–1356
14. Skog I, Haendel P (2006) Calibration of MEMS inertial unit. In: Proceedings of the IXVII IMEKO world congress on metrology for a sustainable development
15. Tomasi C, Shi J (1994) Good features to track. In: IEEE computer vision and pattern recognition 1994
16. Welch G, Bishop G (2006) An introduction to the Kalman filter, Technical Report TR 95-041. Department of Computer Science, University of North Carolina at Chapel Hill

Inferring Heading Direction from Silhouettes

Amina Bensebaa, Slimane Larabi and Neil M. Robertson

Abstract Due to the absence of features that may be extracted from face, heading direction estimation for low resolution images is a difficult task. For such images, estimating heading direction requires to taking into account all information that may be inferred from human body in image, particularly its silhouette. We propose in this paper a set of geometric features extracted from shape shoulders-head, feet and knees shapes which jointly allow the estimation of body direction. Other features extracted from head-shoulders are proposed for the estimation of heading direction based on body direction. The constraint of camera position related to proposed features is discussed and results of experiments conducted are presented.

1 Introduction

Heading direction estimation is one of challenging tasks for computer vision researchers especially in case of low resolution images. In case of high and medium resolution images, many approaches has been proposed to solve this problem. A survey may be found in [11]. All of these approaches try to find the most discriminate set of facial features which permit to estimate the pose. The objective to reach for any proposed technique is to verify a set of criteria such as: Accuracy, Monocular, Autonomous, Multi-person, Identity and Lighting invariant, Resolution independent, Full range of head motion and Real time [11].

Face extraction in low-resolution images is an important task in the process of heading direction estimation. Few works have been devoted for this purpose and

A. Bensebaa (✉) · S. Larabi
Computer Science Department, USTHB University, BP 32 El Alia, Algiers, Algeria
e-mail: bensebaa.amina@gmail.com

S. Larabi
e-mail: slarabi@usthb.dz

N. M. Robertson
Edinburgh Research Partnership in Engineering and Mathematics, Heriot-Watt University, Edinburgh, EH14 4AS, UK
e-mail: n.m.robertson@hw.ac.uk

J. M. R. S. Tavares, R. Natal Jorge (eds.), *Developments in Medical Image Processing and Computational Vision,* Lecture Notes in Computational Vision and Biomechanics 19,
DOI 10.1007/978-3-319-13407-9_19

all present difficulties for detecting faces when the resolution of images decreases [18]: Labeled training examples of head images are used to train various types of classifiers such as support vector machines, neural networks, nearest neighbor and tree based classifiers [3, 4, 13]. The disadvantage of these methods is the requirement of all combinations of lighting conditions and skin/hair colour variations in order to estimate an accurate classification.

Contextual features has been used in addition to visual ones in order to improve the quality of heading direction estimation [1, 8, 9]. Using multiple views camera, Voit et al. [17] estimate head pose for low resolution image by appearance-based method. The head size varies around 20×25 and the obtained results are satisfactory due to the use of multiple cameras. Additional contextual information: multiple calibrated camera and a specific scene allows estimating of absolute coarse head pose for wide-angle overhead cameras by integrating 3D head position [16].

Head-shoulders shape has been studied and many methods have been proposed for the purpose of human detection in images using wavelet decomposition technique and support vector machine [14] or background subtraction algorithm [12]. In other side, Head-shoulders shape has been used for human tracking and head pose estimation. In [12], the direction of head movements is detected and tracked throughout video frames. Templates are captured for a specific position of the camera (mounted sufficiently high above to provide a top-view of the scene) and do not use all positions of the head pose. Shape context is used but this descriptor is sensitive to the locations of pixels of the shape outline.

Another important feature that may contribute for heading-direction estimation is the legs shape. However, the use of detectors on the lower parts of the body has been introduced in many works for human body pose calculation and human action recognition [15]. Legs shape has been also used for human segmentation. Lin et al. [10] modeled the parts of the body particularly the legs in order to detect and segment human. The proposed approach is based on the matching of part-template tree images hierarchically proposed and used initially in [6, 7].

The problem or heading for low-resolution images without adding contextual information requires yet more contributions in order to deal with complex scenes where human are relatively far from the camera. The performance of proposed methods are principally limited because they are based on extracted features from the head which are very dependent on camera placement and the chosen texture and skin color models depend on the resolution of the head in the image and therefore doesn't work for lower resolution.

In this paper, we investigate what can be done from shoulders-head and legs shapes for heading direction estimation in case of low-resolution images. Firstly, a set of features are extracted from shoulders-head and legs shapes and used for inferring body direction. In the next, heading direction is estimated using body direction and features extracted from head-shoulders shape. Section 2 covers the theoretical aspects of body and heading direction estimation based on features extracted from shoulders-head and legs shapes. Experiments are conducted to validate our approach and obtained results are presented in Sect. 3.

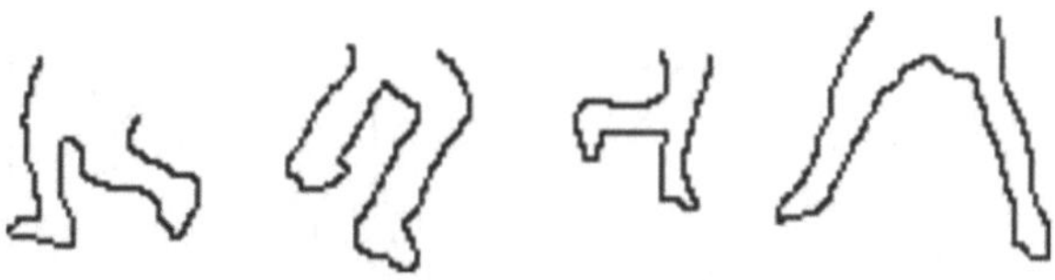

Fig. 1 Some shapes of legs for which it is easy to infer body direction

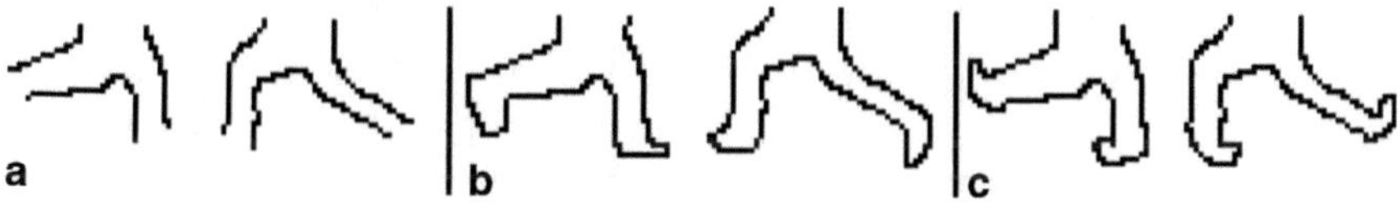

Fig. 2 Shapes of legs with inflected knee

2 Basic Principle of the Method

Assuming that silhouettes of humans are extracted from images of low resolution, our aim is to estimate body and heading directions. Geometric features are extracted from silhouette due to the absence of other features that may be extracted from the face for such images. We will focus in this paper on the parts head, shoulders, knees and feet shapes which may be considered as a good features to achieve this task. Body direction is firstly estimated using features extracted from head and shoulders, knees and feet shapes. Secondly, heading direction is inferred from estimated body direction and features of head and shoulders shape.

2.1 Features Extraction from Silhouette

A shape leg is a part of human silhouette which plays a dominant role in the process of inferring body direction from image. Indeed, our visual system is able to infer body direction seeing only the outline shape legs (see Fig. 1). We propose three determinant cues of shapes legs and head-shoulders that allow inferring body direction when they are extracted from outline shape. These features cannot be computed for a fixed top down camera because head-shoulders are confused with body silhouette.

The **first one** is the inflections of the knees. When a leg is well separated from the other and the knee is inflected, a coarse body direction can be inferred without ambiguity. Figure 2a illustrates an example of shape legs where feet are cut. Our visual system can easily give an estimate of body direction because the feet have limited possibilities of poses due to the geometry of one leg (high inflexion). Figure 2b illustrates the correct poses and the directions can be inferred using the feet shapes, however Fig. 2c shows impossible situation. The directions of the lines joining inflexion points of the same leg are used to infer the body direction.

The **second one** is the direction of shape foot. Indeed, our visual system encounters difficulties by looking at legs shapes without feet and cannot estimate body direction for many configurations even if the body is moving and legs are well separated but without inflexion of knees. For example, seeing to the outlines of Fig 3a, without

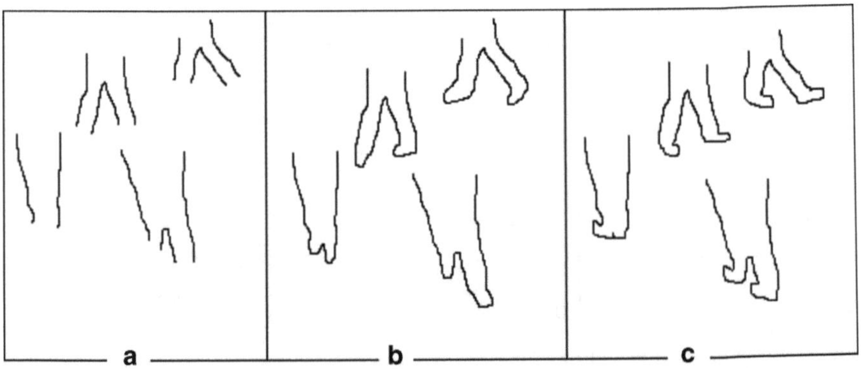

Fig. 3 Ambiguity in body direction estimation in case of missed shape feet

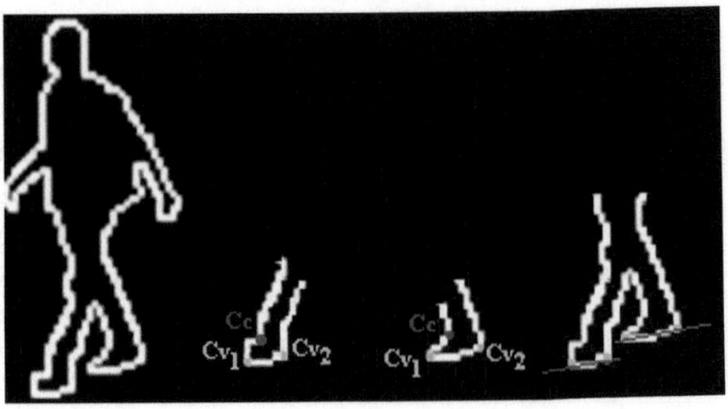

Fig. 4 Steps of body direction estimation based on foot directions

feet we cannot recognize to what direction body is moving. This ambiguity is clear seeing at the original shapes (see Fig. 3b) and at new shapes obtained drawing feet (see Fig. 3c). The base lines of the feet are good features because they indicate the body direction. Their use is explained in Sect. 2.2.

The **third feature** concerns the variation of silhouette's width along the shape head-shoulders and the length of each shoulder. The ratio of the width of the upper part (head) and the lower part (shoulders) with the varying of the shoulders length are related to the angle of rotation. We noticed that there's an opposite relationship between the ratio and the orientation angle.

2.2 *Inferring Body Direction*

Body Direction Estimation Using Feet's Features: This task consists to split the lower human shape into separated legs, separated lower legs or grouped legs (The two first cases include the case where the knee of one leg is inflected). We associate to each foot a **base line** defined by two extremities of the foot located between the heel and the toes. The outline of lower part is processed in order to determine the baseline of the feet located between the heel and the toes. Firstly, high convexities points Cv_1 and Cv_2 characterizing the outline foot are located (see Fig. 4). Secondly,

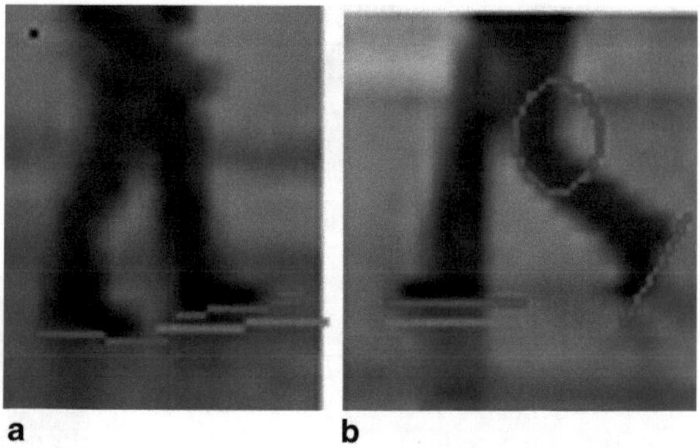

Fig. 5 Body orientation from feet (In *red color* the feet orientations of foot and in *blue* the body orientation)

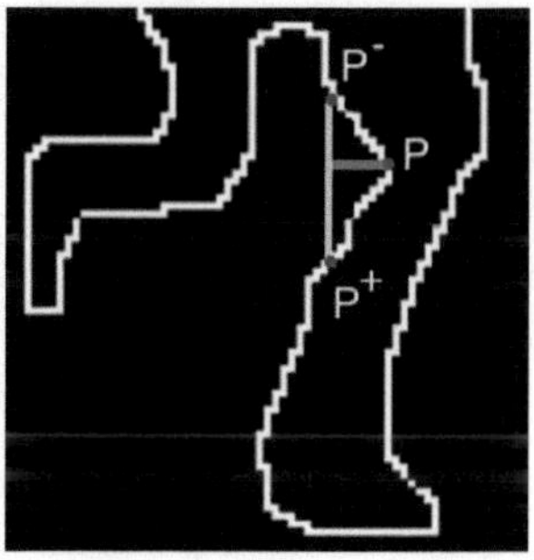

Fig. 6 Location of inflection points on outline legs

the last point of interest Cc representing a high concavity on this outline is located, such as the distances $CcCv_2$ is minimal. The convex point that represents toes, will be the closest point to the concave point of the feet outline, the other convex point will obviously correspond to the heel. Thus the base line joins the two convexities of the foot and the orientation of feet corresponds to the vector carried by the feet base line.

Applying the 2D quasi-invariant, the angle between the two vectors measured in 3D-space varies slowly in the image as viewpoint varies [2]. As in the scene the disposition of foot vectors is restricted by the human physic constraints, it will be the same case in image plane; the body direction is inferred as the average of foot directions. Once the base lines of feet are extracted, body orientation is computed as the resultant vector of the two orientations (see Fig. 5a). When one foot is not put on the ground, which correspond to a high inflection of the knee, the resultant vector will have the direction of the base line of the other foot (see Fig. 5b).

Body Direction Estimation Using Knee's Features: Extraction of inflection points consists to find the best concave or convex pixels of the lower part of the silhouette using the Chetverikov's algorithm [5]. Among the selected points of inflection p, p^* which is the farthest to the line binding p^- and p^+ is chosen. The position of p^-, p^+ to p^* is a parameter (see Fig. 6).

Many types of knees inflexion may be located (see Fig. 7). The direction of the body follows the direction of the inflected knee considered as the direction of the

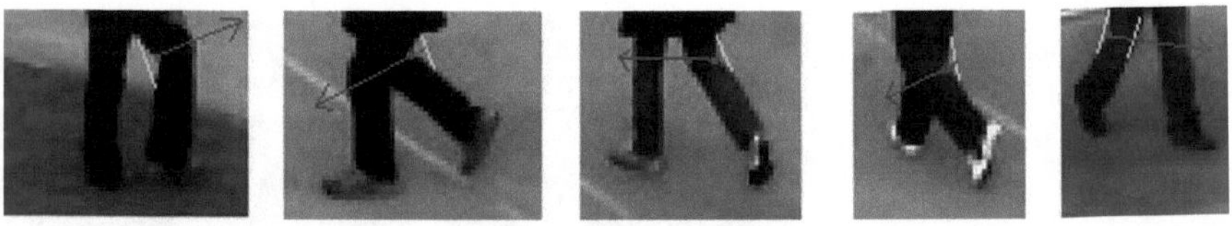

Fig. 7 Some cases of knee inflexion and the inferred direction of them

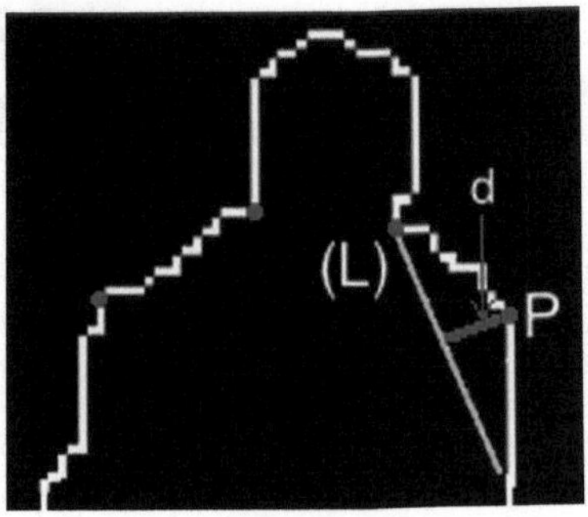

Fig. 8 The pixel p is the farthest from the line L

Table 1 Body direction inferred from head-shoulders features

Body direction	Ratio R_w
$[0°, 15°]$	≥ 1.82
$[15°, 30°]$	$[1.70, 1.81]$
$[30°, 45°]$	$[1.61, 1.69]$
$[45°, 60°]$	$[1.51, 1.60]$
$[60°, 75°]$	$[1.36, 1.5]$
$[75°, 90°]$	$[1.4, 1.5]$

line joining the concave point to the convex one. Only the direction left towards right and inversely will be considered.

Body Direction Estimation Using Head-Shoulders Features: Applying the algorithm of D. Chetverikov [5], the two concave points (left and right) delineating the head and the two convex points (left and right) extremities of shoulders are located. Head is separated by locating the pixel having the minimum angle among the selected point candidates. The two convex pixels are located based on high curvature. Each pixel is characterized by the fact that it is the farthest from the line (L) connecting the beginning of the shoulder and the end pixel of the head-shoulders outline (see Fig. 8).

When human is in the centre of field view of the camera, the average of computed ratios R_w (ratio of the widths of head and shoulders) estimated are given by Table 1 and the Fig. 9 illustrates an example corresponding to the rotation of a person towards the left using the ratio R_w of head-shoulders.

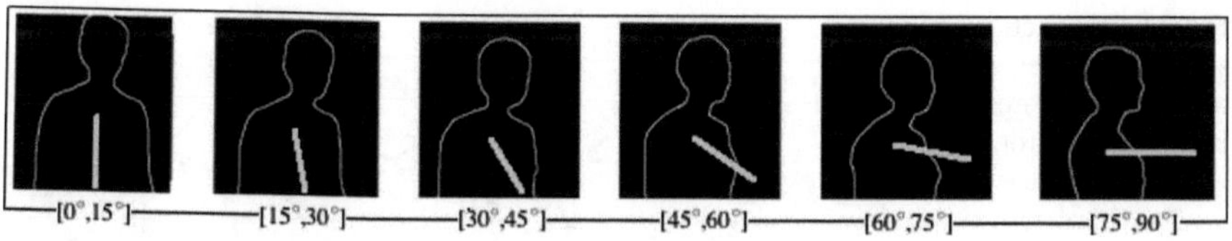

Fig. 9 Estimating body direction using the ratio R_w

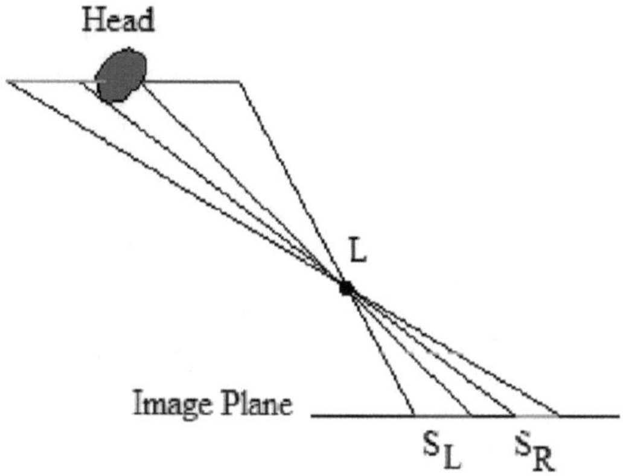

Fig. 10 Case of occlusion of shoulder by head

2.3 *Inferring Head Direction from Shoulders-Head Shape*

We assume now that body direction is estimated based on the three features proposed above (head-shoulders, knee inflexion and feet). In order to estimate the heading direction, we will base our approach on two features extracted from head-shoulders outline.

Features Extraction The **first feature** concerns the lengths of shoulders S_L and S_R on shape head-shoulders. In some cases, the end of the neck is not visible on one side due to head occlusion. In this case, it will be replaced by the point of high curvature on head-shoulders outline.

The lengths of shoulders are important cues for both head and body directions estimation and the difference between lengths of S_L and S_R arises from one of the following configurations:

- Depending on the camera and body positions, the head can occlude a part of one shoulder and then decreases the shoulder length. For example, when the camera is on top at the right or at the left of the person (see Fig. 10).
- When human body is rotating, one of shoulders becomes less visible. This occurs for example when the camera is on top even if the person is in front of the camera. In this case, length of one shoulder decreases until that the two sides of the shape head-shoulders do not correspond to shoulders.

Consequently, when the direction of body and head is in front to the camera, the lengths $L(S_L)$, $L(S_R)$ of shoulders are identical. Otherwise, when the head is rotating or when body is at the lateral side of the camera, this equality is not verified because

Fig. 11 Intersection of shoulders in case where **a** body and head are in front, **b** body and head rotating

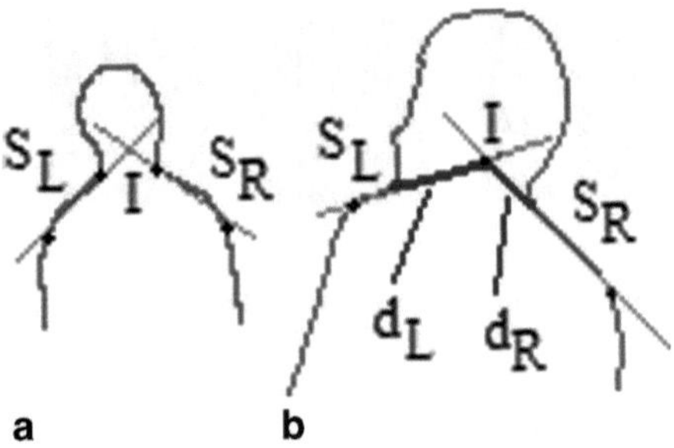

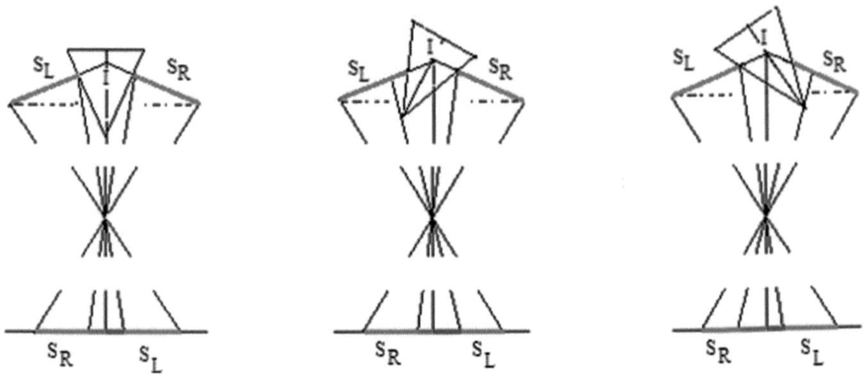

Fig. 12 Different poses of head where d_R, d_L are illustrated with *blue* and *red color* in case of human is in the *center* of the field of view

in both cases the head occludes a part of one shoulder (see Fig. 10). We proved geometrically that without occlusion by head, the lengths of one shoulder decreases when body is rotating.

The **second feature** which completes the first one, concerns the occluded parts of shoulders that permit to estimate head rotation. Let I be the intersection point of the lines joining extremities of shoulders S_L and S_R (see Fig. 11). When body and head are in front to the camera, the distances $d_L$and d_R from I to shoulders are identical in the scene and in image plane. However, when head or body are rotating, these distances are different in image because a part of shoulder is occluded by head and thus in image the distance d_L or d_R includes the occluded segment of the shoulder and a part of the neck. The distances d_L, d_R will be used to infer the heading direction.

Coarse Estimation of Head Direction Heading direction is estimated assuming that in previous steps, the body orientation, the difference ΔL between the lengths of shoulders (S_L) and (S_R) and the difference Δd between the distances d_L and d_R are computed. We distinguish three cases: body is in the center, at the left, or at right of the view field. For the two first cases, We give in Table 2 the results obtained of heading direction applying a geometric reasoning depending on the values of ΔL and δd and body direction. The third case is symmetrical to the second one. Figure 12 illustrates the variation of ΔL and δd in case where human in the center of the field of view of the camera.

Table 2 Heading direction inferred in cases where body is in front and at the left

Body in the center	$\delta d = 0$	$\delta d > 0$	$\delta d < 0$
$\Delta L = 0$	Head in Front	Not possible	Not possible
$\Delta L < 0$	Not possible	Rotation to left	Not possible
$\Delta L > 0$	Not possible	Not possible	Rotation to right
Body at the left			
$\Delta L = 0$	Low Rotation to right	Not possible	Not possible
$\Delta L < 0$	Not possible	Head in front or rotating to left	Not possible
$\Delta L > 0$	Not possible	Not possible	Hight rotation to right

2.4 *Study of the Camera Position Constraint*

As we are interested in this work to images of low resolution which means a far field of view, the camera may be:

- Fixed at the top and far from the scene. In this case, none from the features: head, shoulders, legs and feet can't be located using the blob representing human.
- Fixed so as its optical axis is oblique or horizontal towards the scene. in this case, whatever the position of the camera relatively to human in the scene: in front or at the lateral position, its head-shoulders, legs and feet are viewed. Consequently, the availability of the proposed features depends only on the pose, which means that inflexion of knees or feet base lines may be missed, what is required is the presence of the head-shoulders outline.

3 Results

We applied our method on PETS data set. Firstly silhouettes are extracted and body direction is firstly computed. In the next, heading direction is estimated. We used all features extracted from head-shoulders, feet and knees outlines.

Figure 13 illustrates some poses, extracted silhouettes and computed body directions. Body direction is computed using the ratio R_w having respectively the values

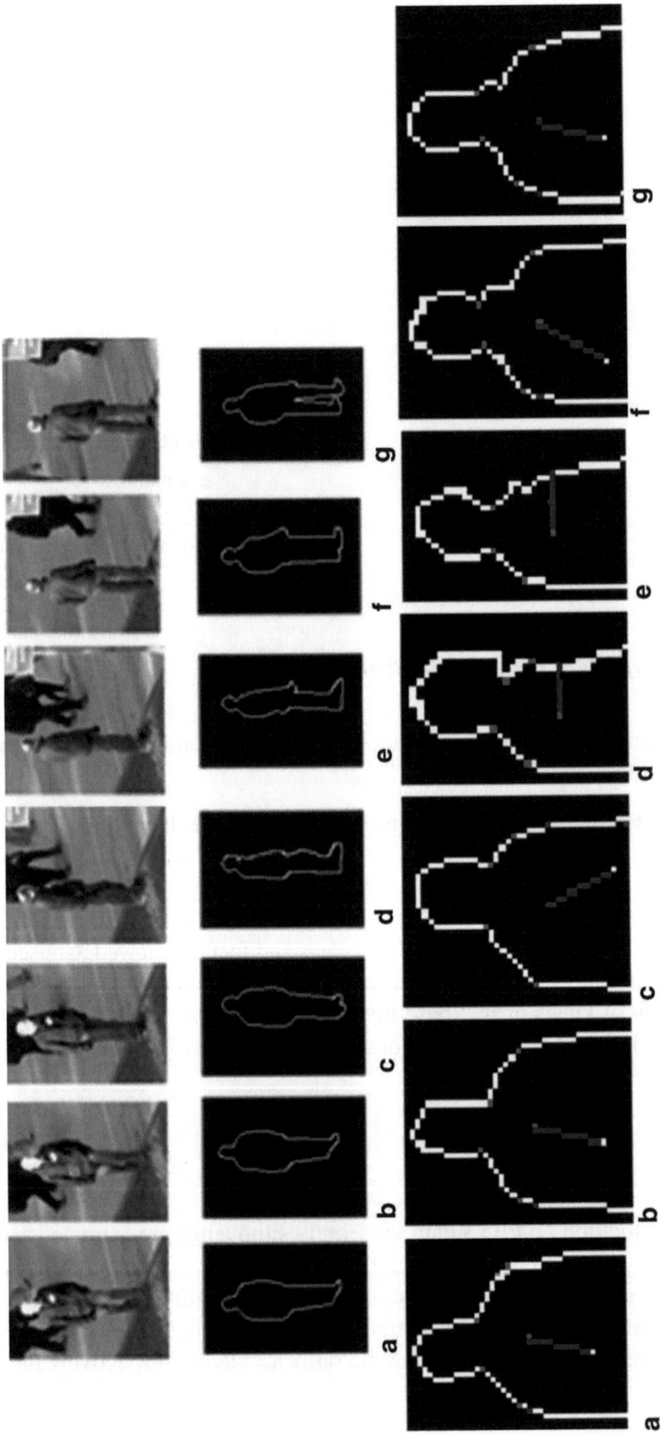

Fig. 13 Some poses and extracted silhouettes and the computed body directions based on R_w values

$2.6, 2.89, 2.25, 1.33, 1.36, 2.27, 2.09$ giving the directions: $[0°, 15°], [0°, 15°], [15°, 30°], [75°, 90°], [75°, 90°], [15°, 30°], [0°, 15°]$. As the computed body direction for the two last poses $(f), (g)$ are done using only the first feature which cannot differentiate if the body is in front or of back with regard to the camera.

The orientation of feet, when are located in the image, eliminates the ambiguity (in front or of back). Figure 14 illustrates some body poses which combine only features of head-shoulders and feet (knees inflexions are not visible).

The combination of features used for body direction depends on what can be extracted in image. The features extracted from feet and knees are more strong than those extracted from head-shoulders which just allows us to calculate the direction. Figure 15 illustrates the results obtained when inflexion of knees are used in addition of the ratio R_w.

Heading direction estimation is based on estimated body direction and the values of d_L, d_R computed using head-shoulders outline. We can see in Figure 16 the use of all presented features for estimating heading direction. Figure 17 summarizes this combination of features and shows that a good estimation is made even if the images are of low resolution.

4 Conclusion

We proposed in this paper a method for heading direction for images based on geometric features which can be extracted from silhouette even if images are of low resolution. Body direction is inferred from features extracted from outlines of knees and feet and head-shoulders. This direction is used in addition to features extracted from outlines of head-shoulders for estimating heading direction. The proposed method has been applied on real images and achieves good estimation of heading direction. Also, the features extracted are independent from camera pose, except the top view where head-shoulders, knees and feet cannot be located on human shape.

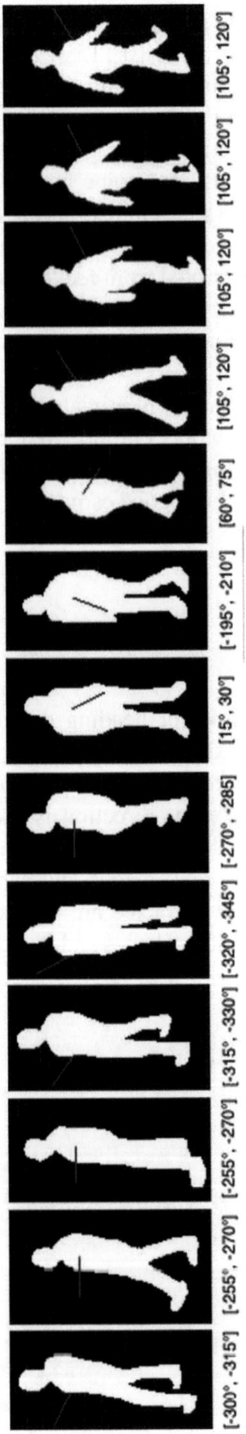

Fig. 14 Body orientation using the features: feet and R_w ratio

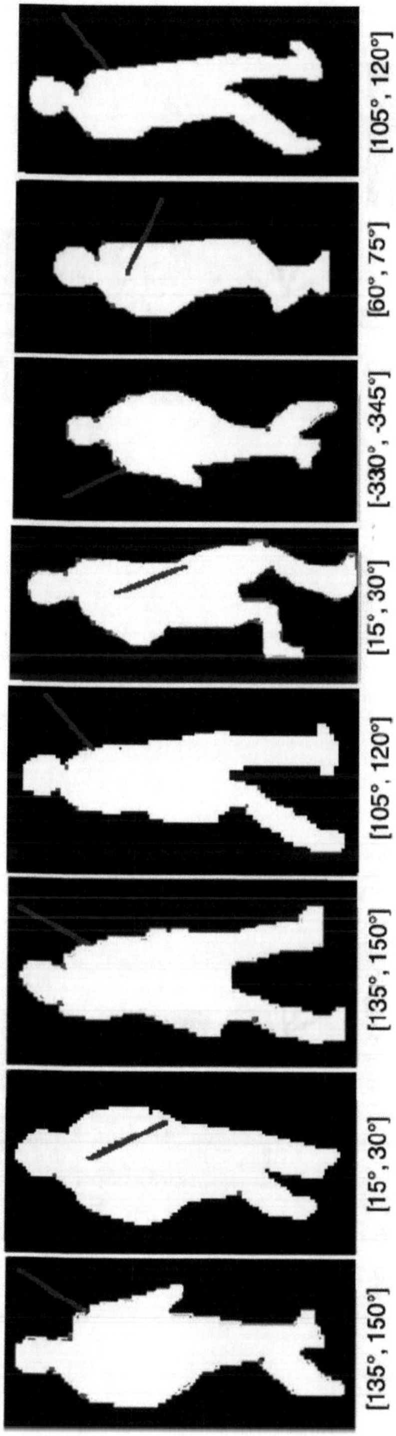

Fig. 15 Body orientation using the features: knee inflexion and R_w ratio

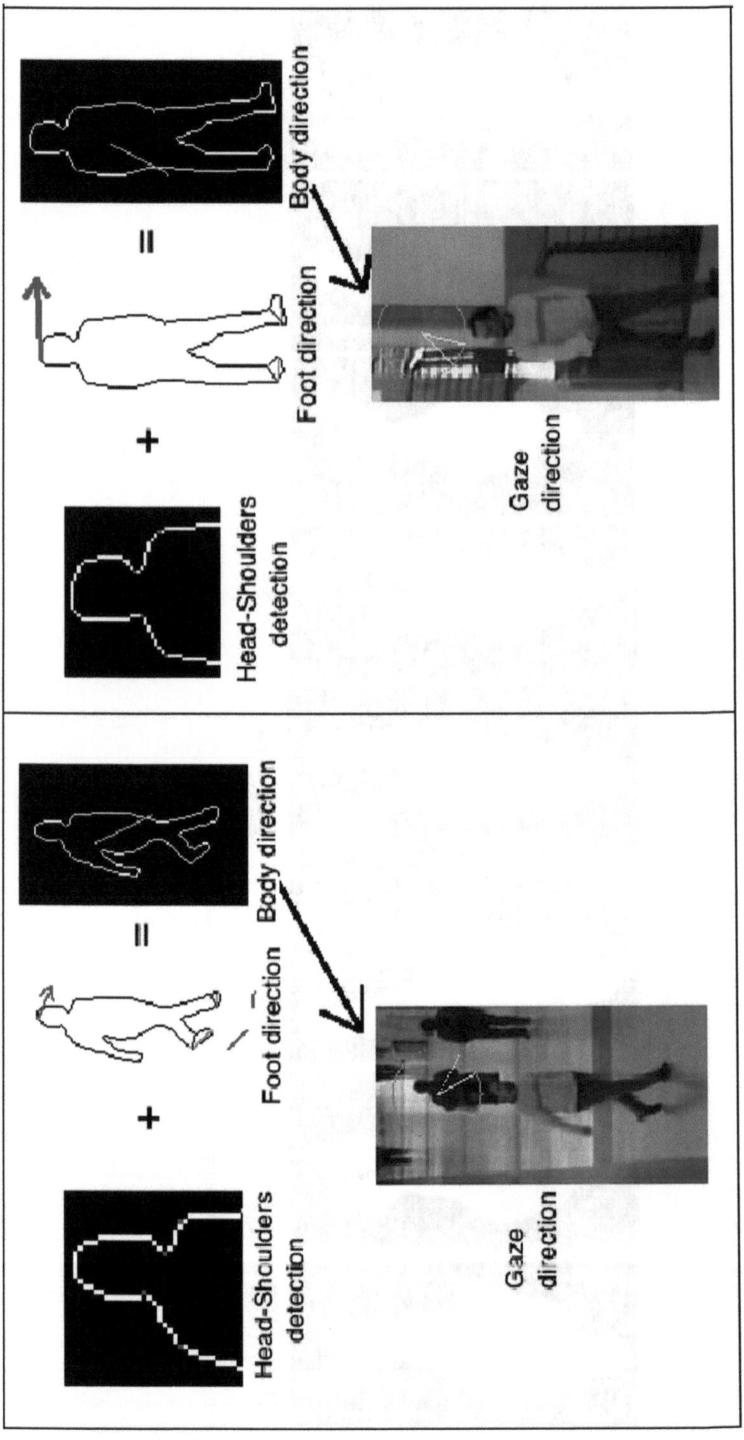

Fig. 16 Step of heading direction estimation

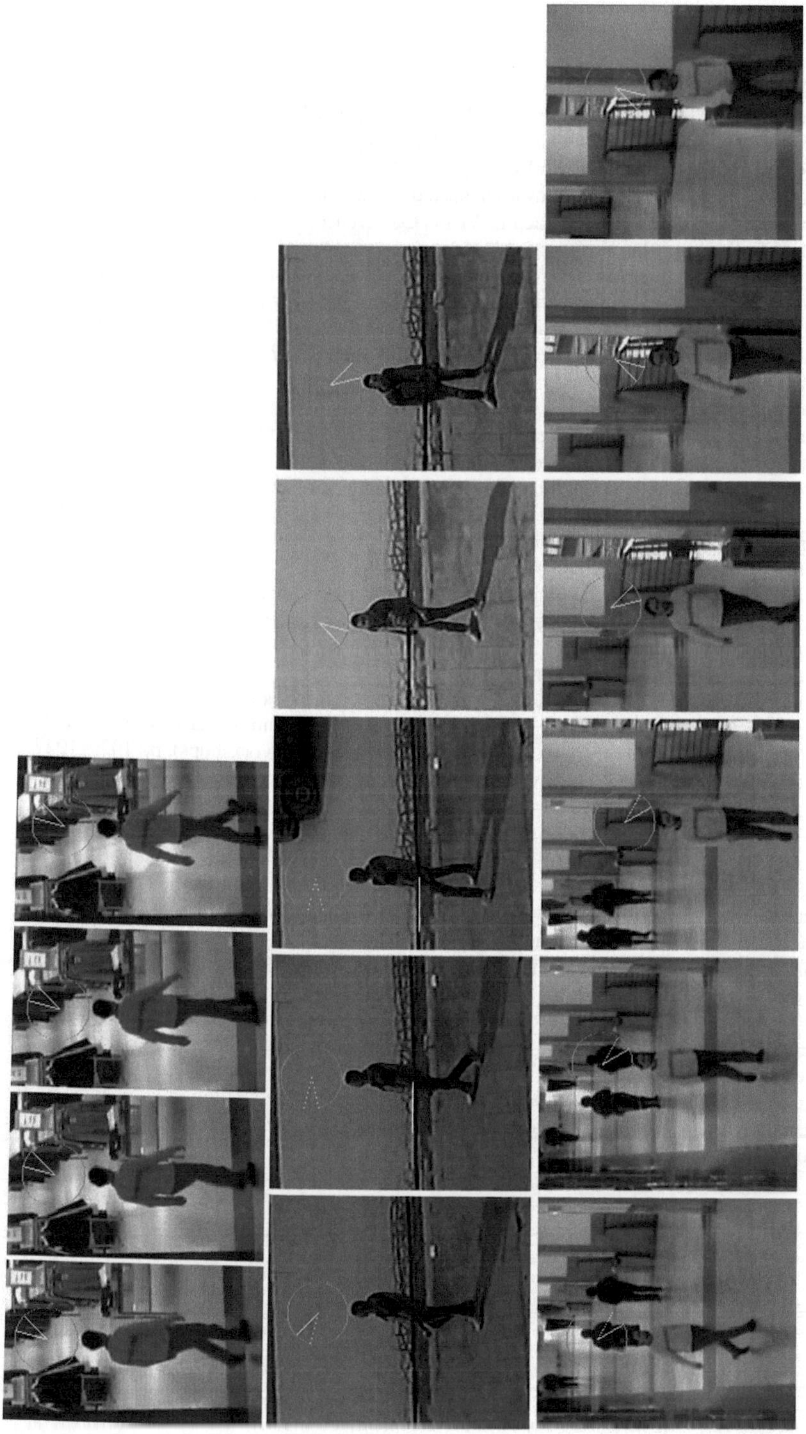

Fig. 17 Heading and body directions from combined features

References

1. Ba SO, Odobez JM (2011) Multiperson visual focus of attention from head pose and meeting contextual cues. IEEE Trans Pattern Anal Mach Intell 33(1):101–116
2. Binford TO, Levitt TS (1993) Quasi-invariants: theory and exploitation. In: Proceedings of DARPA Image Understanding Workshop, pp 819–829
3. Benfold B, Reid I (2008) Colour invariant head pose classification in low resolution video. In: Proceedings of the 19th British Machine Vision Conference
4. Benfold B, Reid I (2011) Unsupervised learning of a scene-specific coarse gaze estimator. In: Proceedings of the International Conference on Computer Vision (ICCV), pp 2344–2351
5. Chetverikov D (2003) A simple and efficient algorithm for detection of high curvature points in planar curves. In: Computer analysis of images and patterns, 10th international conference, CAIP 2003, Groningen, the Netherlands, August 2003, pp 25–27
6. Gavrila DM (1999, Jan) The visual analysis of human movement: a survey. Comput Vis Image Underst 73(1):8298
7. Gavrila DM (2007) A bayesian, exemplar-based approach to hierarchical shape matching. IEEE Trans Pattern Anal Mach Intell 29(8):1408–1421
8. Lanz O, Brunelli R (2008) Joint Bayesian tracking of head location and pose from low-resolution video. In: Multimodal technologies for perception of humans, pp 287–296
9. Launila A, Sullivan J (2010) Contextual features for head pose estimation in football games. In: International conference on pattern recognition (ICPR 2010), Turkey, pp 340–343
10. Lin Z, Davis LS (2010) Shape-based human detection and segmentation via hierarchical part-template matching. IEEE Trans Pattern Anal Mach Intell 32(4):604–618
11. Murphy-Chutorian E, Trivedi MM (2009, April) Head pose estimation in computer vision: a survey. Pattern Anal Mach Intell, IEEE Trans 31(4):607–626
12. Ozturk O, Yamasaki T, Aizawa K (2009) Tracking of humans and estimation of body/head orientation from top-view single camera for visual focus of attention analysis. In: IEEE 12th international conference on computer vision workshops (ICCV workshops), pp 1020–1027
13. Robertson NM, Reid ID (2006) A general method for human activity recognition in video. Comput Vis Image Underst 104(2–3):232–248
14. Sun Y, Wang Y, He Y, Hua Y (2005) Head-and-shoulder detection in varying pose. In: Advances in natural computation, first international conference, ICNC, Changsha, China, pp 12–20
15. Singh VK, Nevatia R, Huang C (2010) Efficient inference with multiple heterogeneous part detectors for human pose estimation. In: Computer vision ECCV 2010, pp 314–327
16. Tian YL, Brown L, Connell C, Sharat P, Arun H, Senior A, Bolle R (2003) Absolute head pose estimation from overhead wide-angle cameras. In: IEEE international workshop on analysis and modeling of faces and gestures, AMFG 2003, pp 92–99
17. Voit M, Nickel K, Stiefelhagen R (2006) A Bayesian approach for multi-view head pose estimation. In: IEEE international conference on multisensor fusion and integration for intelligent systems, pp 31–34
18. Zheng J, Ramirez GA, Fuentes O (2010) Face detection in low-resolution color images. In: Proceedings of the 7th international conference on image analysis and recognition, ICIAR'10, Portugal, pp 454–463

A Fast and Accurate Algorithm for Detecting and Tracking Moving Hand Gestures

Walter C. S. S. Simões, Ricardo da S. Barboza, Vicente F. de Jr Lucena and Rafael D. Lins

Abstract Human vision plays a very important role in the perception of the environment, communication and interaction between individuals. Machine vision is increasingly being embedded in electronic devices, as cameras are used with the function of perceiving the environment and identifying the elements inserted in a scene. Real-time image processing and pattern recognition are processing intensive tasks, even with the technology of today. This chapter proposes a vision system that recognizes hand gestures combining motion detection techniques, detection of skin tones, and classification using a model based on the Haar Cascade and CamShift algorithms. The new algorithm presented is 29 % faster than its competitors.

1 Introduction

The evolution of computing devices made possible new types of man-machine interaction. Touch screens, voice recognition, and motion detection are amongst the main representatives of such new interfaces. Motion detection systems are becoming more popular every day and either use controls with markers or cameras for modern gesture recognition. Motion recognition systems provide a very flexible and flexible way to allow users to control equipments and softwares without using of traditional devices such as keyboards, mice and remote controls.

Walter C. S. S. Simões (✉) · Vicente F. de J. Lucena
Universidade Federal do Amazonas, Amazonas, Brazil
e-mail: waltersimoes@gmail.com

Vicente F. de J. Lucena
e-mail: vicente@ufam.edu.br

Ricardo da S. Barboza · Rafael D. Lins
Universidade Federal de Pernambuco, Pernambuco, Brazil
e-mail: rsbarboza@gmail.com

Rafael D. Lins
e-mail: rdl@cin.ufpe.br

J. M. R. S. Tavares, R. Natal Jorge (eds.), *Developments in Medical Image Processing and Computational Vision*, Lecture Notes in Computational Vision and Biomechanics 19,
DOI 10.1007/978-3-319-13407-9_20

Real-time recognition and tracking of gestures only recently became viable; it opens new frontiers for man-machine interaction. Active markers emit their location to a receiver that maps the input coordination onto the application. In general, active markers are used to analyze the movement of very complex objects, such as modeling the movements of the human body to detect problems. For instance, to analyze the instability of the walk of some elderly patients a set of markers is glued in strategic parts of the body. The precise coordinates provided by the markers allows the creation of a 3D-model of the body of the patient and to analyze its dynamic in movement. The larger the number of markers used, the more precise the model to be developed. On the other hand, the markers need to be placed onto the object somehow and this imposes applicability limitations. The use of cameras to capture gestures removes the inconvenience of having to place markers but brings the necessity to process the entire image to extracting the data that is important to coordinate the application. The equipment must have processing power and enough memory to handle the captured images in real-time meeting the demands of the application. Several approaches have been proposed in this direction, but the high resource consumption of processor and memory may force users to purchase special equipments such as video game consoles as the Xbox with Kinect [4], which is the main representative of this technology or using ordinary cameras associated with simpler and less accurate software.

This chapter presents a way of recognizing hand gestures that can be detected quickly and accurately, using techniques of Motion Detection and Skin Detection eliminating pixels that are not important in the identification of the coordinate gestures and to leave only pixels that bring a standard tone of human skin to the Haar Cascade for gesture recognition. Besides that, the new algorithm also delivers to CamShift an image that is faster tracked than the one that is produces using Haar Cascade only. The proposed algorithm is suitable for applications such as controlling TV-sets advantageously replacing infrared remote control devices.

2 Related Works

This chapter presents a gesture recognition algorithm that combines techniques that seek to reduce the consumption of hardware resources and increase the efficiency of gesture tracking. Thus, the works related to this article address the steps necessary to the construction of a faster and more efficient algorithm for human gesture tracking to "navigate" on a computer screen.

The difficulty in recognizing a color pattern, complicated by the "noise" inserted by uneven illumination of the environment and the throughput limitations of the embedded system was addressed in reference [18].

The image processing strategy of reducing the image resolution and yielding only the silhouette of the original image that contains only the parts that moved was described in reference [17].

The work [19] exploits the classification model based on gestures of a tree of features proposed in reference [9], working with images of size 640 × 480 and the classifier generated from a set of 300 images containing a gesture with its variations. The method proposed in [9] was initially used to detect faces, but could be trained to detect any object that has features that could be distinguished from the background.

To allow users to interact with computing devices over larger distances, for example, for handling an iDTV (interactive Digital TV) set with a distance between device and spectator over 3 m, the images need to have quality and definition enough to meet the requirements of the gesture recognition algorithm. The work [20] deals with the construction of a strong cascade type classifier, formed from a set of 2000 gesture images. The approach applied in that work combines the techniques of motion detection to reduce the observation area on the image, detecting skin tones to restrict gestures and search only on elements that have moved and have a skin color pattern, followed by the classification of gestures using the model described in reference [9].

3 The New Algorithm

This chapter builds upon the work developed in [20], replacing the Haar classifier in the step of tracking by CamShift—Continuously Adaptive Mean Shift [1]. The AdaBoost Haar classifier needs to search for the information in each frame to identify the object of interest at each stage and such information is used in each of the cascaded features.

Detecting a hand moving over a relatively constant background seems to be a simple task at first glance, but in reality that is a complex process. The major problem faced is the large amount of input information available. Another problem addressed in computer vision is the poor reliability and instability in object tracking, due to, among other things, changes in lighting, occlusion, motion and noise in the capture equipment. The human vision system integrates several features that are analyzed in parallel, such as motion, color, contour, etc. Thus, with the acquired "knowledge of the surrounding world", one is able to easily deal with identification problem, most of times. Accomplishing those tasks in a computer is not an easy task, however [12].

When developing a computer vision application, one must first define how to capture gestures. In this chapter the optical model [16] was adopted. Such model uses cameras that receive images and deliver them to the algorithm without physical markers to assist in the process of searching for patterns in the images. This step is important because the extracted features are used to train the gesture recognition tool.

Two tasks are of paramount importance in gesture recognition: the construction of the classifier, which serves as a knowledge base system and the image processing application. The group of acquired images must undergo a noise reduction process and elimination of unnecessary data before "feeding" the classifier. Such was the strategy used in reference [20] and maintained in the present chapter in order to have a common comparison basis for the results obtained when the Haar classifier is replaced by the CamShift one in the process of tracking gestures.

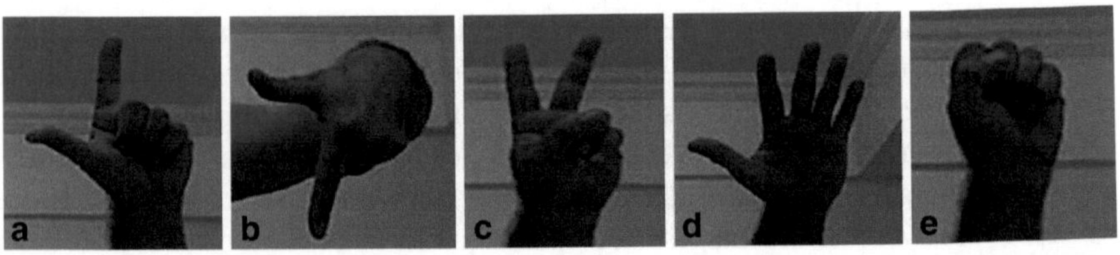

Fig. 1 Gestures suggested by the group of people after a questionnaire, using techniques of usability engineering [11, 16]

3.1 Gesture Classifiers

Classifiers are responsible for the clustering of the input space. This clustering process is carried out to determine the class of each object from its features. Such clustering process can be of two types: supervised and unsupervised. In supervised feature clustering, during training, the test samples are accompanied by annotations indicating the actual class of the sample. The unsupervised classifier must infer N divisions in the group data from relations between the characteristics of the samples, the number of divisions normally specified by the developer. Among the methods using unsupervised classification learning there are decision trees [9] and Boosting [5].

Many algorithms use only the decision tree to get the features of the objects in the images, because each node is associated with a measure that represents the ratio between the amounts of each class of object in the tree node. This measure can be modified through breaks (splits), which are performed on the dataset from restrictions on the values of certain features in order to reduce the combination of different classes in the same node. This clustering mode has the disadvantage that characteristics may be sensitive to overfitting, and if incorrectly trained the classifier may be incorrectly set up. Overfitting occurs when the statistical model used describes a random error or noise instead of the desired object or gesture.

The Boosting technique allows building a strong classifier on top of a number of weak classifiers, though the combination of their results. In particular AdaBoost—Adaptive Boosting [2, 5, 11], which extended the original Boosting method to make it adaptive, needs special attention. This method represents each weak classifier by a small decision tree, which normally comprises only a break (Split). As the algorithm progresses, the weak classifiers focus on points that the previous step had the worst results, incrementally improving the quality of the final response. For this reason, this chapter uses AdaBoost based classifiers.

The gestures (Fig. 1) that were mapped to the construction of classifiers were defined from a study in [20].

To build an AdaBoost classifier it is necessary to choose two sets of images: the positive, which contains the object one wants to map and the negative, which contains other objects. After defining those two groups of images, three algorithms provided by the set of OpenCV libraries [2] are used. They are: *Objectmarker*, *CreateSamples* and *Traincascade*

Objectmarker is responsible for scoring the positive images of the objects of interest, creating a file containing the image name and the coordinates of the marking area. Such text file is converted into a vector through the tool CreateSamples that while standardizing brightness, lighting, and suitably scaling the window to the size for the images to be cropped from the group of positive images. The default size chosen for the images of this chapter is 20 by 20 pixels. The greater the number of images and variations regarding illumination, reflection, backgrounds, scaling, rotation, etc. in this step, the more accurate is the resulting classifier.

According to reference [9], each stage of the cascading should be independent of the others, allowing creating a simple tree. When it is necessary to increase the accuracy of the classifier, more images or more stages to the tree must be added. Many references, such as [13, 14, 22, 23], suggest that in order to reach an accurate classifier about 10,000 images are necessary.

This project made use of 2000 images acquired through an image capture software written in Java. Such number of images was empirically defined by tuning the number of images for the tree construction features. The process started with 500 images, and it was found that increasing number of images, each stage became stronger, improving the classifier eventually.

Another relevant feature that must be observed is the resolution of the images used. While the literature indicates the use of images with dimensions of 640 $\times$ 480 pixels, this study used images with resolution 320 $\times$ 240 pixels, obtained from a camera with native resolution of 12 mega pixels, which greatly increased the number of perceived characteristics at each stage and a performance far superior to that obtained with images of 640 $\times$ 480 pixels.

Finally, after these two steps, the vector of positive images and folder containing the negative images are submitted to the algorithm Traincascade that performs the training and the creation of the cascade of classifiers. This algorithm compares the positive and negative images, used as a background, attempting to find edges and other features [17]. This is the step that is more time intensive to execute, thus it was important to monitor the estimates that are displayed on the screen and see if the classifier would be either effective or not based on the successes and false alarm rates at each stage. Reference [9] indicates that it takes at least 14 steps to start the process of recognition of some object.

The Traincascade algorithm trains the classifier with the submitted sample, and generates a cascade using Haar-type features. Despite the importance of determining the texture, the detection of the shape of an object is a recurring problem in machine vision. Reference [9, 11] proposed the use of rectangular features, known as Haar-like, rather than the color intensities to improve the inference to the shape of an object and increase the accuracy of the classifier from a concept called integral image. From the integral image it is possible to calculate the sum of values in a rectangular region in constant time, simplifying and speeding up the feature extraction in image processing.

An image is composed of pixels containing information of the intensities of its layers of colors, ranging from 0 (darker) to 255 (lighter) for each color channel. The most widely used color systems have three components, such as RGB and HSV [21]. Those representation modes require a higher computational effort and more storage space than binary ones. Thus, the use of binary vision systems, if proven adequate, allows much faster processing and more compact representation. Such images are extremely important for real time applications, in which it is necessary to speedily process the feature extraction to deliver the results to the recognition algorithm. In general, binary vision systems are useful in cases where the contour contains enough information to allow recognizing objects even in environments with uneven lighting. The vision system typically uses a binary threshold to separate objects from the background. The appropriate value of such threshold depends on the lighting and the reflective characteristics of the objects. The effective object-background separation claims that the object and background have sufficient contrast and that the intensity levels of both objects and the background are known [21].

In order to create an integral image, reference [9] used binarized images to simplify the description of the features. The result of the cascaded process is saved in a file with Extensible Markup Language (XML).

3.2 *Image Processing*

A software module was developed to enable the camera to capture images, process them, and submit them to the classifier. Multiple gestures recognition was achieved through the use of threads.

To increase the possibility of using the algorithm in different environments, various methods of image processing were used to minimize the noise level and also elements that do not make gestures mapped to classifiers. Overall, the technical literature divides a recognition system of objects and gestures into four parts [7]: *Pre-processing*; *Segmentation*; *Feature extraction* and *Statistical Classification*. The following sub-sections describe the main features of each of them.

3.2.1 Pre-Processing

System calibration tasks, geometric distortion correction, and noise removal take place in the pre-processing stage. One of the concerns in the pre-processing is the removal of noise caused by many factors, such as resolution of the equipment used, lighting, distance from the object or gesture over the camera, etc. *Salt-and-pepper* noises often appear in the images. The white pixels scattered in the image, called salt noises, are the pixels of a particular image region that have high value surrounded by low value pixels. The pepper noise is the opposite situation to that of salt noise. There are two ways to process those noises: using morphological transformations or

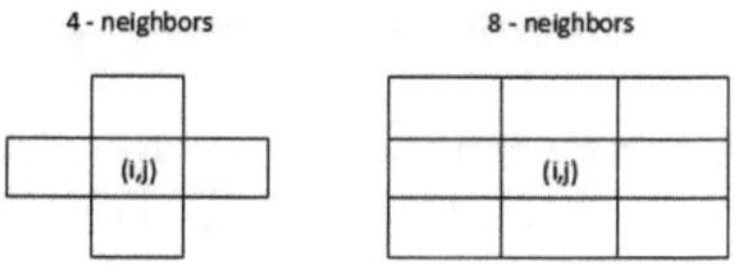

Fig. 2 Pixel neighborhood

applying Gaussian smoothing methods to approximate the values of the pixels and decreasing the perception of such noises.

In a digital image represented on a grid, a pixel has a common border with four pixels and shares a common corner with four additional pixels. It is said that two pixels are 4-neighbors if they share a common border. [8, 10] Similarly, two pixels are 8-neighbors if they share at least one corner. For example, a pixel at location [i, j] is 4-neighbors [i + 1, j], [i-1, j], [i, j + 1] and [i, j-1]. The 8-neighbors of the pixel including the four-nearest neighbor [i + 1, j + 1], [i + 1, j-1] [i-1, j + 1] and [i-1, j-1]. Figure 6 shows how the pixels are presented in order neighbors and 4-8-neighbors. (Fig. 2)

The morphological operations used in this study were erosion, which removed the pixels that did not meet the minimum requirements of the neighborhood and dilation, which entered pixels in the image is crafted by erosion, also according to a pre-determined neighborhood. After applying the morphological transformation, a smoothing operation takes place. Such transformation performs the approximation of the values of the pixels, attempting to blur or to filter out the noise or other fine-scale or dispersed structures. The model used in this project was the 3 $\times$ 3 Gaussian Blur, also known as Gaussian smoothing. The visual effect of such technique is a blurred soft similar to display the image on a translucent screen.

3.2.2 Segmentation

Image segmentation consists in the extraction and identification of objects of interest contained in the image, where the object is the entire region with semantic content relevant to the desired application. After segmentation, each object is described by their geometric and topological properties, for example, attributes such as area, shape and texture of objects can be extracted and used later in the analysis process. Image segmentation can be performed by the basic properties of gray level values, detecting discontinuities or similarities. The discontinuities may be dots, lines, edges, which one can apply a mask to highlight the type of discontinuity that may exist.

After, filters are used to detect similarity, merging them as edges. The first filter used was Sobel, which is an operator that calculates the finite difference, giving an approximation of the gradient of intensity of image pixels. The second filter used was Canny [3] that smoothen the noise and finds edges by combining a differential operator with a Gaussian filter.

3.2.3 Feature Extraction

A feature extractor is used to reduce the space of the significant image elements, that is, a facilitator of the classification process and is often applied not only for the recognition of objects, but also to group together similar characteristics in the image segmentation process [24]. Therefore feature extraction is a way to achieve dimensional reduction. This task is especially important in real-time applications because they receive a stream of input data that must be processed immediately. Usually, there is a high degree of redundancy is such data stream (much data with repeated information) and need to be reduced to a set of representative features. If the extracted features are carefully chosen, this set is expected to bring relevant information to perform a task. The steps taken here to sieve the significant pixels in the data stream were *Motion detection* and *Skin detection*, which are detailed next.

3.2.4 Motion Detection

The technique chosen to perform the motion detection consisted in making a background subtraction, removing the pixels that have not been altered from the previous frame, thereby decreasing the number of pixels to be subjected to the subsequent process of gesture recognition. The algorithm performed the following steps:

- Capture two frames;
- Compare the colors of the pixels in each frame;
- If the color is the same, replace the original color by a white pixel. Otherwise leave it unchanged.

This algorithm, while reducing the amount of pixels in the image that will be presented to the process of gesture recognition can still display some elements that do not relate to the gesture itself, such as the clothing of the user or other object that may be moving the captured images and that will only increase the need of processing without the end result being of any relevance.

A second way to reduce the amount of pixels is applying a color filter. As the goal is to track gestures, the choice was Skin detection.

3.2.5 Skin Detection

There may be many objects in the environment that have the same color as the human skin, which varies in color, hues, color, intensity and position of the illumination source, the environment the person is in, etc. In such cases, even a human observer cannot determine whether a particular color was obtained from a region of the skin or an object that is in the image without taking into account contextual information. An effective model of skin color should solve this ambiguity between skin colors and other objects.

It is not a simple task to build a model of skin color that works in all possible lighting conditions. However, a good model of skin color must have some kind of robustness to succeed even in varying lighting conditions. A robust model requires an algorithm for color classification and a color space in which all objects are represented. There are many algorithms, including multilayer perceptrons [15], self-organizing maps, linear decision boundaries [6, 15], and based on the probabilistic density estimation [24]. The choice of color space is also varied: RGB [21] YCbCr [6], HSV [6], CIE Luv [24] Farnsworth UCS [15], and normalized RGB [21].

Some problems can be solved more easily by using the HSV representation [21], formed by the components Hue, Saturation and Value. The hue is the type of color ranging from red to violet, and from 0 to 360. The saturation indicates how much the color is gray, the lower the value the greater the amount of gray. Finally, the value defines the brightness of the color, ranging between 0 and 100 %. Due to this characteristic, HSV allows more easily to express certain types of image characteristics. The HSV format simplified pattern detection channel saturation and hue, for skin tones to be performed regardless of ethnic variation, therefore the value associated with skin color. No specific method is required for the extraction techniques to detect only certain patterns of colors. Thus, the color model of human skin used in this chapter is the HSV.

The steps of the algorithm for detecting skin are described below. Steps 1–2 are responsible for detecting skin color. Steps 3–4 are for segmentation using skin color and edge. Step 5 is post-processing.

Step 1 Convert the image from RGB to HSV to enhance skin tones. Apply a median filter (smoothing) of size 3×3 to soften and make the most homogeneous possible skin tone present in the image.

Step 2 Apply a threshold of skin tones, containing a minimum and a maximum for each color layer. This threshold should provide all possible kinds of skin tones, even though still remaining after certain objects in the image that are not skin.

Step 3 Apply canny edge detector and Sobel on color channels of the input image to find the edge pixels. The two edge filters are required as the canny edge detector is suitable for detecting strong edges between homogeneous regions, while the Sobel is better in the detection of non-homogeneous blocks within a region of skin color.

Step 4 Remove regions that are smaller than 1 % of the larger region, and regions whose area is reduced to less than 5 % after a morphological erosion operation.

Step 5 Rewrite the output of these algorithms in the original image by removing objects that do not fit this pattern.

A single color filter usually is not enough to detect objects in uncontrolled environments. For this reason this project adopted motion detection as an initial step to perform the elimination of pixels of no interest to the recognition process.

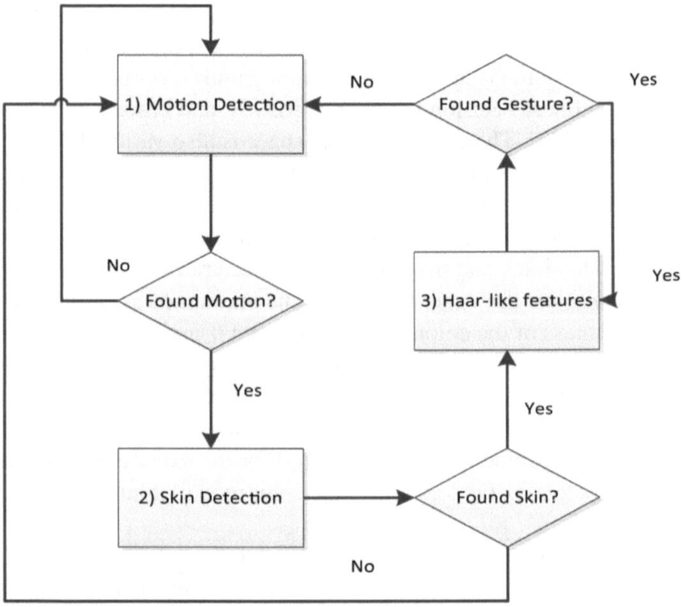

Fig. 3 Diagram of the process of gesture recognition using motion detection, skin and Haar cascade [20]

3.3 Classifiers in Action

The detection of gestures using the Haar classifier is done by sliding a search window across the image and checking whether a region of the image in a certain location can be classified as a gesture. In uncontrolled environments, gestures can be presented to the different distances that were used to build the classifier. For such reason, the method proposed here uses Haar scaling to modify the size of the detector rather than scaling the image.

The initial size of the detector is 20×20 pixels, and after each scanning of the sliding window over the entire frame containing the image, the scale of the detector is increased by α. The search process defined by the values in the image classifier can be affected both in efficiency and in performance, because if the scale s, the detector window is configured to $[s\Delta]$, where [ ] represents the rounding operation. The choice of the factor α affects both the speed of the detection process for accuracy. Such a value has to be carefully chosen in order to obtain a better relationship between accuracy and processing time. The factor α applied in this project is $10\,\%$.

The developed system received 800×600 images containing hand gestures. The assessment of the classifier showed that it could process 20 frames per second and correctly detected 89 % of the input frames, executing on a machine with a processor Intel i5 2.27 GHz M430.

The diagram in Fig. 3 shows the complete flow of the image processing technique presented in [20], from image capture to gesture recognition, in which the key steps

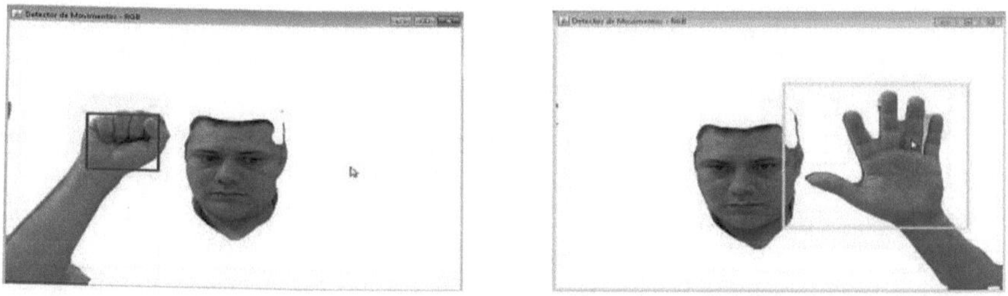

Fig. 4 Detection of the open right hand and left hand in hand after the steps of skin detection and motion detection, passing the resulting vector to the classifier

were already outlined. Figure 4 shows the open right hand and left hand being detected.

3.4 *Camshift*

CamShift is a method of object tracking, which is a modification of the method MeanShift. The Mean-Shift algorithm is a robust non-parametric technique used to find the mode in a probability distribution [1, 2].

In CamShift, the MeanShift algorithm is modified so that it can handle the changing dynamics of the probability distribution of color taken from the images submitted to the process [18]. The CamShift is an algorithm that starts with the selection of a target region defined manually by a user, with little care or certainty that this is the best area to be used for screening of a gesture or object. This uncertainty when defining rectangles for the object or gesture can result in errors yielding a decrease in the robustness of the method. As in the selection of the region of interest, in each frame there is a lot of background information included; these will also be information to be tracked by the process of search.

The CamShift algorithm can be summarized by the following steps:

1. Definition of the initial region of interest that contains the object one wants to track.
2. Creating a color histogram of the region containing the object.
3. Make a probability distribution of the frame using the color histogram.
4. Based on the image of probability distribution, find the center of mass of the search window using the method MeanShift.
5. Center of the search window to the point of taken over from step 4 and performing loops from step 4 until convergence.
6. Process the next frame with the position of the search window from step 5.

The CamShift algorithm tracks the gesture from a color image, it is designed to work with images with the HSV color system, requiring only the Hue component for the construction of the histogram.

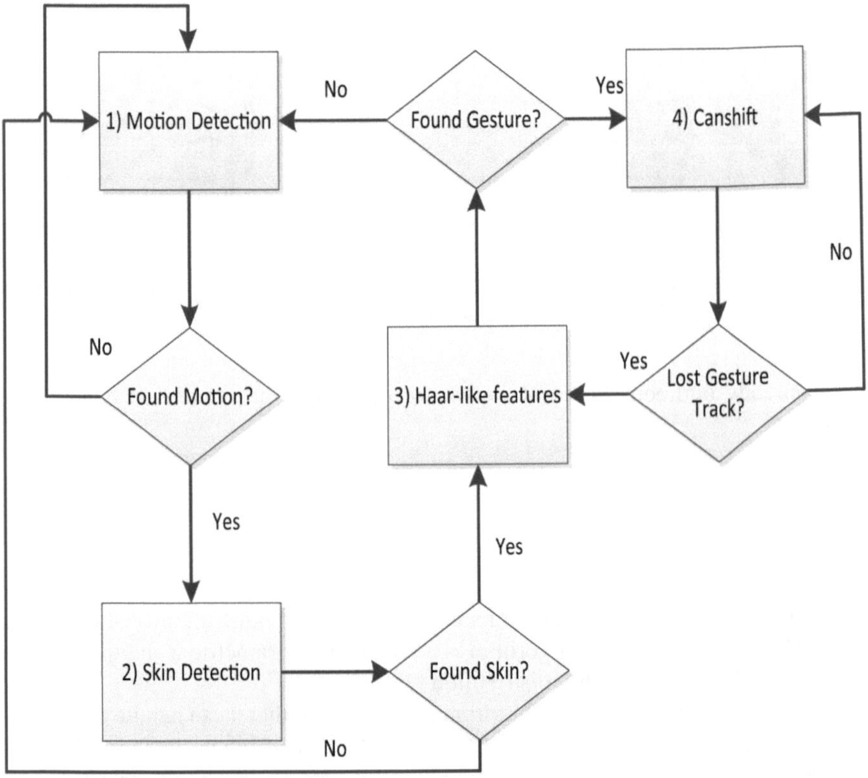

Fig. 5 Diagram of the gesture recognition process using motion, skin, Haar cascade and CamShift

In this project, the CamShift procedure receives a defined region from the Haar classifier as input. At this stage the CamShift is no longer receiving ROIs of motion and skin detection, so the images that are passed to it does not contain pixels that have a component H with a value less than 60, thus only the most relevant pixels are processed.

The addition of the CamShift procedure and removal of the Haar transform after the positive gesture identification yielded a throughput of 28 frames per second with a correct detection rate of 94 %, thus a performance gain of 29 and 5.6 % efficiency over the algorithm presented in [20].

The diagram in Fig. 5 shows the complete flow of the image processing technique developed in this chapter.

4 Results and Discussion

To benchmark the efficiency of the classifier built here recognition tests were performed using an image database with 1000 files for each gesture. Such files were generated together with 2000 files used to build the classifier encompassing people

Table 1 Results obtained in the efficiency tests for the classifiers developed

Gesture	True positive (%)	False positive (%)
a	80	20
b	78	22
c	93	11
d	91	9
e	93	7

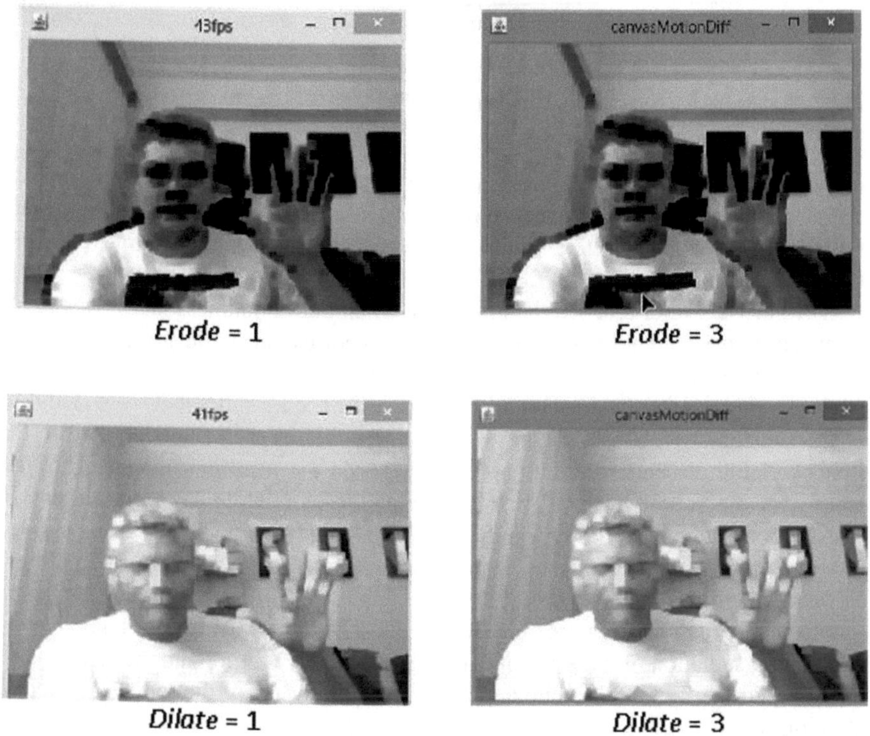

Fig. 6 Testing images applying erosion and dilatation filters

of different skin color using non-uniform varied backgrounds under several illumination scenarios. Such test files were not used for training the classifiers, being kept only for benchmarking purposes of gesture recognition accuracy.

Table 1 presents the results of the classifiers for each of the gesture. The average accuracy of the proposed classifier for gesture recognition reached 87 %.

To assess the efficiency of the each of the processing phases of the images used in this work, specific tests were made to analyze the preprocessing, segmentation, feature extraction and the classification performance.

In the preprocessing phase the values of the components of the morphological transformation were varied and it was observed if the recognition algorithm still succeeded in correctly detecting a gesture. Figure 6 shows the variation of the values

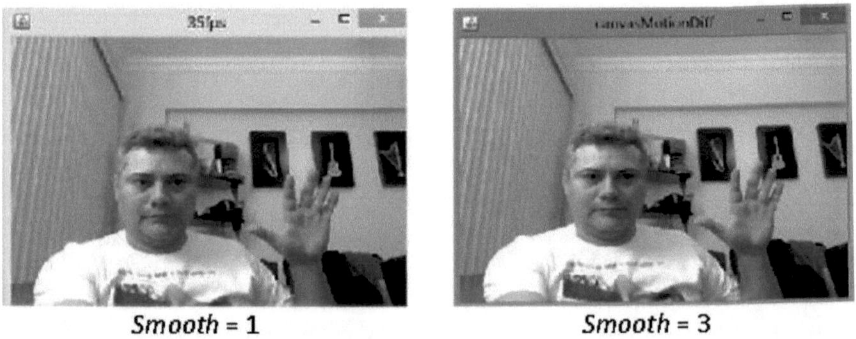

Fig. 7 Results obtained using image smoothening filters

of the erosion and dilatation component. The best configuration observed was the one that used the erosion factor equal to three and dilatation factor also equal to three. Other values for such factors would eliminate parts that were relevant to gesture detection.

The gaussian filter reached the best value when the smoothness factor was equal to five, because it did not eliminate the pixels that correspond to the gestures, making the other pixels more uniform as may be seen in Fig. 7.

The parameters of the edge recognition filters of Canny and Sobel were analyzed in the segmentation phase. Figure 8 shows the effect of such filters applied to the images yielding a better definition of the edges in the resulting images. The best setting for the Sobel filter was with factor equal to two, while for Canny filter that was 120, both with the minimum number of edges equal to three. Such setting yielded a "strengthen" in the edges of the gesture parts, eliminating the elements that did not fit such pattern.

Feature extraction made use of two techniques: Motion Detection and Skin Detection. The association of those two techniques attempted to eliminate the static pixels and that did not fit the minimum and maximum thresholds of the ranges defined as skin tones.

Two techniques were used in Motion Detection: the border and internal pixel detection, the latter also known as *gaussian mixture*. Some of the results of the tests performed over the parameters of such two techniques are shown in the images of Fig. 9.

The best configuration to the Motion Detection algorithm used a frame distance factor equal to three and a Gaussian mixture with a morphological transformation factor of five and a smoothness factor of three, because those were the parameters that kept at minimum the variation of the quantity of moving pixels.

The Skin Detection algorithm used as lower thresholds in its components $r = 25$, $g = 55$ and $b = 5$ and the upper thresholds of $rr = 160$, $gg = 255$, $bb = 190$ (Fig. 10).

After the tests that used only the Haar-like classifiers other resources were tested to assess the result of feature extraction with the techniques of Motion Detection, Skin Detection and CamShift. The results obtained are shown in Fig. 11.

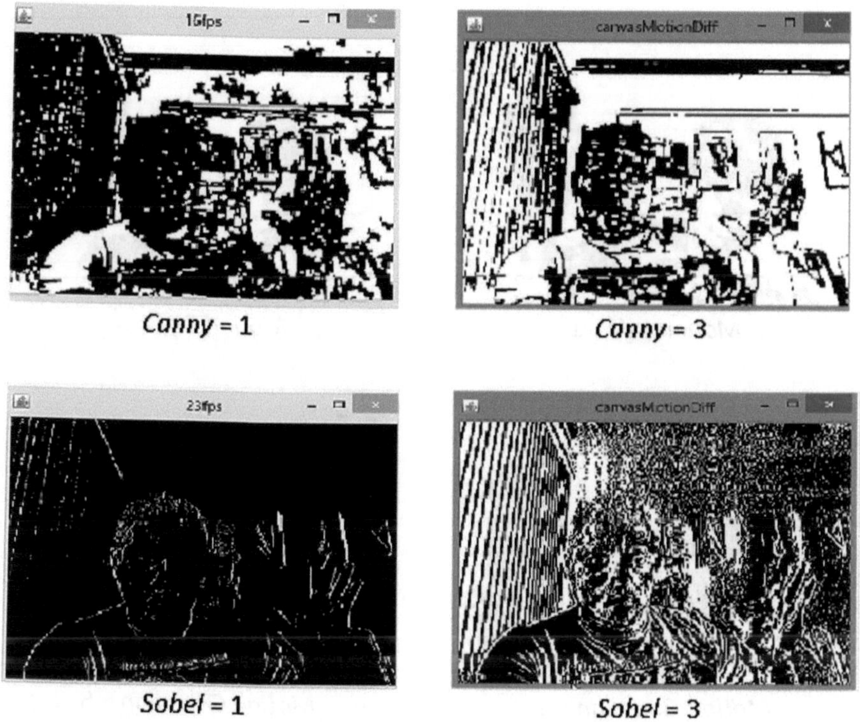

Fig. 8 Results of the application of Canny and Sobel filters

One must remark that using a Haar-like classifier there was a high processing effort involved in the task of tracking the gesture. That fact was observed by counting the number of frames per second in the classifier that were able to be processed using each of the methods described. Such processing effort was made lower with the association of techniques of Motion and Skin Detection, which reduced the quantity of bits that was submitted to the comparison process with the classifier, but that was still far behind of the throughput of the camera. Besides the performance factor, the classifier had its performance degraded with the variation in the illumination, and changes in angles and rotation of the gestures presented. As the real performance bounds in real-time image processing is the throughput of the capture device, CamShift was used as it is a technique that is a gesture or object tracking scheme that has constant-time performance after that the Haar-like classifier has performed the mapping of the gestures onto the classifiers. The addition of CamShift, removing the tracking task of the Haar-like scheme presented a processing performance of 26 frames per second.

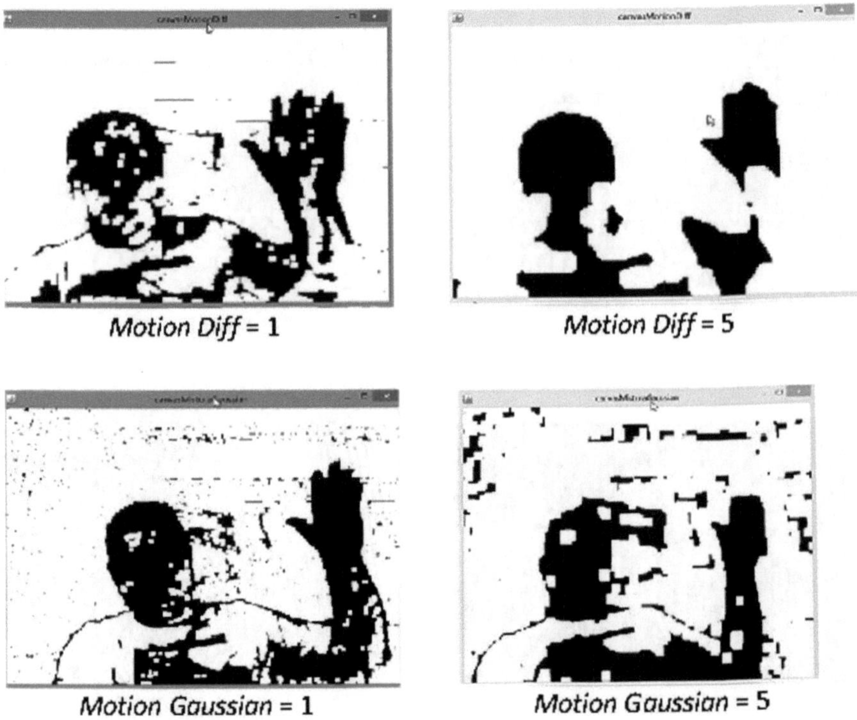

Fig. 9 Results for the movement detection application

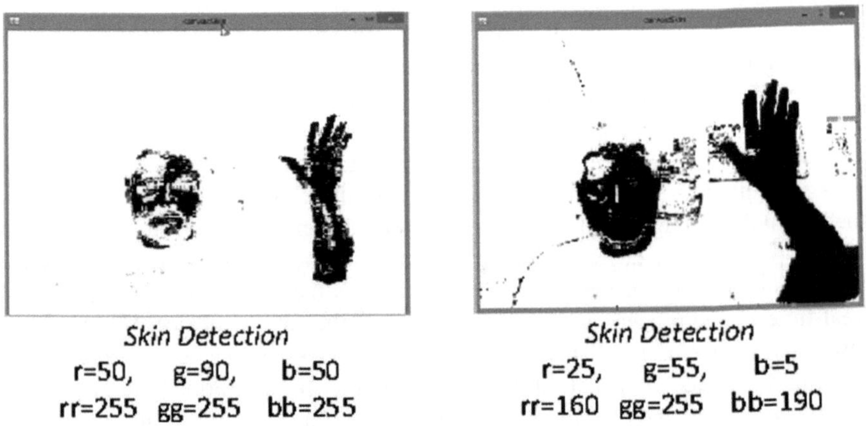

Fig. 10 Tests for skin detection

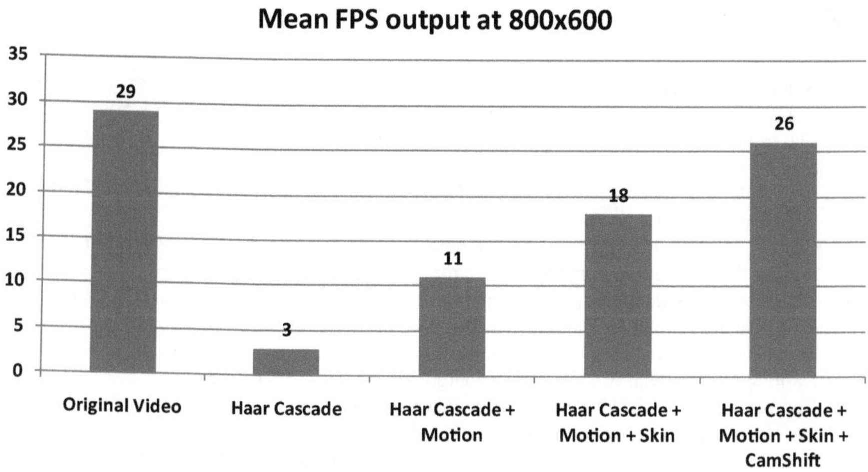

Fig. 11 Diagram comparing the several methods to the one proposed in this project (rightmost bar)

5 Conclusions

Real-time gesture recognition widens the frontiers of man-machine interaction and is becoming an area of growing interest. It is a task that requires intensive computational resources, thus it is important to find more efficient algorithms to reach the maximum performance of the equipment used. The combination of motion and skin detections, and the use of various image processing operations are important to improve the perception of gestures that will be delivered to the classifier, but those are not sufficient to ensure good performance.

The Haar classifier presents a feature that must be modified to make efficiency and performance meet. In general, to increase the efficiency in pattern recognition one has also to increase the processing time and vice versa, leaving the designer to find out what the best trade-off values.

The use of CamShift, despite having some difficulty in effectively locating gestures in an environment that has a similar color background to the color of the skin of the hand of the user, has proved to be efficient in tracking gestures in real time even in noisy environments.

The algorithm presented here lost only 3 frames in identifying gestures using a camera operating at 29 frames per second. It was also able to correctly identify 87 % of the gestures presented to it.

References

1. Allen JG, Xu RYD, Jin JS (2004) Object tracking using camshift algorithm and multiple quantized feature spaces. In: VIP '05: Proceedings of the Pan-Sydney area workshop on Visual information processing, pp 3–7, Darlinghurst, Australia, Australia, Australian Computer Society, Inc.
2. Bradski G, Kaehler A (2008) Learning OpenCV: computer vision with the OpenCV library. O'Reilly Media Inc., pp 415–453
3. Canny J (1986) Uma aproximação computacional para afiar a detecção, transporte de IEEE. Análise do teste padrão e inteligência da máquina 8:679–714
4. DU Heng, TszHang TO (2011) Hand gesture recognition suing Kinect. Department of Electrical and Computer Engineering, Boston University, Boston, USA
5. Freund Y, Schapire RE (1996) Experiments with a new boosting algorithm. In machine learning-international workshop then conference, pp 148–156. Citeseer
6. Garcia C, Tziritas G (1999) Face detection using quantized skin color regions merging and wavelet packet analysis. IEEE Multimedia 1(3):264–277
7. Gonzalez RC, Woods, RE (2008) Digital image processing, 3rd edn. Prentice Hall, Upper Saddle River
8. Handenberg C (2001) Finger tracking and hand posture recognition for real-time human-computer interaction, master these at Fachbereich Elektrotechnik und Informatik der Technischen Universität Berlin
9. Jones M, Viola P (2001) Rapid object detection using a boosted cascade of simple features. IEEE CVPR
10. Kulesa T, Hoch M (1998) Efficient color segmentation under varying illumination conditions. Academy of media arts, Peter-Welter—Platz 2. Venue tenth IEEE image and multidimensional digital signal processing (IMDSP) workshop, Germany
11. Lienhart R, Kuranov A, Pisarevsky V (2002) Empirical analysis of detection cascades of boosted classifiers for rapid object detection. MRL Technical Report, May 2002
12. Miranda LC, Hornung HH, Baranauskas MCC (2009) Prospecting a gesture based interaction model for iDTV. In: IADIS international conference on interfaces and human computer interaction (IHCI)/IADIS multi conference on computer science and information systems (MCCSIS), 2009, Algarve, Portugal. Proceedings of the IADIS international conference on interfaces and human computer interaction. Lisbon, Portugal: IADIS Press. pp 19–26
13. Monteiro G, Peixoto P, Nunes U (2006) Vision-based pedestrian detection using Haar-like features. Institute of Systems and Robotic. Coimbra—Portugal
14. Phillip Ian W, Fernandez Dr J (2009) Facial feature detection using Haar classifiers. Texas A & M University—Corpus
15. Phung L, Chai D, Bouzerdoum A (2001) A universal and robust human skin color model using neural networks. In: Proceeding IJCNN'01, July 2001, pp 2844–2849
16. Silva FWSV da Motion capture: introdução à tecnologia, Rio de Janeiro. http://www.visgraf.impa.br/Projects/mcapture/publ/mc-tech/. Accessed 30 March 2014
17. Simoes WCSS, Lucena Jr V (2011) Remoção do Fundo da cena para Detecção da Silhueta da Mão Humana e Detecção de Movimentos. I SIGES—I Simpósio de Informática e Geotecnologia de Santarém. Santarém (ISSN: 2237–3519)
18. Simoes WCSS, Lucena Jr V, Collins E, Albuquerque W, Padilla R, Valente R (2010) Avaliação de ambientes de desenvolvimento para automação do problema do cubo mágico para o robô Lego Mindstorms NXT. V CONNEPI—Congresso Norte-Nordeste de Pesquisa e Inovação, Maceió (ISBN: 978-85-64320-00–0)
19. Simoes WCSS, Lucena Jr V, Leite J C, Silva CA de S (2012) Visíon por computador para manos a base de reconocimiento de gestos para la interacción com los sistemas operativos de escritório Windows y Linux. XXXIII UPADI—Convención Panamericana de Ingenierías. La Habana

20. Simoes WCSS, Barboza R da S, Lucena Jr V, Lins RD (2013) Use of hand gestures as interface for interaction between multi-users and the IDTV. XI EuroITV—European Interactive TV Conference. Como
21. Smith AR (1978) Color gamut transform pairs. In: proceedings of the 5th annual conference on computer graphics and interactive techniques, p 19. ACM
22. Wilson PI, Fernandez J (2009) Facial feature detection using Haar classifiers. Texas A & M University, Corpus Christi
23. Xiang S W G, Xuan Y (2009) Real-time follow-up head tracking in dynamic complex environments. J Shanghai Jiaotong Univ (Sci) 14:593–599 DOI 10.1007/s12204-009-0593-2
24. Yang M-H, Ahuja N (1999) Gaussian mixture model for human skin color and its applications in image and video databases. In: Proceedings SPIE Storage and Retrieval for Image and Video Databases, Jan 1999, pp 458–466

Hand Gesture Recognition System Based in Computer Vision and Machine Learning

Paulo Trigueiros, Fernando Ribeiro and Luís Paulo Reis

Abstract Hand gesture recognition is a natural way of human computer interaction and an area of very active research in computer vision and machine learning. This is an area with many different possible applications, giving users a simpler and more natural way to communicate with robots/systems interfaces, without the need for extra devices. So, the primary goal of gesture recognition research applied to Human-Computer Interaction (HCI) is to create systems, which can identify specific human gestures and use them to convey information or controlling devices. For that, vision-based hand gesture interfaces require fast and extremely robust hand detection, and gesture recognition in real time. This paper presents a solution, generic enough, with the help of machine learning algorithms, allowing its application in a wide range of human-computer interfaces, for real-time gesture recognition. Experiments carried out showed that the system was able to achieve an accuracy of 99.4 % in terms of hand posture recognition and an average accuracy of 93.72 % in terms of dynamic gesture recognition. To validate the proposed framework, two applications were implemented. The first one is a real-time system able to help a robotic soccer referee judge a game in real time. The prototype combines a vision-based hand gesture

P. Trigueiros (✉)
Insituto Politécnico do Porto, IPP, Porto, Portugal
e-mail: pjt@iscap.ipp.pt

P. Trigueiros · F. Ribeiro
DEI/EEUM—Departamento de Electrónica Industrial, Escola de Engenharia, Universidade do Minho, Guimarães, Portugal
e-mail: fernando@dei.uminho.pt

L. P. Reis
DSI/EEUM—Departamento de Sistemas de Informação, Escola de Engenharia, Universidade do Minho, Guimarães, Portugal
e-mail: lpreis@dsi.uminho.pt

P. Trigueiros · F. Ribeiro · L. P. Reis
Centro Algoritmi, Universidade do Minho, Guimarães, Portugal

L. P. Reis
LIACC—Laboratório de Inteligência Artificial e Ciência de Computadores, Porto, Portugal

J. M. R. S. Tavares, R. Natal Jorge (eds.), *Developments in Medical Image Processing and Computational Vision,* Lecture Notes in Computational Vision and Biomechanics 19, DOI 10.1007/978-3-319-13407-9_21

recognition system with a formal language definition, the *Referee CommLang*, into what is called the *Referee Command Language Interface System* (ReCLIS). The second one is a real-time system able to interpret the Portuguese Sign Language. Sign languages are not standard and universal and the grammars differ from country to country. Although the implemented prototype was only trained to recognize the vowels, it is easily extended to recognize the rest of the alphabet, being a solid foundation for the development of any vision-based sign language recognition user interface system.

1 Introduction

Hand gesture recognition for human computer interaction is an area of active research in computer vision and machine learning [19]. One of the primary goals of gesture recognition research is to create systems, which can identify specific gestures and use them to convey information or to control a device. Though, gestures need to be modelled in the spatial and temporal domains, where a hand posture is the static structure of the hand and a gesture is the dynamic movement of the hand. Being hand-pose one of the most important communication tools in human's daily life, and with the continuous advances of image and video processing techniques, research on human-machine interaction through gesture recognition led to the use of such technology in a very broad range of possible applications [3, 22], of which some are here highlighted:

- **Virtual reality**: enable realistic manipulation of virtual objects using ones hands [5, 43], for 3D display interactions or 2D displays that simulate 3D interactions.
- **Robotics and Tele-presence**: gestures used to interact with robots and to control robots [34] are similar to fully-immersed virtual reality interactions, however the worlds are often real, presenting the operator with video feed from cameras located on the robot. Here, for example, gestures can control a robots hand and arm movements to reach for and manipulate actual objects, as well as its movement through the world.
- **Desktop and Tablet PC Applications**: In desktop computing applications, gestures can provide an alternative interaction to mouse and keyboard [16, 17, 37, 41]. Many gestures for desktop computing tasks involve manipulating graphics, or annotating and editing documents using pen-based gestures.
- **Games**: track a player's hand or body position to control movement and orientation of interactive game objects such as cars, or use gestures to control the movement of avatars in a virtual world. Play Station 2 for example has introduced the Eye Toy [14], a camera that tracks hand movements for interactive games, and Microsoft introduced the Kinect [9] that is able to track users full body to control games.
- **Sign Language**: this is an important case of communicative gestures. Since sign languages are highly structural, they are very suitable as test-beds for vision-based algorithms [12, 26, 32, 44].

There are areas where this trend is an asset, as for example in the application of these technologies on interfaces that can help people with physical disabilities, or areas where it is a complement to the normal way of communicating. Sign language, for example, is the most natural way of exchanging information among deaf people, although it has been observed that they have difficulties in interacting with normal people. Sign language consists of a vocabulary of signs in exactly the same way as spoken language consists of a vocabulary of words. Sign languages are not standard and universal and the grammars differ from country to country. The Portuguese Sign Language (PSL), for example, involves hand movements, body movements and facial expressions [39]. The purpose of Sign Language Recognition (SLR) systems is to provide an efficient and accurate way to convert sign language into text or voice has aids for the hearing impaired for example, or enabling very young children to interact with computers (recognizing sign language), among others. Since SLR implies conveying meaningful information through the use of hand gestures [38], careful feature selection and extraction are very important aspects to consider

In terms of hand gesture recognition, there are basically two types of approaches: vision-based approaches and data glove methods. This paper focuses on creating a vision-based approach, to implement a system capable of performing posture and gesture recognition for real-time applications. Vision-based hand gesture recognition systems were the main focus of the work since they provide a simpler and more intuitive way of communication between a human and a computer. Using visual input in this context makes it possible to communicate remotely with computerized equipment, without the need for physical contact or any extra devices [8, 35].

As Hasanuzzaman [11] argue, it is necessary to develop efficient and real time gesture recognition systems, in order to perform more human-like interfaces between humans and robots. Although it is difficult to implement a vision-based interface for generic usage, it is nevertheless possible to design this type of interface for a controlled environment [13, 25]. Furthermore, computer vision based techniques have the advantage of being non-invasive and based on the way human beings perceive information from their surroundings [36]. However, to be able to implement such systems, there are a number of requirements that the system must satisfy, in order to be implemented in a successful way [25], which are:

- **Robustness**: the system should be user independent and robust enough to factors like visual noise, incomplete information due for example to occlusions, variations of illumination, etc.
- **Computational efficiency**: vision based interaction requires real-time systems, so the algorithms and learning techniques should be the most effective possible and computational cost effective.
- **Error tolerance**: mistakes on vision-based systems should be tolerated and accepted. If some mistake is made, the user should be able to repeat the command, instead of letting the system make wrong decisions.
- **Scalability**: the system must be easily adapted and configured so that it can serve a number of different applications. The core of vision based applications for human computer interaction should be the same, regardless of the application.

Also, we need to have systems that allow training gestures and learn models capable of being used in real-time interaction systems. These systems should be easily configurable in terms of the number and type of gestures that they can train, to ensure the necessary flexibility and scalability.

The rest of this paper is as follows. First we present the Vision-based Hand Gesture Recognition System Architecture in Sect. 2, where the modules that constitute it are described. In this section, the problem of hand detection and tracking are addressed, as well as the problem of hand segmentation. Also, hand posture classification and dynamic gesture classification implementations are described. In Sect. 3, the Referee Command Language Interface System (ReCLIS), built to validate the proposed framework and able to help a robotic soccer referee judge a game in real time is described. This section also discusses the problem of modelling the command semantics for command classification. Section 4 presents the Sign Language Recognition prototype architecture and discusses its implementation. The prototype can be used to supplement the normal form of communication for people with hearing impairment. Conclusions and future work are drawn in Sect. 5.

2 Vision-Based Hand Gesture Recognition System Architecture

The design of any gesture recognition system essentially involves the following three aspects: (1) *data acquisition and pre-processing*; (2) *data representation or feature extraction* and (3) *classification or decision-making*. Taking this into account, a possible solution to be used in any human-computer interaction system is represented in the diagram of Fig. 1. As it can be seen in the diagram, the system first detects and tracks the user hand, segments the hand from the video image and extracts the necessary hand features. The features thus obtained are used to identify the user gesture. If a static gesture is being identified, the obtained features are first normalized and the obtained instance vector is then used for classification. On the other hand, if a dynamic gesture is being classified, the obtained hand path is first labelled according to the predefined alphabet, giving a discrete vector of labels, which is then translated to the origin and finally used for classification. Each detected gesture is used as input into a module that builds the command sequence, i.e. accumulates each received gesture until a predefined sequence defined in the *Command Language* is found. The sequence thus obtained is classified into one of a set of predefined number of commands that can be transmitted to a Generic System Interface (GSI) for robot/system control.

In the following sections we will describe the problems of hand posture classification and dynamic gesture classification.

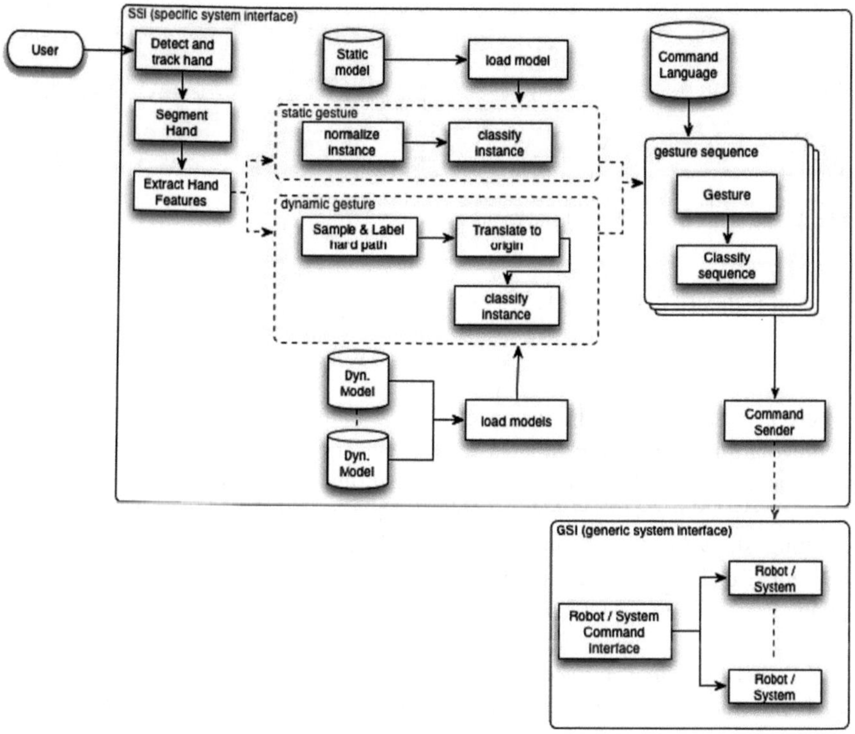

Fig. 1 Vision-based hand gesture recognition system architecture

2.1 *Hand Posture Classification*

For hand posture classification, hand segmentation and feature extraction is a crucial step in vision-based hand gesture recognition systems. The pre-processing stage prepares the input image and extracts features used later with classification algorithms [36]. The proposed system uses feature vectors composed of centroid distance values for hand posture classification. The centroid distance signature is a type of shape signature [36] expressed by the distance of the hand contour boundary points, from the hand centroid (x_c, y_c) and is calculated in the following manner:

$$d\,(i) = \sqrt{(x_i - x_c)^2 + (y_i - y_c)^2},\; i = 0, \ldots ., N - 1 \qquad (1)$$

This way, a one-dimensional function representing the hand shape is obtained. The number of equally spaced points N used in the implementation was 16. Due to the subtraction of centroid from the boundary coordinates, this operator is invariant to translation as shown by Rayi Yanu Tara [32] and a rotation of the hand results in a circularly shift version of the original image. All the features vectors are normalized, using the *z-normalization,* prior to training, by subtracting their mean and dividing

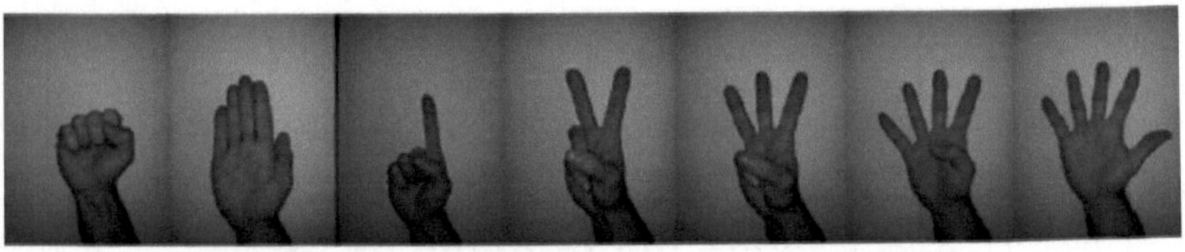

Fig. 2 The defined and trained hand postures

by their standard deviation [1, 23] as follows,

$$Z = \left(a_{ij} - \bar{a}\right) / \sigma \quad (2)$$

where $\bar{a}$ is the mean of the instance *i,* and σ is the respective standard deviation, achieving this way scale invariance as desired. The vectors thus obtained have zero mean and a standard deviation of 1. The resulting feature vectors are used to train a multi-class Support Vector Machine (SVM) that is used to learn the set of hand postures shown in Fig. 2, and used in the Referee Command Language Interface System (ReCLIS) and the hand postures shown in Fig. 3 used with the Sign Language Recognition System. The SVM is a pattern recognition technique in the area of supervised machine learning, which works very well with high-dimensional data. SVM's select a small number of boundary feature vectors, *support vectors,* from each class and builds a linear discriminant function that separates them as widely as possible (Fig. 4)—*maximum-margin hyperplane*[40]. Maximum-margin hyperplanes have the advantage of being relatively stable, i.e., they only move if training instances that are support vectors are added or deleted. SVM's are non-probabilistic classifiers that predict for each given input the corresponding class. When more than two classes are present, there are several approaches that evolve around the 2-class case [33]. The one used in the system is the one-against-all, where *c* classifiers have to be designed. Each one of them is designed to separate one class from the rest.

2.1.1 Model Training

For feature extraction, model learning and testing, a C++ application was built with openFrameworks [18], OpenCV [4], OpenNI [27] and the Dlib machine-learning library [15]. OpenCV was used for some of the vision-based operations like hand segmentation and contour extraction, and OpenNI was responsible for the RGB and depth image acquisition. Figure 5 shows the main user interface for the application, with a sample vector (feature vector) for the posture being learned displayed below the RGB image.

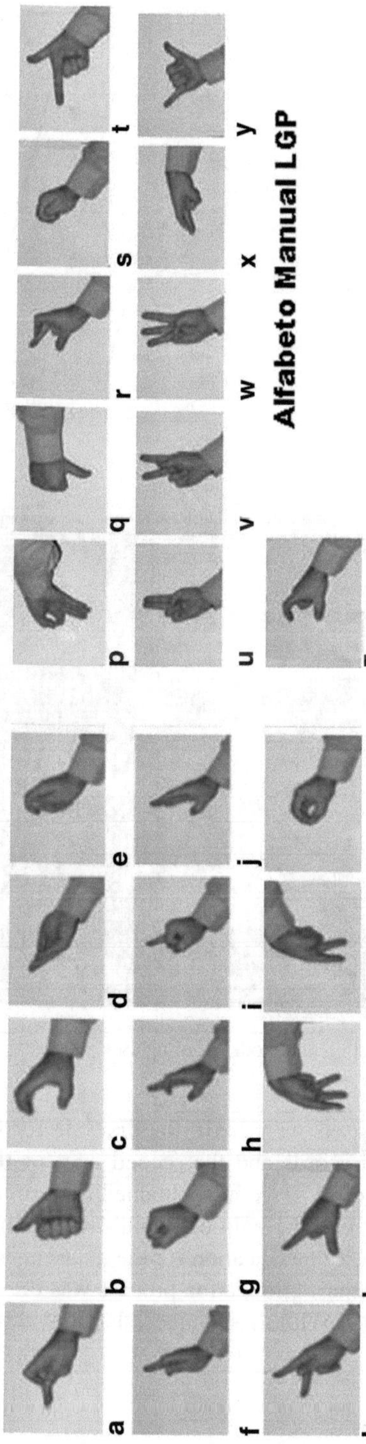

Fig. 3 Manual alphabet for the Portuguese Language

Fig. 4 SVM: support vectors representation with maximum-margin hyperplane [31]

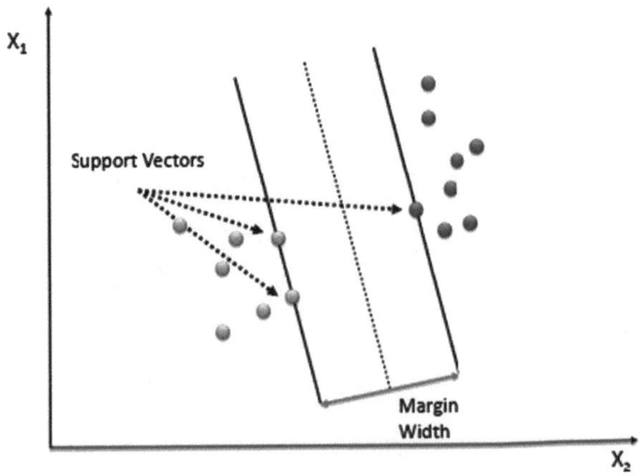

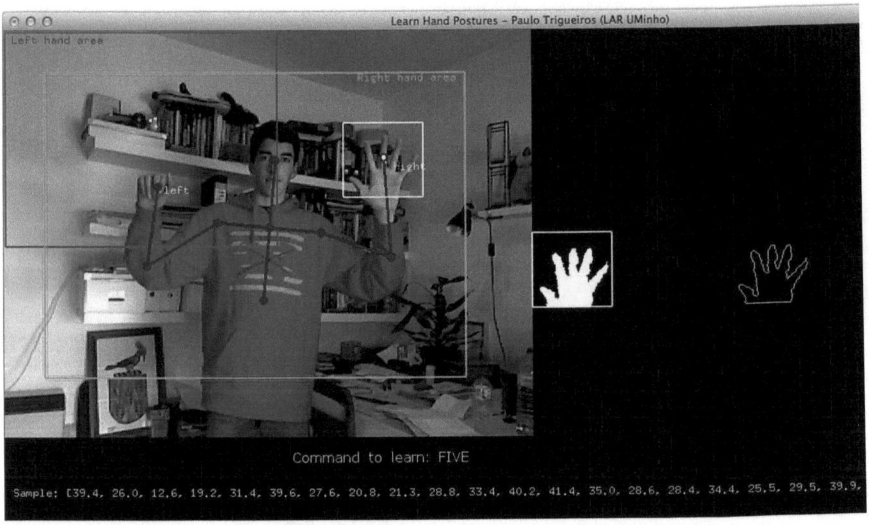

Fig. 5 Static gesture feature extraction and model learning user interface

Two centroid distance datasets were built: the first one for the first seven hand postures defined, with 7848 records and the second one for the Portuguese Sign Language vowels with a total of 2170 records, obtained from four users. The features thus obtained were analysed with the help of RapidMiner (Miner) in order to find the best kernel in terms of SVM classification for the datasets under study. The best kernel obtained with a parameter optimization process was the *linear kernel* with a *cost parameter* ***C*** equal to one. With these values, the final achieved accuracy was 99.4 %.

Table 1 Confusion matrix for the seven hand postures trained

	Actual class						
Predicted class	1	2	3	4	5	6	7
1	**602**	0	0	0	0	0	0
2	2	**712**	0	0	1	0	1
3	0	1	**578**	1	0	0	0
4	0	0	12	**715**	3	0	0
5	0	1	1	13	**542**	1	3
6	1	2	0	1	5	**701**	12
7	0	0	0	2	0	1	**751**

Table 2 Confusion matrix for the Portuguese Sign Language vowels

	Actual class				
Predicted class	1	2	3	4	5
1	**455**	0	0	2	0
2	0	**394**	1	1	0
3	0	0	**401**	1	0
4	4	2	0	**382**	0
5	0	0	1	0	**439**

In order to analyse how classification errors were distributed among classes, a confusion matrix for the two hand posture datasets was computed with the final results shown in Tables 1 and 2.

2.2 *Dynamic Gesture Classification*

Dynamic gestures are time-varying processes, which show statistical variations, making Hidden Markov Models (HMMs) a plausible choice for modelling the processes [29, 42]. A Markov Model is a typical model for a stochastic (i.e. random) sequence of a finite number of states [10]. When the true states of the model $S = \{s_1, s_2, s_3, \ldots, s_N\}$ are hidden in the sense that they cannot be directly observed, the Markov model is called a Hidden Markov Model (HMM). At each state an output symbol $O = \{o_1, o_2, o_3, \ldots, o_N\}$ is emitted with some probability, and the state transitions to another with some probability, as shown in Fig. 7. With discrete number of states and output symbols, this model is sometimes called a "*discrete HMM*" and the set of output symbols the *alphabet*. In summary, an HMM has the following elements:

Fig. 6 Gesture path with respective feature vector

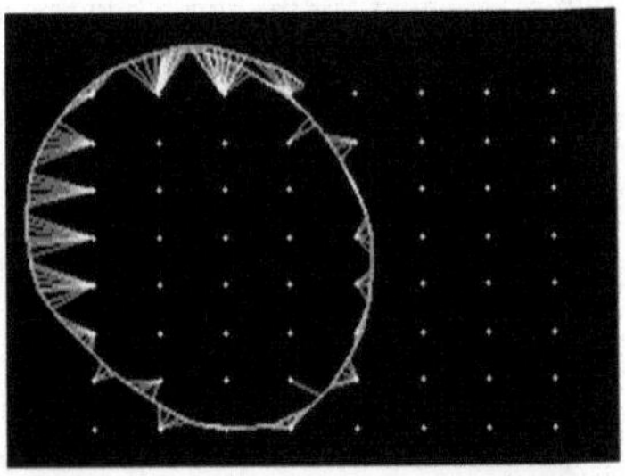

[1 2 2 2 3 3 4 4 4 5 6 13 13 14 14 14 14 14 14 14 13 13 20 19 19 18 18 17 24 23 22 22 22 22 22 29 29 29 29 29 29 29]

- **N**: the number of states in the model $S = \{S_1, S_2, \ldots, S_N\}$;
- **M**: the number of distinct symbols in the alphabet $V = \{v_1, v_2, \ldots, v_M\}$;
- State transition probabilities:

$$\boldsymbol{A} = \left[a_{ij}\right] \; where \; a_{ij} \equiv P\left(q_{t+1} = S_j | q_t = S_i\right) \; and \; q_t \; is \; the \; state \; at \; time \; t;$$

- Observation probabilities:

$$\boldsymbol{B} = \left\{b_j\left(m\right)\right\} \; where \; b_j\left(m\right) \equiv P\left(O_t = v_m | q_t = S_j\right)$$
$$and \; O \; is \; the \; observation \; sequence;$$

- Initial state probabilities: $\boldsymbol{\Pi} = [\pi_i] \; where \; \pi_i \equiv P\left(q_1 = S_i\right)$;

and is defined as $\lambda = (A, B, \Pi)$, where N and M are implicitly defined in the other parameters. The transition probabilities and the observation probabilities are learned during the training phase, with known data, which makes this is a supervised learning problem [36].

In this sense, a human gesture can be understood as a HMM where the true states of the model are hidden in the sense that they cannot be directly observed. So, for the recognition of dynamic gestures a HMM model was trained for each possible gesture. HMMs have been widely used in a successfully way in speech recognition and hand writing recognition [28]. In the implemented system, the 2D hand trajectory points are used and labelled according to the distance to the nearest centroid, based on Euclidean distance. The resulting vector is then translated to origin resulting in a discrete feature vector like the one shown in Fig. 6.

The feature vectors thus obtained are used to train the different HMMs and learn the model parameters. In the recognition phase an output score for the sample gesture is calculated for each model, given the likelihood that the corresponding model generated the underlying gesture. The model with the highest output score represents the recognized gesture. The implemented system uses a Left-Right (LR) HMM [1, 7], like the one shown in Fig. 7. This kind of HMM has the states ordered in time so that as time increases, the state index increases or stays the same. This topology has been chosen, since it is perfectly suitable to model the kind of temporal gestures used.

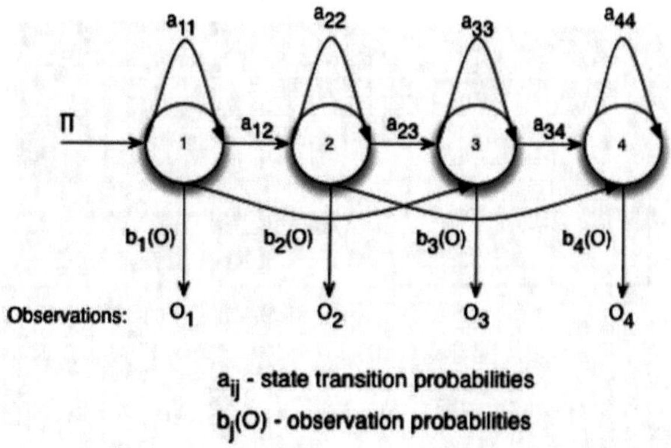

Fig. 7 A 4-state Left-Right HMM model

2.2.1 Model Training

For dynamic gesture model training, a C++ application for the acquisition of hand motion sequences (dynamic gestures) for each of the defined gestures, feature extraction and model training and testing was implemented. This application uses the same libraries as the previous application and an openFrameworks [18] add-on implementation of the HMM algorithm for classification and recognition of numeric sequences. This add-on is a C++ porting implementation of a MATLAB code from Kevin Murphy [24].

Figure 8 shows the main user interface for the application, with a hand path drawn on top of the centroids with the corresponding path distance to centroids drawn as white lines. For each gesture that required training, a dataset was built and the system trained in order to learn the corresponding model parameters. The number of observation symbols defined and implemented was 64 with 4 hidden states. Several values for the number of observations in the set $\{16, 25, 36, 49, 64, 81\}$, and hidden states, ranging from 2 to 12 were tried out during the experiments, without significant improvements for values greater than the selected ones.

For model testing, a new set of datasets were built with data from four different users with a total of 25 per gesture and per user, totalling 1100 records for the predefined 11 gestures (Fig. 9).

These datasets were analysed with the previous obtained models and the final accuracy results obtained with Eq. 3 are represented in Table 3.

$$accuracy = \frac{\#\, correctly\ predicted\ class}{\#\, total\ testing\ class} \times 100\% \qquad (3)$$

So, for the dynamic gesture recognition, with the obtained HMM models, an average accuracy of 93.72 % was achieved.

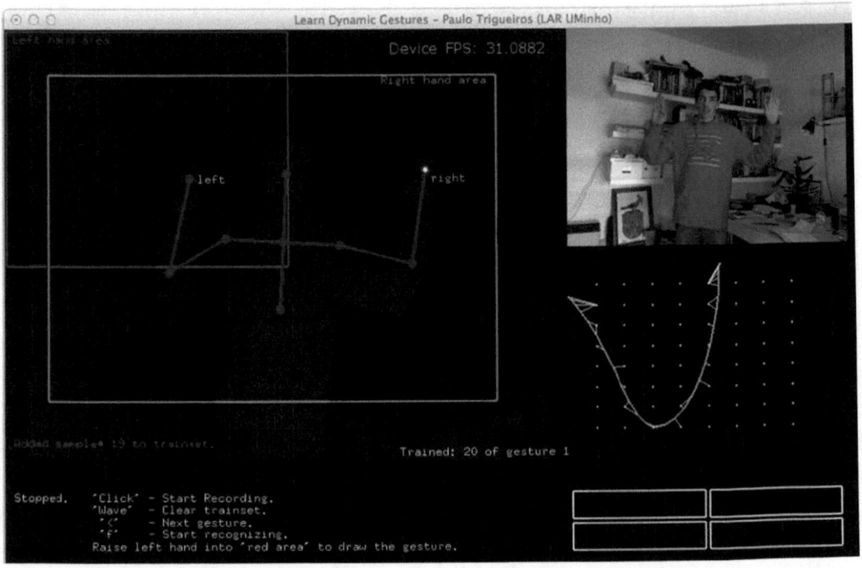

Fig. 8 Dynamic gestures feature extraction and model training user interface

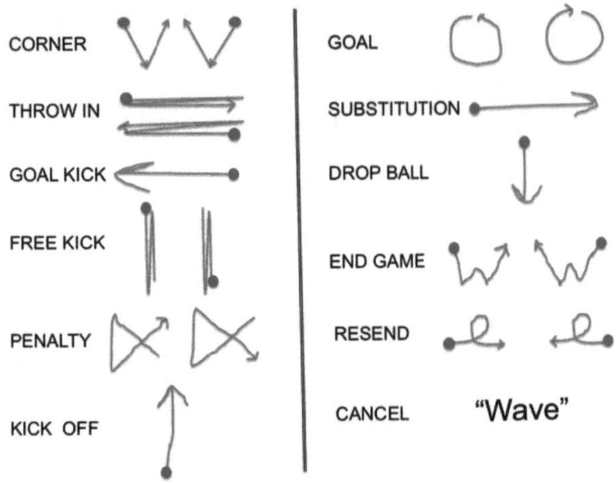

Fig. 9 The set of dynamic gestures defined and used in the Referee CommLang

Table 3 Hidden Markov Models accuracy for each gesture defined

Gesture	1	2	3	4	5	6	7	8	9	10	11
Accuracy (%)	75	100	100	100	92	88	92	100	100	96	88

3 Referee Command Language Interface System

To validate the proposed framework, an online system able to help a robotic soccer game referee judge a game in real time was implemented. The proposed solution combines a vision-based hand gesture recognition system with a formal language definition, the *Referee CommLang*, into what is called the *Referee Command Language Interface System* (ReCLIS). The system builds a command based on system-interpreted static and dynamic referee gestures, and is able to send it to a computer interface, which can then transmit the proper commands to the robots. The commands were defined in a new formal language described in Sect. 3.1. With the proposed solution, there is the possibility of eliminating the assistant referee, thereby allowing a more natural game interface.

The system uses only one camera, a Kinect camera [9], and is based on a set of assumptions, hereby defined:

1. The user must be within a defined perimeter area, in front of the camera.
2. The user must be within a defined distance range, due to camera limitations. System defined values are 0.7 m for the near plane and 3 m for the far plane.
3. Hand pose is defined with a bare hand and not occluded by other objects.
4. The system must be used indoor, since the selected camera does not work well under sun light conditions.

The following sections describe the Referee Command Language Definition and the Referee CommLang Prototype implementation.

3.1 *The Referee Command Language Definition*

This section presents the *Referee CommLang* keywords with a syntax summary and description. The *Referee CommLang* is a new and formal definition of all commands that the system is able to identify. As in [30], the language must represent all the possible gesture combinations (static and dynamic) and at the same time be simple in its syntax. The language was defined with BNF (Bakus Normal Form or Bakus-Naur Form) [2]:

- Terminal symbols (keywords and operator symbols) are in a constant-width typeface.
- Choices are separated by vertical bars '|' and in greater-than and less-than symbols (<choice>).
- Optional elements are in square brackets ([optional]).
- Sets of values are in curly braces ({set}).
- A syntax description is introduced with:: = .

The language has three types of commands: **Team commands**, **Player commands** and **Game commands.** This way, a language is defined to be a set of commands that can be a TEAM_COMMAND, a GAME_COMMAND or a PLAYER_COMMAND.

The TEAM_COMMAND is composed of the following ones: KICK_OFF, CORNER, THROW_IN, GOAL_KICK, FREE_KICK, PENALTY, GOAL or DROP_BALL.

A GAME_COMMAND can be the START or STOP of the game, a command to end the game (END_GAME), cancel the just defined command (CANCEL) or resend the last command (RESEND).

For the END_GAME command, it is necessary to define the game part, identified by PART_ID with one of four commands—1ST, 2ND, EXTRA or PEN (penalties).

```
<LANGUAGE>::={<COMMAND>}
<COMMAND>::=<TEAM_COMMAND> | <GAME_COMMAND> | <PLAYER_COMMAND>
<TEAM_COMMAND>::=<KICK_OFF> | <CORNER> | <THROW_IN> | <GOAL_KICK> | <FREE_KICK> |
      <PENALTY> | <GOAL> | <DROP_BALL>
<GAME_COMMAND>::=<START> | <STOP> | <END_GAME> | <CANCEL> | <RESEND>
<PLAYER_COMMAND>::=<SUBSTITUTION> | <PLAYER_IN> | <PLAYER_OUT> | <YELLOW_CARD> |
      <RED_CARD>
```

For the TEAM_COMMANDS there are several options: KICK_OFF, CORNER, THROW_IN, GOAL_KICK, FREE_KICK, PENALTY and GOAL that need a TEAM_ID (team identification) command, that can be one of two values - CYAN or MAGENTA, and finally the DROP_BALL command.

```
<KICK_OFF> ::= KICK_OFF <TEAM_ID>
<CORNER> ::= CORNER <TEAM_ID>
<THROW_IN> ::= THROW_IN <TEAM_ID>
<GOAL_KICK> ::= GOAL_KICK <TEAM_ID>
<FREE_KICK> ::= FREE_KICK <TEAM_ID>
<PENALTY> ::= PENALTY <TEAM_ID>
<GOAL> ::= GOAL <TEAM_ID>
<DROP_BALL> ::= DROP_BALL
```

For the PLAYER_COMMAND, first there is a SUBSTITUTION command with the identification of the player out (PLAYER_OUT) and the player in (PLAYER_IN) the game with the PLAYER_ID command.

The PLAYER_ID can take one of seven values (PL1, PL2, PL3, PL4, PL5, PL6, PL7). For the remaining commands: PLAYER_IN, PLAYER_OUT, YELLOW_CARD or RED_CARD, it is necessary to define the TEAM_ID as explained above, and the PLAYER_ID.

```
<SUBSTITUTION> ::= SUBSTITUTION <PLAYER_IN> <PLAYER_OUT>
<PLAYER_IN> ::= PLAYER_IN <TEAM_ID> <PLAYER_ID>
<PLAYER_OUT> ::= PLAYER_OUT <TEAM_ID> <PLAYER_ID>
<YELLOW_CARD> ::= YELLOW_CARD <TEAM_ID> <PLAYER_ID>
<RED_CARD> ::= RED_CARD <TEAM_ID> <PLAYER_ID>
<START> ::= START
<STOP> ::= STOP
<END_GAME> ::= END_GAME <PART_ID>
<CANCEL> ::= CANCEL
<RESEND> ::= RESEND
<TEAM_ID > ::= CYAN | MAGENTA
<PLAYER_ID> ::= PL1 | PL2 | PL3 | PL4 | PL5 | PL6 | PL7
<PART_ID> ::= 1ST | 2ND | EXTRA | PEN
```

3.2 *Referee CommLang Prototype Implementation*

The Human-Computer Interface (HCI) for the prototype was implemented using the C++ language, and the *openFrameworks* toolkit [18] with the OpenCV [4] and the OpenNI [27] add-ons.

The proposed system involves three modules as can be seen in the diagram of Fig. 10:

1. Data acquisition, pre-processing and feature extraction.
2. Gesture and posture classification with the models obtained in Sect. 2.1 and Sect. 2.2.
3. Gesture sequence construction or command classification.

As explained in Sect. 3, a referee command is composed by a set of dynamic gestures (Fig. 9) and hand postures (Fig. 2). The hand postures are used to identify one of the following commands: *team number*, *player number* or *game part*.

The problems of data acquisition, pre-processing, feature extraction and gesture classification were discussed in Sect. 2. The following section will describe the problem of modelling the command semantics for command classification.

3.3 *Command Classification*

Since the system uses a combination of dynamic and static gestures, modelling the command semantics became necessary. A Finite State Machine is a usually employed technique to handle this situation [6, 20]. In the implemented system, the FSM shown in the diagram of Fig. 11 and described in the state transition Table 4 was implemented to control the transition between three possible defined states: DYNAMIC, STATIC and PAUSE. A *state transition table*, as the name implies, is a table that describes all the conditions and the states those conditions lead to. A

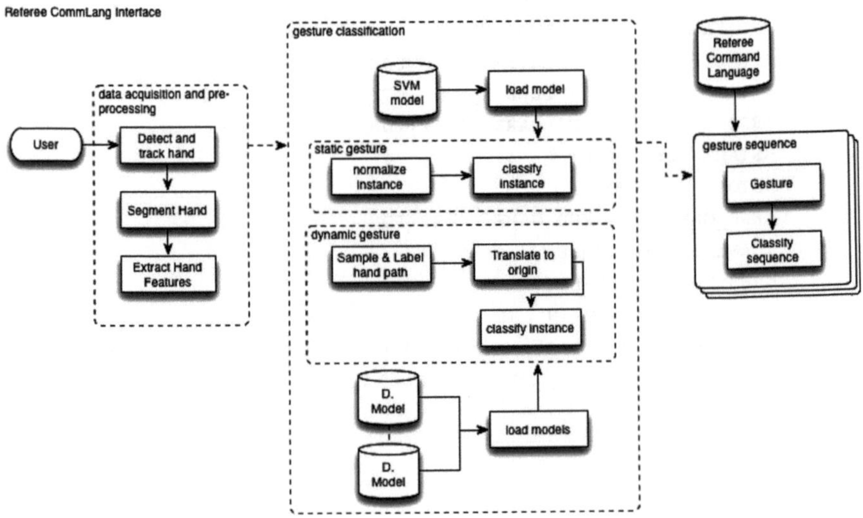

Fig. 10 Referee CommLang Interface diagram

Fig. 11 The Referee Command Language System finite state machine (FSM)

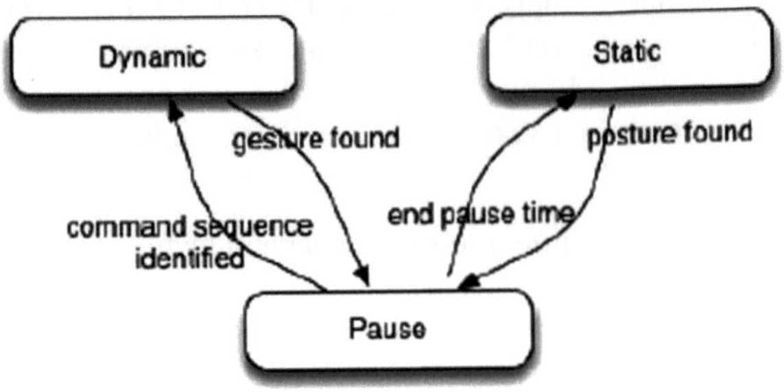

Table 4 The Referee CommLang state transition table

Current State	Condition	Sate transition
Dynamic	Found gesture	Pause
Static	Found posture	Pause
Pause	End pause time	Static
Pause	Command sequence identified	Dynamic

PAUSE state is used to control the transitions between user postures and gestures and somehow eliminate all unintentional actions between DYNAMIC/STATIC and STATIC/STATIC gestures. This state is entered every time a gesture or hand posture is found, and exited after a predefined period of time or when a command sequence is identified, as can be seen in the state transition table.

The following sequence of images, Fig. 12, Fig. 13 and Fig. 14, shows the Referee Command Language user interface with the "GOAL, TEAM1, PLAYER2" sequence of commands being recognized.

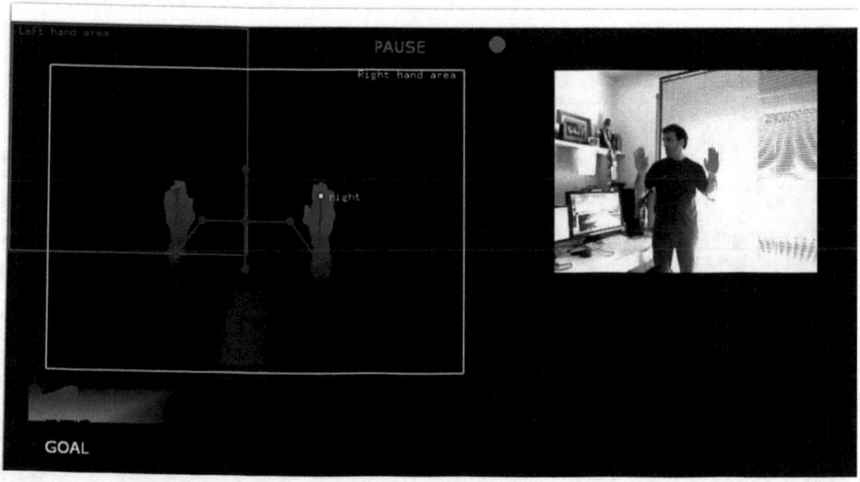

Fig. 12 The "GOAL" gesture recognized

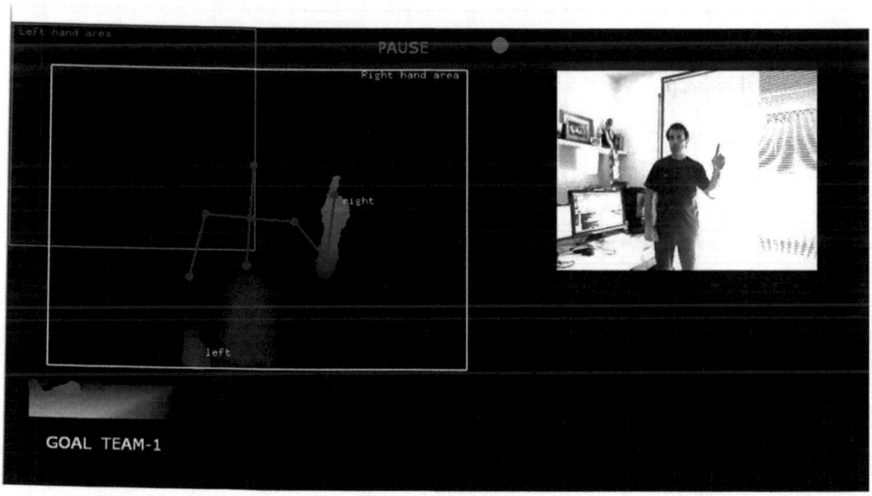

Fig. 13 The "GOAL, TEAM1" sequence recognized

4 Sign Language Recognition Prototype

The *Sign Language Recognition Prototype* is a real-time vision-based system whose purpose is to recognize the Portuguese Sign Language given in the alphabet of Fig. 3. The purpose of the prototype was to test and validate the proposed framework applied to the problem of real-time sign language recognition. For that, the user must be positioned in front of the camera, doing the sign language postures, that will be

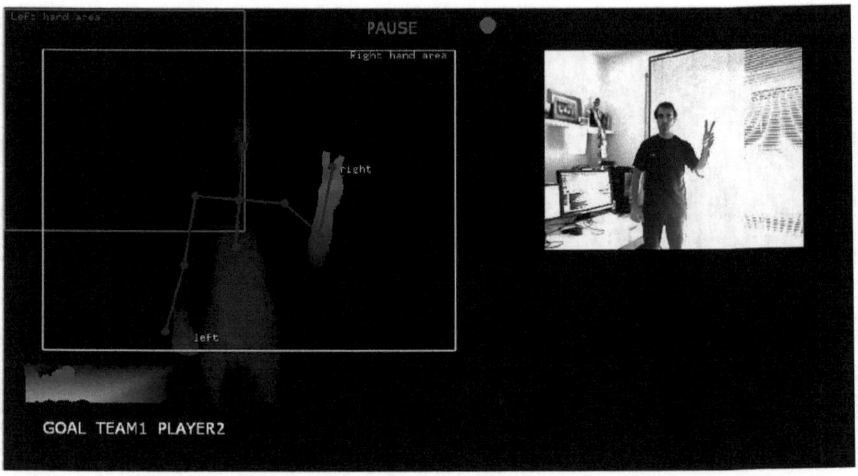

Fig. 14 The "GOAL, TEAM1, PLAYER2" sequence recognized

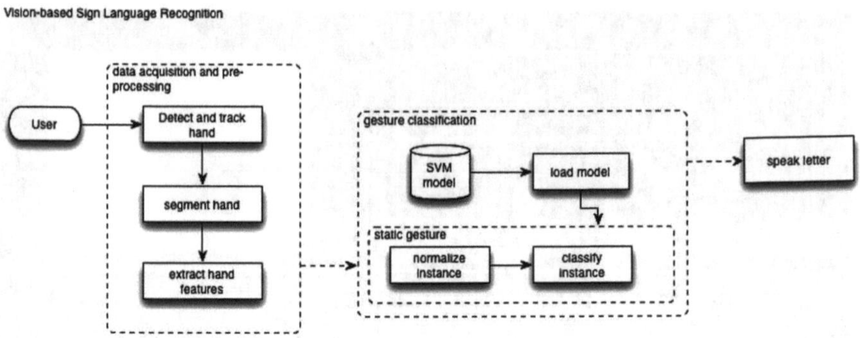

Fig. 15 Sign Language Recognition Prototype diagram

interpreted by the system and their classification will be displayed and spoken by the interface.

The diagram of Fig. 15 shows the proposed system architecture, which consists of two modules, namely: the *data acquisition, pre-processing and feature extraction model* and the *sign language posture classification model*.

In the first module, the hand is detected, tracked and segmented from the video images. From the obtained segmented hand, features are extracted, as explained in Sect. 2, for posture classification.

4.1 Prototype Implementation

The Human-Computer Interface (HCI) for the prototype was developed using the C++ language, and the openFrameworks toolkit [18] with the OpenCV [4] and the

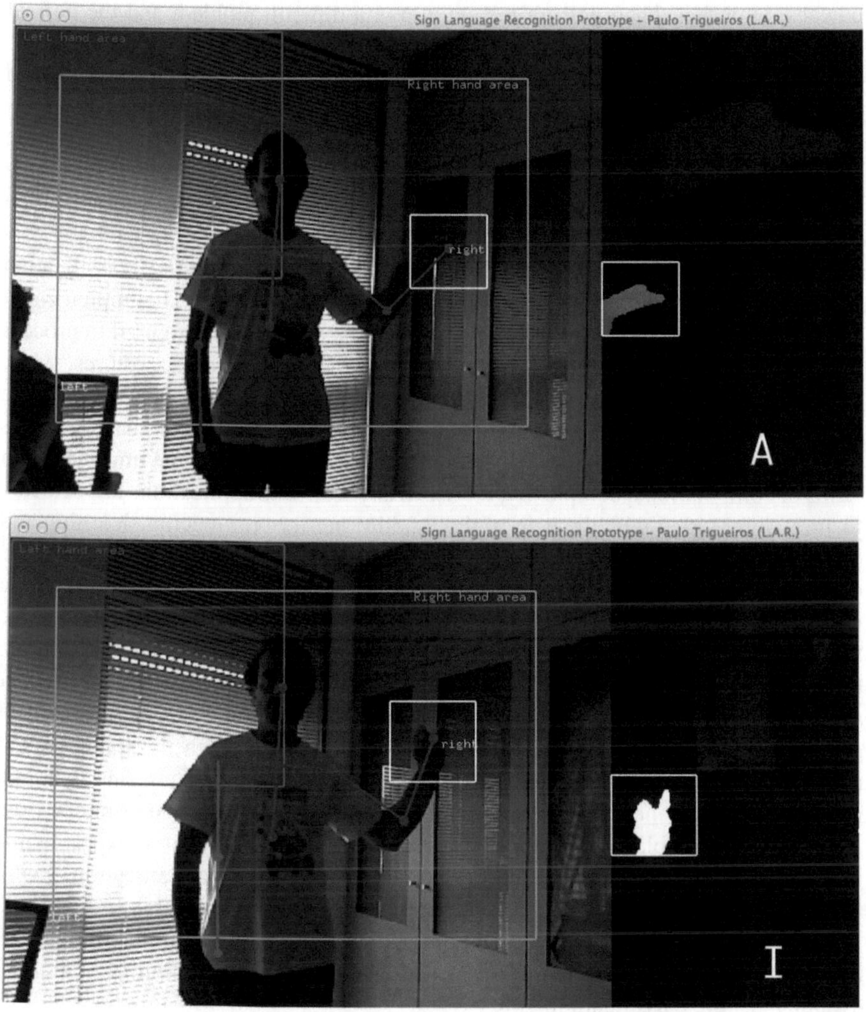

Fig. 16 Sign Language prototype interface wit two vowels correctly classified

OpenNI [27] add-ons, ofxOpenCv and ofxOpenNI respectively. In the following two images it is possible to see the Sign Language Prototype with two vowels correctly classified and displayed on the right side of the user interface (Fig. 16).

5 Conclusions and Future Work

Hand gestures are a powerful way for human communication, with lots of potential applications in the area of human computer interaction. Vision-based hand gesture recognition techniques have many proven advantages compared with traditional devices. However, hand gesture recognition is a difficult problem and the current work is only a small contribution towards achieving the results needed in the field.

The main objective of this work was to study and implement solutions that could be generic enough, with the help of machine learning algorithms, allowing its application in a wide range of human-computer interfaces, for online gesture and posture recognition. To achieve this, a set of implementations for processing and retrieving hand user information, learn statistical models and able to do online classification were created. The final prototype is a generic solution for a vision-based hand gesture recognition system, which is able to integrate posture and gesture classification and that, can be integrated with any human-computer interface. The implemented solutions, based on supervised learning algorithms, are easily configured to process new hand features or to learn different hand postures and dynamic gestures, while creating statistical models that can be used in any real-time user interface for online gesture classification. For the problem of hand posture classification, hand features that give good classification results were identified, being at the same time simple in terms of computational complexity, for use in any real-time application. The selected features were tested with the help of the RapidMiner tool for machine learning and data mining. That way, it was possible to identify a learning algorithm that was able to achieve very good results in terms of pattern classification, and that was the one used in the final solution. For the case of dynamic gesture recognition, the choice fell on Hidden Markov Models, due to the nature of the data, gestures, which are time-varying processes. This type of models has proven to be very effective in other areas of application, and had already been applied successfully to the problem of gesture recognition. The evaluation of the trained gestures with the implemented prototypes proved that, it was possible to successfully integrate static and dynamic gestures with the generic framework and use them for human/computer interaction.

It was also possible to prove through this study, and with the various experiments, which were carried out, that proper feature selection for image classification is vital for the future performance of the recognition system. It was possible to learn and select sensible features that could be effectively used with machine learning algorithms in order to increase the performance and effectiveness of online static and dynamic gesture classification.

To demonstrate the effectiveness of our vision based gesture recognition system, the proposed methods were evaluated with two applications: the Referee CommLang Prototype and the Sign Language Recognition Prototype. The first one is able to interpret user commands defined in the new formal language, *the Referee CommLang*, created with the aim of interpreting a set of commands made by a robotic soccer referee. The second one is able to interpret Portuguese sign language hand postures.

An important aspect to report on the implemented solutions has to do with the fact that new users were able to learn and adapt to the systems very quickly and were able to start using them in a normal way after a short period of time, making them solutions that can be easily adapted and applied to other areas of application.

As future work and major development prospects it is suggested:

- Explore other machine learning algorithms applied to the problem of hand gesture classification and compare obtained results.
- Include not only the possibility of 3D gestures but also to work with several cameras to thereby obtain a full 3D environment and achieve view-independent recognition, thus eliminating some limitations of the current system.
- Explore the possibility of applying stereo vision instead of only depth range cameras, applied to human/computer interaction and particularly to hand gesture recognition.
- Introduce gesture recognition with both hands, enabling the creation of more natural interaction environments.
- Investigate and try to find more reliable solutions for the identification of the beginning and end of a gesture.
- Build systems that are able to recognize continuous gestures, i.e., without the need to introduce pauses for gesture or command construction.
- Explore reinforcement learning as a way to start with a reduced number of hand features per gesture, reducing the time to learn the models, and be able to learn with user interaction, possibly using multimodal dialog strategies.
- Explore unsupervised learning applied to gesture recognition. Give the robot/system the possibility to learn by interaction with the user, again with the possibility of multimodal strategies.

As a final conclusion one can say that although there is still much to do in the area, the implemented solutions are a solid foundation for the development of generic gesture recognition systems that could be used with any interface for human computer interaction. The interface language can be redefined and the system can be easily configured to train different set of postures and gestures that can be easily integrated with any desired solution.

Acknowledgments The authors wish to thank all members of the Laboratório de Automação e Robótica (LAR), at University of Minho, Guimarães. The authors would like to thank also, everyone who contributed to the hand data features acquisition phase, without which it would have been very difficult to carry out this study. Also special thanks to the Polytechnic Institute of Porto, the ALGORITMI Research Centre and the LIACC Research Center, for the opportunity to develop this research work.

References

1. Alpaydin E (2004) Introduction to machine learning. MIT Press, Cambridge
2. Backus JW, Bauer FL, Green J, Katz C, Mccarthy J, Perlis AJ, Rutishauser H, Samelson K, Vauquois B, Wegstein JH, Wijngaarden AV, Woodger M (1960) Revised report on the algorithmic language ALGOL 60. Communications of the ACM. ACM
3. Bourennane S, Fossati C (2010) Comparison of shape descriptors for hand posture recognition in video. SIViP 6:147–157
4. Bradski G, Kaehler A (2008) Learning OpenCV: computer vision with the OpenCV library. O'Reilly Media, Sebastopol

5. Buchmann V, Violich S, Billinghurst M, Cockburn A (2004) FingARtips: gesture based direct manipulation in augmented reality. 2nd International Conference on Computer Graphics and Interactive Techniques in Australasia and South East Asia. ACM, Singapore
6. Buckland M (2005) Programming game AI by example. Wordware Publishing, Inc.
7. Camastra F, Vinciarelli A (2008) Machine learning for audio, image and video analysis. Springer, London
8. Chaudhary A, Raheja JL, Das K, Raheja S (2011) Intelligent approaches to interact with machines using hand gesture recognition in natural way: a survey. Int J Comp Sci Eng Survey 2:122–133
9. Chowdhury JR (2012) Kinect sensor for Xbox gaming. M. Tech CSE, IIT Kharagpur
10. Fink GA (2008) Markov models for pattern recognition—from theory to applications. Springer, Berlin
11. Hasanuzzaman M, Ampornaramveth V, Zhang T, Bhuiyan Ma, Shirai Y, Ueno H (2004) Real-time vision-based gesture recognition for human robot interaction. IEEE International Conference on Robotics and Biomimetics, August 22–26. Shenyang. IEEE, pp 413–418
12. Holt GAT, Reinders MJT, Hendriks EA, Ridder HD, Doorn AJV (2010) Influence of handshape information on automatic sign language recognition. 8th International Conference on Gesture in Embodied Communication and Human-Computer Interaction, February 25–27. Bielefeld. 2127632: Springer-Verlag, pp 301–312
13. Huang T, Pavlovic VH (1995) Gesture modeling, analysis, and synthesis. In Proc. of IEEE International Workshop on Automatic Face and Gesture Recognition, pp 73–79
14. KIM T (2008) In-depth: eye to eye—the history of Eyetoy [online]. http://www.gamasutra.com. http://www.gamasutra.com/php-bin/news_index.php?story=20975. Accessed 29 March 2013
15. King DE (2009) Dlib-ml: a machine learning toolkit. J Mach Learn Res 10:1755–1758
16. Kratz S, Rohs M (2011) Protractor3D: a closed-form solution to rotation-invariant 3D gestures. 16th International Conference on Intelligent User Interfaces. ACM, Palo Alto
17. LI Y (2010) Protractor: a fast and accurate gesture recognizer. Conference on Human Factors in Computing Systems. ACM, Atlanta
18. Lieberman Z, Watson T, Castro A (2004) OpenFrameworks [online]. http://www.openframeworks.cc/ (2011)
19. Maung THH (2009) Real-time hand tracking and gesture recognition system using neural networks. Proc World Acad Sci: Enginee Tech 50:466–470
20. Millington I, Funge J (2009) Artificial intelligence for games. Elsevier, USA
21. Miner R (2006) RapidMiner: report the future [online]. http://rapid-i.com/. Accessed Dec 2011
22. Mitra S, Acharya T (2007) Gesture recognition: a survey. IEEE transactions on systems, man and cybernetics. IEEE
23. Montgomery DC, Runger GC (1994) Applied statistics and probability for engineers. Wiley, USA
24. Murphy K (1998) Hidden Markov Model (HMM) toolbox for Matlab [online]. http://www.cs.ubc.ca/~murphyk/Software/HMM/hmm.html (2012)
25. Murthy GRS, Jadon RS (2009) A review of vision based hand gestures recognition. Int J Info Technol Knowl Manag 2:405–410
26. Ong SC, Ranganath S (2005) Automatic sign language analysis: a survey and the future beyond lexical meaning. IEEE Trans Pattern Anal Mach Intell 27:873–891
27. OPENNI (2013) The standard framework for 3D sensing [online]. http://www.openni.org/
28. Rabiner LR (1989) A tutorial on Hidden Markov Models and selected applications in speech recognition. Proc IEEE 77:257–286
29. Rabiner LR, Juang BH (1986) An introduction to Hidden Markov Models. IEEE ASSp Magazine
30. Reis LP, Lau N (2002) COACH UNILANG—a standard language for coaching a (robo) soccer team. In: Birk A, Coradeschi S, Tadokoro, S (eds) RoboCup 2001: Robot Soccer World Cup V. Springer Berlin Heidelberg
31. Sayad DS 2010. Support Vector Machine—Classification (SVM) [online]. http://www.saedsayad.com/support_vector_machine.htm. Accessed 8 Nov 2012

32. Tara RY, Santosa PI, Adji TB (2012) Sign language recognition in robot teleoperation using centroid distance Fourier descriptors. Int J Comput Appl 48(2):8–12
33. Theodoridis S, Koutroumbas K (2010) An introduction to pattern recognition: a Matlab Approach. Academic, Burlington
34. Trigueiros P, Ribeiro F, Lopes G (2011) Vision-based hand segmentation techniques for human-robot interaction for real-time applications. In: Tavares JM, Jorge RMN (eds) III ECCOMAS thematic conference on computational vision and medical image processing, 12–14 De Oubtubro 2011 Olhão. Taylor and Francis, Publication pp 31–35
35. Trigueiros P, Ribeiro F, Reis LP (2012) A comparison of machine learning algorithms applied to hand gesture recognition. 7th Iberian Conference on Information Systems and Technologies, 20–23 July. Madrid, pp 41–46
36. Trigueiros P, Ribeiro F, Reis LP (2013) A comparative study of different image features for hand gesture machine learning. 5th International Conference on Agents and Artificial Intelligence, 15–18 February. Barcelona
37. Vatavu R-D, Anthony L, Wobbrock JO (2012) Gestures as point clouds: a $P recognizer for user interface prototypes. 14th ACM International Conference on Multimodal Interaction. ACM, Santa Monica
38. Vijay PK, Suhas NN, Chandrashekhar CS, Dhananjay DK (2012) Recent developments in sign language recognition: a review. Int J Adv Comput Eng Commun Technol 1:21–26
39. Wikipedia (2012) Língua gestual portuguesa [online]. http://pt.wikipedia.org/wiki/Lingua_gestual_portuguesa. (2013)
40. Witten IH, Frank E, Hall MA (2011) Data mining—practical machine learning tools and techniques. Elsevier
41. Wobbrock JO, Wilson AD, Li Y (2007) Gestures without libraries, toolkits or training: a $1 recognizer for user interface prototypes. Proceedings of the 20th Annual ACM Symposium on User Interface Software and Technology. ACM, Newport
42. Wu Y, Huang TS (1999) Vision-based gesture recognition: a review. Proceedings of the International Gesture Workshop on Gesture-Based Communication in Human-Computer Interaction. Springer-Verlag.
43. Yoon J-H, Park J-S, Sung MY (2006) Vision-Based bare-hand gesture interface for interactive augmented reality applications. 5th International Conference on Entertainment Computing, September 20–22. Cambridge. 2092520: Springer-Verlag, pp 386–389
44. Zafrulla Z, Brashear H, Starner T, Hamilton H, Presti P (2011) American sign language recognition with the kinect. 13th International Conference on Multimodal Interfaces. ACM, Alicante

3D Scanning Using RGBD Imaging Devices: A Survey

Eduardo E. Hitomi, Jorge V. L. Silva and Guilherme C. S. Ruppert

Abstract The capture and digital reconstruction of tridimensional objects and scenarios are issues of great importance in computational vision and computer graphics, for the numerous applications, from navigation and scenario mapping, augmented reality to medical prototyping. In the past years, with the appearance of portable and low-cost devices such as the Kinect Sensor, which are capable of acquiring RGBD video (depth and color data) in real-time, there was a major interest to use these technologies, efficiently, in 3D surface scanning. In this paper, we present a survey of the most relevant methods from recent literature on scanning 3D surfaces using these devices and give the reader a general overview of the current status of the field in order to motivate and enable other works in this topic.

1 Introduction

Tridimensional scanning and reconstruction are processes related to the scan of intrinsic characteristics of objects surfaces or scenarios, like shape and appearance. While scanning deals with the capture of data on a surface and creation of a point cloud from the geometric samples collected, the process of reconstruction uses the point cloud data to extrapolate the surface shape. The use of these data is increasing in prototyping, navigation, augmented reality, quality control, among others and intense by the entertainment industry, motivating many research in computational vision and computer graphics.

G. C. S. Ruppert (✉) · E. E. Hitomi · J. V. L. Silva
Center for Information Technology Renato Archer, Campinas, SP, Brazil
e-mail: guilherme.ruppert@cti.gov.br

E. E. Hitomi
e-mail: eduardoe.hitomi@gmail.com

J. V. L. Silva
e-mail: jorge.silva@cti.gov.br

J. M. R. S. Tavares, R. Natal Jorge (eds.), *Developments in Medical Image Processing and Computational Vision,* Lecture Notes in Computational Vision and Biomechanics 19,
DOI 10.1007/978-3-319-13407-9_22

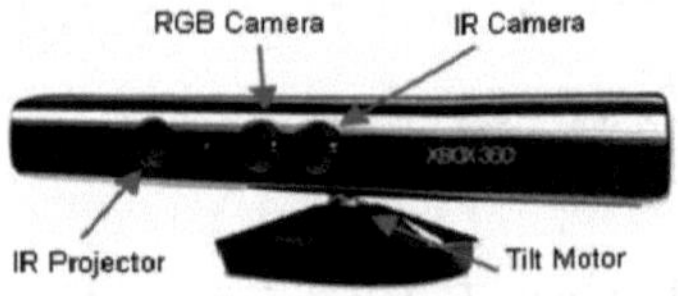

Fig. 1 Kinect main components

The processes of scanning and reconstruction are often combined and seen as a single pipeline, consisting basically of: acquiring the data map, translating it to point-cloud, allocation in a single coherent system of reference (also called alignment), and fusion of different captures in a single global solid model.

Although the 3D scanning technologies are not novel, they went through a revolution with the launch of the Kinect device, in 2010. This occurred by the presentation of the integrated depth camera with very low cost when compared to the existing high density scanners, and also for capturing with convincing quality, the geometry and colors of the objects and scenarios in real time.

The Kinect Sensor (Fig. 1) was launched initially as a accessory of the XBox360 game console, serving as a touchless joystick. The device is composed basically by a RGB camera, an infrared-based depth camera (then the D from the RGBD term), both with 640×480 resolution and frame rate of 30 fps, a set of microphones and a motor controlling the tilt of the device.

In particular, the depth sensor is comprised by an IR camera and an IR dotted pattern projector, and uses a computer vision technology developed by PrimeSense. It has an approximately range of 30 cm–6 m, and it allows building depth maps of 11-bit depth resolution. Open-source drivers (such as Libfreenect and Avin2/OpenNI) as well as the Microsoft Kinect SDK allow this product to be connected to a computer and to be used in many other applications other than gaming, such as: robotics, surveillance systems, intra-operatory medical imaging systems, accessibility, among others.

Other similar devices were also released, such as the Asus Xtion, Primesense Carmine and Panasonic D-Imager, but the Kinect remained as the most popular and reference device.

This work presents a survey of the main recent works from the literature related to 3D scanning using RGBD cameras, in special, the Kinect Sensor. The goal is to provide a wide survey of the area, providing references and introducing the methodologies and applications, from the simple reconstruction of small static objects to the constantly updated mapping of dense or large scenarios, in order to motivate and enable other works in this topic.

2 Methods

In this Section, we present the survey of methods found on the literature. For each method, we present: references, the responsible institution, release date, availability of the software or source-code, a general overview and a brief description of the method.

It is necessary to take into consideration the high rate of improvements and innovations in this topic currently, therefore, the methods in this section are limited to the progress of the new technologies until the time of conclusion of this work.

2.1 *Kinectfusion*

References: [1, 2]
Developed at: Microsoft Research Cambridge
Released in: October 2011
Availability: There is an open-source implementation in C++, called Kinfu, in the PCL (Point Cloud Library) project [3]. An implementation within Microsoft's Kinect for Windows SDK [4] will be released.

General Description In this method, only the depth image is used to track the sensor position and reconstruct 3D models of the physical scenario in real-time, limited to a fixed resolution volume (typically 512^3), through a GPU implementation. The RGB camera information is only used in the case of texture mapping. Although the approach aims at speed efficiency to explore real-time rates, it is not GPU memory efficient, requiring above 512 MB of capacity and 512 or more float-point colors, for an implementation using 32-bit voxels.

The authors show some potential applications of the KinectFusion modifying or extending the GPU pipeline implementation to use in 3D scanning, augmented reality, object segmentation, physical simulations and interactions with the user directly in the front of the sensor. Because of the speed and accuracy, the method has generated various other improved extensions for different applications.

Approach Basically, the system continually tracks the six degrees of freedom (DOF) pose of the camera and fuses, in real time, the camera depth data in a single global 3D model of a fixed size 3D scene. The reconstruction is incremental, with a refined model as the camera moves, even by vibrating, resulting in new viewpoints of the real scenario revealed and fused into the global model.

The main system of the GPU pipeline consists of four steps executed concurrently, using the CUDA language:

1. *Surface measurement:* the depth map acquired directly from the Kinect is converted in a vertex map and a normal map. Bilateral filtering is used to reduce the inherent sensor noise. Each CUDA thread works in parallel in each pixel of the depth map and projects as a vertex in the coordinate space of the camera, to generate a vertex map. Also each thread computes the normal vector for each vertex, resulting in a normal map.
2. *Camera pose tracking:* the ICP (Iterative Closest Point) algorithm, implemented in GPU, is used in each measurement in the 640 × 480 depth map, to track the camera pose at each depth frame, using the vertex and normal maps. Therefore, a 6-DOF rigid transformation is estimated for approximate alignment of the

oriented points with the ones from the previous frame. Incrementally, the estimated transformations are applied to the transformation that defines the Kinect global position.
3. *Volume integration:* a 3D fixed resolution volume is predefined, mapping the specific dimensions of a 3D fixed space. This volume is subdivided uniformly in a 3D grid of voxels. A volumetric representation is used to integrate the 3D global vertices of the conversion of the oriented points in global coordinates from the camera global position, into voxels, through a GPU implementation of the volumetric TSDF (Truncated Signed Distance Functions). The complete 3D grid is allocated in the GPU as linear aligned memory.
4. *Surface prediction:* raycasting of the volumetric TSDF is performed at the estimated frame to extract views from the implicit surface for depth map alignment and rendering. In each GPU thread, there is a single ray and it renders a single pixel at the output image.

The rendering pipeline allows conventional polygon-based graphics to be composed in the raycasting view, enabling the fusion of real and virtual scenes, including shadowing, all through a single algorithm. Moreover, there is data generation for better camera tracking by ICP algorithm.

2.2 *Moving Volume Kinectfusion*

References: [5] and website[1]
Developed at: Northeastern University/CCIS
Released in: September 2012
Availability: implementation to be included in the PCL project.

General Description Moving Volume KinectFusion is an extension of KinectFusion, with additional algorithms, to allow the translation and rotation of the 3D volume, fixed in the basis approach, as the camera moves. The main goal is the application in mobile robotic perception in rough terrain, providing simultaneously visual odometry and a local scenario dense map.

The implementation was based on the open-source Point Cloud Library (PCL)'s Kinfu [3] by Willow Garage organization and these modifications were submitted to be available at the project.

The requirements for the processing are similar to those of the original implementation and the authors used for tests, Intel Xeon W3520 processor (4 cores, 12 GB RAM, 2.8 GHz) and NVidia GeForce GTX580 GPU (512 cores, 3 GB RAM, 1.5 GHz).

Approach The method performs simultaneously the global camera pose tracking and the building of the local surroundings spatial map.

[1] http://www.ccs.neu.edu/research/gpc/mvkinfu/index.html.

Considering the KinectFusion approach after the tracking step, it is determined if a new volume frame is needed, calculating the linear and angular offsets, relative to the camera local pose.

To introduce a new volume frame, it is used remapping, that interpolates the TSDF values at the previous volume in the grid of corresponding points to the samples of the new rotated and translated volume. A swap buffer is kept in the GPU memory of the same size as the TSDF buffer and buffer swap is performed after remapping. Therefore, defining a new volume transformation.

A fast memory displacement re-sampling algorithm is used. During the re-sampling, a search is done at the closest neighbor, and if it is in the interval of truncation, a trilinear interpolation is performed.

2.3 *Kintinuous*

References: [6, 7] and website[2]
Developed at: National University of Ireland Maynooth and CSAIL/MIT
Released in: July 2012 (first version - RSS Workshop on RGBD:Advanced Reasoning with Depth Cameras), September 2012 (current version—submitted to ICRA'13).
Availability: implementation to be included in the PCL project.

General Description Kintinuous is another KinectFusion extension with the aim of mapping large scale scenarios in real time. The algorithm is modified so that the fixed volume to be mapped in real-time can be dynamically changed, with the corresponding point-cloud continuously incremented for triangular mesh representation.

As well as the Moving Volume KinectFusion, the authors here have also used the Kinfu implementation from PCL as basis. The hardware used for evaluation tests was a Intel Core i7- 2600 3.4 GHz CPU, 8 GB DDR 1333 MHz RAM and NVidia GeForce GTX 560 Ti 2 GB GPU, performed in 32-bit Ubuntu 10.10.

Approach The method is an extension of the KinectFusion method, in the sense that the same original algorithm is used in the region bounded by the threshold. However several modifications were incorporated:

- *Continuous representation:* It is allowed to the mapped area by the TSDF to move along the time, in tracking and reconstruction. The basic process of the system is: (i) Determine the camera distance to the origin: if above a specific threshold, translate virtually the TSDF to centralize the camera. (ii) Add the surface excluded from the TSDF region into a position graph, and initialize a new region entering the TSDF, as not mapped.
- *Implementation:* (i) A cyclic vector of TSDF voxels is used. (ii) Surface points are extracted by orthogonal raycasting through each TSDF slice, which are zeroed

[2] http://www.cs.nuim.ie/research/vision/data/rgbd2012

after that, where the zero-crossings are extracted as reconstructed surface vertices. (iii) A voxel grid filter is applied to remove the possible duplicate points in the orthogonal raycasting.

- *Pose graph representation:* The pose graph representation is used to represent the external meshes, where each position stores a surface slice.
- *Mesh generation:* Uses the greedy mesh triangulation algorithm described by Marton et al. [8].
- *Visual odometry:* The ICP odometry estimation is replaced by a GPU implementation of the dense odometry algorithm based in RGB-D presented by Steinbruecker et al. [9] integrated to the KinectFusion GPU pipeline.

2.4 RGB-D Mapping

References:[10, 11] and website[3].
Developed at: University of Washington
Released in: December 2010 (ISER—first version)/March 2012 (current version)
Availability: No implementation available.

General Description The RGB-D Mapping method is a complete 3D mapping system that aims the 3D reconstruction of interior scenarios, building a global model using surfels to enable compact representations and visualization of 3D maps. It provides a new joint optimization algorithm that combines visual characteristics and alignment based in shapes. The system is implemented using the Robot Operating System (ROS) framework [12].

Approach The method basically consists of:

1. Use of FAST (Features from Accelerated Segment Test) characteristics and Calonder descriptors to extract sparse visual characteristics of two frames and associate them with their respective depth values to generate characteristics points in 3D.
2. For the correspondences between two RGB-D frames, it uses the RGB-D ICP algorithm of two stages: sparse characteristic points extraction to visual appearance incorporation and correspondence by RANSAC (Random Sample Consensus).
3. Alignment between two frames using the implemented algorithm of joint optimization over appearance and shape correspondences.
4. Loop closure detection corresponding data frames to a previously collected set of frames.
5. Sparse Bundle Adjustment (SBA) is used for global optimization and incorporation of ICP restrictions in SBA.

[3] https://www.cs.washington.edu/node/3544/

2.5 RGB-DSLAM

References: [13, 14] and website[4]
Developed at: University of Freighburg/TUM.
Released in: April 2011. (RGB-D Workshop on 3D Perception in Robotics at the European Robotics Forum, 2011)
Availability: open-source implementation available[5].

General Description This method allows a robot to generate 3D colored models of objects and interior scenarios. The approach is similar to the RGB-D Mapping. It won the first prize in the "most useful" category at the ROS 3D challenge organized by Willow Garage.

Approach The method consists of four steps:

1. SURF (Speeded Up Robust Feature) characteristics extraction from the RGBD input images and its correspondence with previous images.
2. Computing the depth images in the local of these characteristic points, a set of 3D punctual correspondences between these two frames is obtained. Based on these correspondences, RANSAC is used to estimate the relative transformation between the frames.
3. Generalized ICP algorithm proposed by Segal et al. [15] is used to improve the initial estimation.
4. Resulting pose graph optimization, using HOG-Man, proposed by Grisetti et al. [16], to take the pose estimations between frames, consistent in the global 3D model.

2.6 Solony et al.

Reference: [17]
Developed at: Brno University of Technology
Released in: June 2011 (STUDENT EEICT)
Availability: No implementation available.

General Description This method aims to build a dense 3D map of interior environments, through multiple Kinect depth images. It can be used to produce effectively dense 3D maps of small workspaces.

The algorithm accumulates errors, caused by small inaccuracies in the camera pose estimation between consecutive frames, since it is not used any loop closure algorithm.

---

[4] http://openslam.org/rgbdslam.html
[5] http://www.ros.org/wiki/rgbdslam

Therefore, when compared to modern algorithms of map construction, this solution is not a SLAM (Simultaneous Localization And Mapping) algorithm, because it does not predict uncertainty in the camera position.

Approach The camera position is initialized in the center of global coordinates and the rotation is aligned with the negative z axis. The sparse set of characteristic points is extracted, and the new position is estimated in the camera tracking:

1. The SURF algorithm is applied to extract the set of visual characteristic points and its descriptors. The correspondence is done heuristically.
2. The RANSAC algorithm and epipolar constraints are used to check the validity of points correspondence.
3. The camera position is found from the valid correspondences, which are used to provide the equations that relate the 3D coordinates with the coordinates of 2D images.

In the map construction process:

1. The depth measurements are used to calculate the points 3d position, which are mapped into the global coordinate system.
2. Overlapping points are checked in the map, and the consecutive frames are processed.

2.7 *Omnikinect*

Reference: [18]
Developed at: ICG, Graz University of Technology
Released in: December 2012 (submitted to VRST).
Availability: No implementation available

General Description The system is a KinectFusion modification to allow the use of multiple Kinect sensors. It proposes hardware configuration and optimized software tools for this system. The tests were executed with Nvidia GTX680 and for comparison, Nvidia Quadro 6000 with 1000×1000 pixel resolution, using 7 Kinects.

Approach The method is composed of five steps, and one additional step (3) related to the KinectFusion implementation, to correct superposition noise and data redundancy:

1. Measurement: vertex and normal map are computed.
2. Pose estimation: predicted and measured surface ICP.
3. TSDF histogram volume: generation of TSDF histogram volume, filtered from TSDF outliers measures before temporal smoothing.
4. Updated reconstruction: surface measure integration in a global TSDF.
5. Surface prediction: TSDF raycast to compute surface prediction.

2.8 Cui et al.

Reference: [19]
Developed at: DFKI, Augmented Vision, University of Kaiserslautern.
Released in: October 2011 (SIGGRAPH)
Availability: No implementation available.

General Description This method aims to scan 3D objects aligning depth and color information. The system is implemented in C++ and evaluated on a Intel Xeon 3520 (2.67 GHz) with 12 GB RAM memory on Windows 7.

Approach The method is based on:

1. Super-resolution: a new super-resolution algorithm is used, similar to the approach of the LidarBoost algorithm by Schuon et al.[20], applied to each set of 10 captured frames. First, all depth maps in the set are aligned to the set center using optical 3D flow. Then, the energy function is minimized to extract a depth and color map without noise.
2. Global alignment: loop closure alignment based on rigid and non-rigid transformation consisting of three steps: (i) Use of ICP register in pairs to calculate corresponding points of two frames. (iii) Label of 'correct' and 'incorrect' using the absolute error. (iii) Compute of the exponential transformation in conformal geometric algebra to each frame using a energy function based on 'correct' correspondences.
3. Non-rigid registration: the global rigid and non-rigid processing is necessary to obtain a 360° model correctly closed.
4. Probabilistic simultaneous non-rigid alignment according to Cui et al. [21] is applied.
5. Finally, a 3D mesh is generated using the Poisson reconstruction method.

2.9 Guo et al.

Reference: [22]
Developed at: State Key Laboratory of Information Engineering in Surveying, Mapping and Remote Sensing, Wuhan University.
Released in: August 2012 (ISPRS).
Availability: no implementation available.

General Description The method is voxel-based, similarly to KinectFusion, but performing automatic re-localization when the tracking fails in cases of excessive slow or fast camera movements.

Approach The method is basically divided in the following steps:

1. Preprocessing: the depth image acquired by Kinect is converted from image coordinates in 3D points and normals into the camera coordinate space.

2. Rigid transformation: a 6 DOF rigid transformation is computed to approximately align the current point cloud with the previous frame. If the Kinect device is moved too slowly, the GPU-based ICP method is used to refine correspondences. If Kinect moves too fast, RGB images are used to extract SIFT (Scalar Invariant Feature Transform) characteristics, and the ICP is used. To determine a subset of characteristic pairs corresponding to a consistent rigid transformation, RANSAC algorithm is executed.
3. Relative transformations: the relative transformations are applied to a single transformation that defines the Kinect global position.
4. Data fusion: voxel-based data fusion is applied to reconstruct incrementally the 3D model of the scenery, using volumetric surface representation based on Curless et al. [23]. Measurement of color similarity is used to evaluate the accuracy of the registered results. If the result is in a predefined threshold, the point clouds can be fused into the 3D model, and it is possible to add the frame in a graph structure. This structure is built to resolve the problem of camera re-localization.

With the dense surface reconstruction and the global camera position, a pixel raycast is performed according to Parker et al. [24]. The corresponding distance to each pixel position, computed with a SDF, is recorded to generate a virtual depth image.

2.10 Neumann et al.

References: [25, 26].
Developed at: Pattern Recognition Lab, Friedrich-Alexander-Universität.
Released in: November 2012 (ICCV).
Availability: no available implementation.

General Description It is proposed a system to map the point cloud in real time in a GPU implementation of the ICP algorithm. The Random Ball Cover (RBC) data structure is explored in GPU for the optimization of the search for the closest neighbor.

The evaluation tests were performed with Intel Core 2 Quad Q9550 and NVIDIA GeForce GTX 460. The GPU framework was implemented using CUDA.

Approach The proposed framework is composed of four stages:

1. The sensor data is transferred to the GPU, where the pipeline is performed.
2. The transformation from the 2D sensor domain into a 3D global coordinate system and data pre-processing are performed.
3. Based on a set of reference points, a ICP photogeometric variant (incorporating geometric and photometric information) is applied, for rigid alignment of 3D point clouds.
4. The current point cloud is attached to the model based on estimated transformation.

The RBC construction and queries to the dataset are done by brute-force (BF) primitives. It is introduced a modification to simplify the RBC construction to a single search by BF, with an approximated search algorithm for the closest neighbor.

To eliminate redundancy and overlapping, the level of overlapping between consecutive frames is measured, computing the distance of its depth histograms. Using the non-similarity metric, the current RGB-D data is discarded for mapping when the distance is below a threshold.

2.11 Stuckler et al.

References: [27].
Developed at: University of Bonn.
Released in: September 2012 (MFI).
Availability: no available implementation.

General Description The aim of this work is to acquire 3D maps from interior scenarios. The approach integrates color and depth data in a multi-resolution representation.

For map representation, multi-resolution surfels map is used. Also, octrees are used to model textured surfaces to multiple resolutions in a probabilistic way.

To register these maps in real-time, used for SLAM, it is performed an iterative refinement process in which, multi-resolution surfels are associated between the maps for each iteration, given the current estimated position. Using these associations, the new position that maximizes the probable correspondence for the maps is determined. Due to the difference of view positions between the images, the scenario content is discretized and to compensate, it is used trilinear interpolation.

In order to add spatial constraints between similar views during the operation in real time, a randomization method is proposed.

2.12 Du et al.

Reference: [28].
Developed at: University of Washington.
Released in: September 2011 (Ubicomp).
Availability: no available implementation.

General Description This method aims the scanning of interior scenarios, although it can be used with near centimeter precision for other applications. The system that can be performed in real time interactively in a laptop.

Approach The system basically follows a well-established structure for 3D mapping: RGB-D frame registration partition in local alignment, or visual odometry, plus global alignment, which uses loop closure information to optimize over the frames and produce camera pose and maps globally consistent. The 3D map is increasingly updated in real time.

In the RGB-D real-time registratio, the 3-point matching algorithm is used to compute 6D transformations between pairs of frames. A new correspondence criteria is used to combine the RANSAC inliers counting with visibility conflict.

Following the RGB-D Mapping alignment, visual characteristics are detected in the color frame using a GPU implementation of the standard SIFT characteristics to eliminate outliers and find the camera pose transformation between two frames.

2.13 KTHRGB

Reference: [29].
Developed at: CVAP, Royal Institute of Technology (KTH).
Released in: 2011
Availability: open-source implementation available[6].

General Description Using the VSLAM (Visual SLAM) process, the aim is to map an environment as closest as real. A mobile robot platform with a Kinect attached is used. Also, different techniques are compared in different stages.

Approach The method basically follows:

1. SIFT or SURF characteristics are extracted, from each frame; for the initial correspondence, a kd-tree id used and the information is integrated to compute the characteristics positions in 3D.
2. From this set of pairs of characteristics, a transformation is computed using the RANSAC algorithm.
3. The initial position is computed and translated into node and edge using the g2o framework [30].
4. Loop closure detection and corresponding edge insertion in the graph.
5. Graph optimization in g2o with the Levenberg-Marquardt (LMA) algorithm with the Cholmod linear solver, and updated camera pose extraction.
6. Reconstruction of the global scenario, generating a point cloud datafile.

2.14 Tenedorio et al.

Reference: [31]
Developed at: Calit2, University of California.
Released in: February 2012 (Proceedings of SPIE).

[6] http://code.google.com/p/kth-rgbd/

Availability: no available implementation.

General Description A novel system of geometry scanning using a 6DOF tracking coupled to the Kinect is introduced in this work. The goal is to obtain triangular models of static objects. Filtering methods are presented, removing scan overlapping or low precision scans. Moreover, it is presented a capture algorithm to scan large areas.

The tests are performed in a prototype implementation in a virtual reality environment, the StarCAVE [32], at the University of California.

Approach The system uses the Kinect calibration method from Nicolas Burrus [33] to associate depth samples with color values.

To obtain a precise camera pose representation in real-time, a tracker is coupled to the top of the Kinect and its position and orientation registered using the AR-Tracking [34], an optical system of wireless tracking. The system uses four infrared cameras to inform the 6DOF position at 60 Hz.

To acquire the camera position and perform scan alignments, it is used the AR-Toolkit [35], an augmented reality library that can compute the relative position between printed markers, searching for images among the video frames.

The library Libfreenect [36] is used to obtain the color and depth images, so that it can put each 3D point in its correct relative position in perspective.

To eliminate 3D redundant data, first the bin-hash data structure is used, allowing the use of OpenGL for rendering, to search new points. A circumference centered between two points is considered, and then a novel algorithm produces a surface of spheres over the scanned points.

A filter is implemented to considerer the majority of points obtained by scanning, orthogonally to the surface. Moreover, the filter removes the depth outlier samples.

Then, texture is applied to the triangle mesh using the Bernadini et al. "ball-pivoting" method [37], implemented using the VCG library [38]. Another method also applied, is Marching Cubes, implemented in CUDA [39], which performs faster and less accurate, with the use of the RANSAC implemented in the Mobile Robot Programming Toolkit [40]. Using image frames from the Kinect RGB camera, a texture is created to each triangle.

Finally, a cleaning scanning mode was implemented to delete any point previously scanned in the field of view.

2.15 Other Methods

The following methods present free and/or commercial implementations, but they do not provide documentation or technical article about the method.

2.15.1 RGBDEMO

Website: http://labs.manctl.com/rgbdemo.
Availability: open-source implementation, with LGPL license (any modification must be shared under the same license).
Platforms: Linux, Windows (32 and 64 bits) and MAC OS X (10.6 or higher).
Description: open-source software initially developed by Nicolas Burrus at RoboticsLab in the Charles III University of Madrid, providing a simple kit for using Kinect data without compiling external libraries. It offers a static scanning system.

2.15.2 SKANECT

Website: http://manctl.com/products.html.
Availability: free.
Platforms: Windows (32 and 64 bits) and MAC OS X (10.6 r higher).
Description: Launched as a product by Manctl, it is based on the RGBDemo implementation.

2.15.3 MATHERIX 3DIFY

Website: http://www.matherix.com.
Availability: copy is available by joining the beta version program.
Platform: Windows 7.
Description: Projected to help artists and designers to build 3D models of real objects.

2.15.4 RECONSTRUCTME

Website: http://reconstructme.net.
Availability: free for non-commercial purposes; 99 Euro for commercial use.
Platform: Windows 7.
Description: some authors, as T. Whelan [6] and Sergey K. (KinectShape), claim that the method is based on the KinectFusion. It is possible that the Master's thesis defended in 2012, "A low-cost real-time 3D Surface Reconstruction System", by Christoph Kopf, one of the method developers, includes a description of the approach. The goal of the method is to reconstruct the objects surfaces.

2.15.5 KIRETU

Website: http://pille.iwr.uni-heidelberg.de/~kinect01/doc/index.html.
Availability: open-source implementation.
Platform: Ubuntu 10.04- 11.04 and LinuxMint 11, both 64 bits.

Description: the Kinect Reconstruction Tutor, Kiretu, was created in a course of the Heidelberg University.

2.15.6 KINECTSHAPE

Website: http://k10v.com/2012/09/02/18.
Availability: open-source implementation.
Description: KinectFusion's minimalist implementation.

2.15.7 KINECT-3D-SLAM

Website: http://www.mrpt.org/Application:kinect-3d-slam.
Availability: open-source implementation.
Platforms: Linux and Windows (32 bits).
Description: the software executes VSLAM with the MRPT libraries, to scan small scenarios.

2.15.8 KINECT TO STL

Website: http://wiki.ultimaker.com/Kinect_2_STL.
Availability: open-source implementation.
Platforms: Linux e Mac OS X.
Description: the software creates STL files for 3D printing.

3 Conclusion

In the present work, we presented a survey of important methods approaches of relative low cost 3D surface scanning, using RGBD imaging devices, in particular the Kinect Sensor. We verified that the objective of the majority of the current methods is building 3D maps of small to medium size interior scenarios. We noticed that there is no method that covers all needs of possible applications, and therefore depends on the compromise desired. On the one hand, there is the speed and user interaction for augmented reality applications. On the other hand, the precise details for 3D modeling for rapid prototyping for example.

It is important to mention that available open-source implementations, such as Kinfu from the PCL project, allow contributions from the community to circumvent the limitations of current algorithms, and can contribute as a starting point for other works.

Acknowledgements This work was supported by the CNPq (Brazilian National Council for Scientific and Technological Development) and the Center for Information Technology Renato Archer.

References

1. Izadi S, Kim D, Hilliges O, Molyneaux D, Newcombe R, Kohli P, Shotton J, Hodges S, Freeman D, Davison A, Fitzgibbon A (2011) KinectFusion: real-time 3D reconstruction and interaction using a moving depth camera. In Proceedings of the 24th annual ACM symposium on user interface software and technology, UIST, pp 559–568
2. Newcombe R, Izadi S, Hilliges O, Molyneaux D, Kim D, Davison A, Kohli P, Shotton J, Hodges S, Fitzgibbon A (2011) KinectFusion: real-time dense surface mapping and tracking. In Proceedings of the 10th IEEE International Symposium on mixed and augmented reality, ISMAR, pp 127–136
3. PCL: Point Cloud Library. http://pointcluds.org. Accessed 28 June 2014
4. Kinect for Windows SDK. http://msdn.microsoft.com/en-us/library/hh855347.aspx. Accessed 28 June 2014
5. Roth H, Vona M (2012) Moving volume KinectFusion. British machine vision conference, BMVC
6. Whelan T, Kaess M, Fallon MF, Johannsson H, Leonard JJ, McDonald JB (2012) Kintinuous: spatially extended kinect fusion. RSS Workshop on RGB-D: advanced reasoning with depth cameras
7. Whelan T, Johannsson H, Kaess M, Leonard J, McDonald JB (2012) Robust tracking for real-time dense rgb-d mapping with kintinuous. Computer science and artificial intelligence laboratory. MIT technical report MIT-CSAIL-TR-2012-031
8. Marton ZC, Rusu RB, Beetz M (2009) On fast surface reconstruction methods for large and noisy datasets. In Proceedings of the IEEE international conference on robotics and automation (ICRA), Kobe, Japan
9. Steinbruecker F, Sturm J, Cremers D (2011) Real-time visual odometry from dense RGB-D images. Workshop on live dense reconstruction with moving cameras at the international conference on computer vision (ICCV)
10. Henry P, Krainin M, Herbst E, Ren X, Fox D (2010) RGB-D mapping: using depth cameras for dense 3D modeling of indoor environments. International symposium on experimental robotics (ISER)
11. Henry P, Krainin M, Herbst E, Ren X, Fox D (2012) RGB-D mapping: using kinect-style depth cameras for dense 3D modeling of indoor environments. Int J Robot Res 31(5):647–663
12. ROS: Robot Operating System. http://www.ros.org/wiki/. Accessed 28 June 2014
13. Endres F, Hess J, Engelhard N, Sturm J, Burgard W (2012) 6D visual slam for RGB-D sensors. Em AT—Automatisierungstechnik 60:270–278
14. Engelhard N, Endres F, Hess J, Sturm J, Burgard W (2011) Real-time 3D visual slam with a hand-held camera. In Proceedings of the RGB-D workshop on 3D perception in robotics at the European Robotics Forum
15. Segal A, Haehnel D, Thrun S (2009) Generalized ICP. In proceedings of robotics: science and systems (RSS)
16. Grisetti G, Kümmerle R, Stachniss C, Frese U, Hertzberg C (2010) Hierarchical optimization on manifolds for online 2D and 3D mapping. In Proceedings of the IEEE international conference on robotics and automation (ICRA)
17. Solony M (2011) Scene reconstruction from kinect motion. In Proceeding of the 17th conference and competition student EEICT 2011, Brno
18. Kainz B, Hauswiesner S, Reitmayr G, Steinberger M, Grasset R, Gruber L, Veas E, Kalkofen D, Seichter H, Schmalstieg D (2012) OmniKinect: Real-time dense volumetric data acquisition and applications. In Proceeding of the 18Th Acm Symposium on virtual reality software and technology (VRST)
19. Cui Y, Stricker D (2011) 3D shape scanning with a kinect. In Proceedings of the ACM SIGGRAPH Posters, art. 57
20. Schuon S, Theobalt C, Davis J, Thrun S (2009) Lidarboost: depth superresolution for tof 3d shape scanning. In proceedings of the CVPR
21. Cui Y, Schuon S, Derek C, Thrun S, Theobalt C (2010) 3d shape scanning with a time-of-flight camera. In proceedings of IEEE CVPR

22. Guo W, Du T, Zhu X, Hu T (2012) Kinect-based real-time RGB-D image fusion method. In international archives of the photogrammetry, remote sensing and spatial information sciences, pp 275–279
23. Curless B, Levoy M (1996) A volumetric method for building com-plex models from range images. In ACM transactions on graphics, SIGGRAPH
24. Parker S, Shirley P, Livnat Y, Hansen C, Sloan P (1998) Interactive ray tracing for isosurface rendering. In proceedings of visualization
25. Neumann D, Lugauer F, Bauer S, Wasza J, Hornegger J (2011) Real-time RGB-D mapping and 3-D modeling on the GPU using the random ball cover data structure. In Proceedings of the 2011 IEEE International Conference on Computer Vision, pp 1161–1167
26. Bauer S, Wasza J, Lugauer F, Neumann D, Hornegger J (2013) Consumer depth cameras for computer vision (Chapter 2). Springer, London, pp 27–48
27. Stückler J, Behnke S (2012) Integrating depth and color cues for dense multi-resolution scene mapping using RGB-D cameras. In Proceedings of the IEEE International Conference on Multisensor Fusion and Information Integration (MFI 2012), Hamburg, Germany
28. Du H, Henry P, Ren X, Chen M, Goldman DB, Seitz SM, Fox D (2011) Interactive 3D modelling of indoor environments with a consumer depth camera. In Proceedings of the 13th international conference on Ubiquitous computing, pp 75–84
29. Hogman V (2011) Building a 3D map from RGB-D sensors. Master's Thesis, KTH Royal Institute of Technology
30. g2o: A general framework for graph optimization. http://openslam.org/g2o.html. Accessed 28 June 2014
31. Tenedorio D, Fecho M, Schwartzhaupt J, Pardridge R, Lue J, Schulze JP (2012) Capturing geometry in real-time using a tracked microsoft kinect. In Proceedings of SPIE 8289, The engineering reality of virtual reality 2012
32. StarCAVE. http://www.andrewnoske.com/wiki/index.php?title=Calit2_-_StarCAVE. Accessed 28 June 2014
33. Nicolas Burrus's Kinect Calibration. http://nicolas.burrus.name/index.php/Research/Kinect-Calibration. Accessed 28 June 2014
34. ART: Advanced realtime tracking. http://ar-tracking.eu. Accessed 28 June 2014
35. ARToolKit. http://www.hitl.washington.edu/artoolkit. Accessed 28 June 2014
36. Libfreenect. https://github.com/OpenKinect/libfreenect. Accessed 28 June 2014
37. Bernardini F, Mittleman J, Rushmeier H, Silva C, Taubin G (1999) The ball-pivoting algorithm for surface reconstruction. In IEEE transactions on visualization computer graphics, vol 5, pp 349–359
38. VCG: Visualization and Computer Graphics Library. http://vcg.isti.cnr.it/vcglib. Accessed 28 June 2014
39. NVIDIA's CUDA Implementation of marching cubes. http://developer.download.nvidia.com/compute/cuda/11/Website/GraphicsInterop.html
40. MRPT: Mobile Robot Programming Toolkit. RANSAC C++ examples. http://www.mrpt.org/tutorials/programming/maths-and-geometry/ransac-c-examples. Accessed 28 June 2014

MIX
Papier aus verantwortungsvollen Quellen
Paper from responsible sources
FSC® C105338

If you have any concerns about our products,
you can contact us on
ProductSafety@springernature.com

In case Publisher is established outside the EU,
the EU authorized representative is:
Springer Nature Customer Service Center GmbH
Europaplatz 3, 69115 Heidelberg, Germany

Printed by Libri Plureos GmbH
in Hamburg, Germany